PRINCIPLES OF CLINICAL TOXICOLOGY

Principles of Clinical Toxicology

Thomas A. Gossel, Ph.D.

*Professor of Pharmacology and Toxicology
Chairman, Department of Pharmacology
and Biomedical Sciences
Ohio Northern University
College of Pharmacy
Ada, Ohio*

J. Douglas Bricker, Ph.D.

*Associate Professor of Pharmacology
and Toxicology
Ohio Northern University
College of Pharmacy
Ada, Ohio*

Raven Press ■ New York

Raven Press, 1140 Avenue of the Americas, New York, New York 10036

Made in the United States of America

International Standard Book Number 0-89004-951-3
Library of Congress Catalog Card Number 82-42594

The material contained in this volume was submitted as previously unpublished material, except in the instances in which credit has been given to the source from which some of the illustrative material was derived.

Great care has been taken to maintain the accuracy of the information contained in the volume. However, Raven Press cannot be held responsible for errors or for any consequences arising from the use of the information contained herein.

Library of Congress Cataloging in Publication Data

Gossel, Thomas A.
    Principles of clinical toxicology.

    Includes bibliographies and index.
    1. Toxicology.   I. Bricker, J. Douglas.   II. Title.
[DNLM: 1. Poisoning.   2. Poisons.   QV 600 G6785p]
RA1211.G6   1984   615.9   84-13238
ISBN 0-89004-951-3

Preface

Toxicology is one of the most rapidly developing sciences in the entire biomedical curriculum. It has evolved over recent years well beyond the boundaries that most authorities envisioned just a decade ago. Today, many students pursuing a degree in one of the health-related areas of the biomedical sciences study the principles of toxicology either in a free-standing format or as a component of their pharmacology sequence.

As is often the case in fields of rapid growth, the literature has not been able to keep up with the developments in toxicology. Specifically, there has not been a textbook written for the sole purpose of aiding the student who is pursuing the contemporary study of clinical toxicology as part of a baccalaureate degree. Although a wide variety of reference books, handbooks, guidelines, and individual articles from the literature is available, none of these presents a comprehensive treatment of the principles of toxicology. Realizing this deficiency we decided to accept the challenge and write an up-to-date toxicology volume.

This book serves a single purpose—to teach the *principles* of clinical toxicology. Principles are rules of action or reasons why certain procedures are undertaken; they are also the foundation of a science. This book adheres to its title in that it is neither a reference book nor a laboratory manual. Rather it is organized around the primary goal of explaining the fundamental principles of clinical toxicology. By understanding the basis for the events that occur and the reasons why a certain treatment is used or perhaps not used, we should then be able to approach any toxic emergency with few problems.

The book consists of two parts. The first part discusses household, occupational, and some common environmental poisons. The second part concentrates on drugs or chemicals that are used intentionally to cause some pharmacologic effect. We have chosen examples of classes of chemicals and drugs that are relatively common causes of poisoning. The uncommonly encountered substances are not included.

Specifically, chapters in this book include discussions of individual classes of toxic agents, their common sources and usual methods of intoxication, incidence and frequency of poisoning, mechanism(s) of action, and clinical signs and symptoms of poisoning, as well as reasons why these are occurring. Other cause-effect relationships are also presented. The management of poisoning is discussed from a descriptive standpoint. Laboratory findings also are included. A list of normal laboratory values comprises Appendix I.

Case studies have been carefully selected for each chapter to further illustrate and reinforce the text discussions of individual classes of poisons. Comments on these studies are presented when appropriate. Each chapter concludes with a list of review questions so that the reader may determine whether the basic concepts have been mastered.

It should be noted that differential diagnoses and prognoses of toxic events are not considered here. Unless otherwise specified, our approach assumes that an accurate diagnosis of the intoxication already has been made; from this point, we proceed to discuss what happens in these specific incidences. Except for a few cases, poisoning discussion is limited to acute exposure (e.g., a single toxic dose, or multiple subtoxic doses within a 24-hour period). The prognosis of any toxic event is highly variable and rarely predictable, unless a complete patient history is available and all of the possible ramifications of the poisoning

v

event are known. Therefore, prognosis is discussed only with reference to making another relevant point.

We have applied a concept-oriented approach, in presenting the information in this text, that emphasizes basic principles and the reasons why things occur rather than merely presenting facts. Facts change often; basic principles remain constant. Furthermore, toxicology is a rapidly changing science. What is true and valid today may be outdated tomorrow.

Throughout this book we state that an event "may" occur, or that something "probably" happens. This is not meant to be elusive; the very nature of toxicology is that we still can only hypothesize regarding some of these areas. Likewise, numerous new methods for antidoting poisonings and new theories about poisoning are being evaluated. As these become known, they will be incorporated into future editions.

Principles of Clinical Toxicology is best utilized after completing courses in organic chemistry, biochemistry, physiology, and an introductory term of pharmacology. Each of these areas of knowledge contributes to clinical toxicology.

No single introductory text can serve as a sole authority. Therefore, we hope that you will continue your search for information using other literature sources. We hope this search will continue throughout your life.

T. A. Gossel
J. D. Bricker

Acknowledgments

We wish to thank our *WIVES*, Phyllis Gossel and Lillian Bricker, for their understanding and patience while this book was being researched and written and for their devotion to spending many hours of unselfish labor in assisting with the manuscript preparation; our *CHILDREN*, for providing us with the initial reasons to secure our own homes against poisoning; our *MENTORS*, from years gone by, who gave so much of themselves to teach us the principles of toxicology; and our *COLLEAGUES*, for their support, suggestions, and critical analysis of various chapters in this book.

Special thanks are offered to Anna Mae Shadley and Peggy Flower for their excellent secretarial services, to Elizabeth Graham and Stewart Graham for their preparation of art work and figures, and to the editorial staff at Raven Press for their careful attention to all phases of preparation of this book.

Most of all, we extend our very special thanks to all of our students, past and present, who have taught us much more than we could ever hope to teach them.

Contents

Toxicology in Perspective

1

INTRODUCTION TO TOXICOLOGY

An introductory chapter in any textbook should provide an overview of the topic and insight into subsequent chapters. We have attempted to do just that. Additionally, we have stressed the point on numerous occasions that toxicology should not be viewed as a free-standing science. Rather, it represents a compilation of many of the basic and clinical sciences, and has developed from input by hundreds of thousands of individuals over the years.

Toxicology, especially clinical toxicology, is still in its formative stages, however. As new concepts and procedures are developed and implemented into clinical practice, it seems that many of them are outmoded even before they have an opportunity to prove their value, as even newer concepts evolve.

But the one basic concept that does remain fairly constant is the premise that there are certain principles of toxicity which do not change. Principles are rules of action, or reasons why certain procedures are conducted. They are also the foundation of a science. We must always keep this in mind as we study toxicology.

Toxicology is not an easy word to define. The term is derived from Greek and Latin origins (L. *toxicum* = poison; Gr. *toxikom* = arrow poison; L. *logia* = science or study) and literally means a study of poisons on living organisms. Therefore, a toxicologist is a person who studies or works in the area of toxicology, but toxicology is not restricted to this narrow definition. Toxicologists do much more than simply work with poisons. In its broadest sense, toxicology traditionally involves all aspects of adverse effects of chemicals on biological systems. This includes their mechanisms of harmful effects and conditions under which these harmful effects occur, socioeconomic considerations, and legal ramifications.

HISTORICAL PERSPECTIVES

Toxicology in its present sense is a relatively new science, having developed over the years from an essence of observation to its current status as an analytical science. This development makes for exciting reading, but an in depth study is beyond the scope of this chapter. Interested students should consult Holmstedt and Liljestrand (5) or Casarett and Bruce (3) for specific details. There is one individual, however, who needs to be cited, for he, more than anyone else, certainly established toxicology as an absolute science.

The father of modern toxicology was Mathieu Joseph Bonaventura Orfila (1787–1853). Orfila was a Spaniard who served as attending physician to Louis XVIII of France, and taught at the University of Paris. During his early professional years, Orfila quickly realized the inadequacy of toxicology as a science, and consequently, in 1815, wrote the first book of general toxicology that was devoted to adverse effects of chemicals (11). Until that time, toxicology had been largely descriptive in nature, and it left wide gaps of information open for broad and often erroneous interpretation. Intuitive hunches often served as the sole basis for determining the cause of a poisoning incidence. Orfila, concerned with legal implications of poisoning, pointed out the importance of determining a chemical analysis to establish a definitive cause of poisoning. He then devised analytical procedures, many of which are still in use today, for detecting specific chemicals. It is reported that he sacrificed over 4,000 dogs to collect the data detailed in his book. Orfila's

book established the basis for all future experimental and forensic toxicological evaluations and, subsequently, was translated into several languages. Orfila eventually followed up on his first book with numerous monographs that discussed, in detail, additional toxicologic information.

More than 165 years have elapsed since Orfila's book appeared. During that time, developments in toxicology were slowly evolving. The bulk of useful information related to modern toxicology only came about since the turn of this century, and most has developed exclusively within the past several decades. Perhaps the most exciting aspect is that the best is yet to come, for toxicology is still in its infancy.

As it developed over the years, toxicology has extracted many of the principles and techniques from many of the basic biological and chemical sciences. For example, Fig. 1 illustrates the progression of information the student of toxicology receives and the basic sciences on which toxicology is based. This is followed at another level by the specific subdisciplines within the science that have evolved over the years, and their specialty areas within those disciplines. We will briefly examine each of these disciplines, first to define the limits of each specialty, then to promote an appreciation of modern toxicology that has, by this point, developed into a very meaningful and necessary science.

DIVERSITY OF TOXICOLOGY

Occupational (industrial) toxicology has grown out of a need to protect the worker from poisonous substances and, in general, to make his working environment safe. The objective, obviously, is to prevent impairment of health of an individual while on the job.

It is the industrial toxicologist's job to define permissible levels (e.g., levels that are safe and do not produce adverse symptoms or disease) of exposure to chemicals as dusts, fumes, particles, etc. As a result of the need for this form of protection and control, the Occupational Safety and Health Act (OSHA) of 1970 was passed.

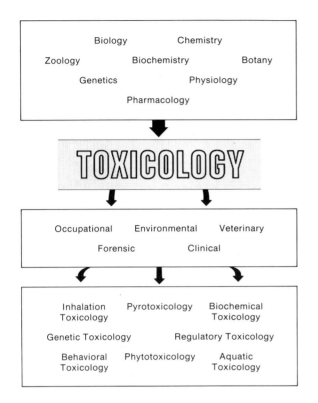

FIG. 1. The evolution of toxicology with its numerous applications.

Under the Secretary of Labor, OSHA was designed to assure that no employee will suffer diminished health, functional capacity, or limited life expectancy as a result of his work experience.

There are two agencies that are critical to the operation of OSHA. One of these is its sister agency, the National Institute for Occupational Safety and Health (NIOSH). This federal agency is charged with developing safety and health standards and is involved in the research aspect of occupational toxicology. It publishes *Criteria Documents* on specific chemicals which state pertinent toxicity and safety information concerning those particular chemicals. For example, NIOSH lists 8-hr exposure limits for chemicals, the immediate first-aid procedures to follow in case of skin or eye exposure, etc.

The other agency is the American Conference of Governmental Industrial Hygienists (ACGIH) which is devoted to setting safety standards for chemicals in the working environment. The research undertaken by this group results in useful data such as threshold limit values (TLV) and maximum allowable concentrations (MAC) of chemicals.

Environmental toxicology is a broad discipline of toxicology which encompasses the study of chemicals that are contaminants of food, water, soil, or the atmosphere.

It was Dr. Harvey Wiley, of the Food and Drug Administration (FDA), who first brought our attention to the problem of food additives (chemical preservatives and dyes), the deplorable conditions of the meat-packing industry, and the many "cure-all" claims for worthless medicines that, in many cases, probably were the cause of death (13). Today, specific information must be supplied to the FDA concerning the use of any substance, as a food additive, before it is released for production. A list of safe food additives is referred to as the GRAS list (Generally Recommended As Safe).

One of the classic incidents that first brought our attention to the problems of air pollution and its consequent toxic sequelae occurred in Donora, Pennsylvania, in 1948. As the result of a temperature inversion in this highly industrialized valley, expulsion into the atmosphere of several pollutants from zinc smelters and steel mills was hindered, and these chemical toxins were literally trapped within the air supply of the valley. This created a pocket of these potentially toxic materials. Consequently, individuals complained of nausea, vomiting, headache, and episodes of syncope. Similar events have occurred for other chemicals in other parts of the country. The most commonly encountered air pollutants are carbon monoxide, sulfur oxides, hydrocarbons, particulate matter, and the nitrogen oxides.

Environmental toxicology is also concerned with toxic substances that may enter the lakes, streams, rivers, and oceans. The most common problems dealt with in this aspect of toxicology are water-borne viruses and bacteria, waste heat from electrical plants, radioactive wastes, sewage eutrophication, and industrial pollutants.

Forensic toxicology is a discipline which combines analytical chemistry with essential toxicological principles in order to deal with the medicolegal aspects of the toxic effects of drugs and chemicals on man. The role of forensic toxicology is to aid in establishing cause-effect relationships between exposure to a drug or chemical and the toxic or lethal effects of the compound. In order to unequivocally confirm a cause-effect relationship, the forensic toxicologist relies on specific and highly sensitive analytical methods which can efficiently isolate, identify, and quantitate the toxic compound in question from biological fluids and tissues.

Clinical toxicology, as might be expected, is involved with the specific diseases caused by toxic substances and how they can be treated. Clinical toxicology encompasses the study of chemicals originating from any and all sources. It is concerned with all aspects of the interaction between these chemicals and people.

Veterinary toxicology is to animals what clinical toxicology is to humans.

TOXICITY: WHEN DOES IT START? WHEN DOES IT END?

When we think of the word *toxic*, or *toxicity*, the first image that often comes to mind is the traditionally-pictured "skull and crossbones." The image of death and destruction is automatically associated with toxicity. But what is a toxic substance? Do all toxic chemicals cause death and destruction? And how about the reverse? Are all chemicals that are usually thought of as being nontoxic safe?

TOXIC SUBSTANCES

A poisonous or toxic substance is any chemical that is capable of producing a detrimental effect on a living organism. As a result of this damage, there is an alteration of structural components or functional processes which may produce injury or even death. Any chemical may be a poison, at a given dose and route of administration. Too much pure oxygen, water, or salt can kill, but even classical toxic chemicals may be ingested in subtoxic quantities as not to cause symptoms of toxicity. Therefore, we cannot segregate those compounds which we generally consider toxic (e.g., cyanide, arsenic, lye, etc.) from the ones we assume are nontoxic. In other words, all chemicals must be assumed to be toxic, under the proper circumstances.

One point we must clarify is that many people consider poisoning to start the moment exposure occurs. While we concur that, in theory, this is true for cases where symptoms develop, it is an incorrect assumption for most toxic exposures. In reality, we are exposed to a wide variety of toxic substances each day from the food and water we ingest, and the air we breathe. We do not display toxic symptoms, so we are not actually poisoned. Thus, it is important to distinguish between poisoning from exposure or ingestion.

Toxicity Values

Another question commonly asked is, when is a chemical considered to be toxic? Or, how much of a substance has to be ingested to cause symptoms? Chemicals produce their toxic effects in a biological system whenever they reach a critical concentration in the target tissues. Toxicity is routinely expressed by the LD_{50} value, or the dose that represents the concentration of chemical required to produce death in 50% of the animals exposed to it. The LD_{50} value is used extensively to categorize the toxic dose of a chemical, and obtaining this value is generally the first experiment conducted on new chemicals.

LD_{50} determinations are plagued with variations, however. For example, species variation, inter-laboratory and intra-laboratory differences in values, and the fact that there is no standardized experimental protocol to calculate it are a few of the variables which make an LD_{50} value only an estimate. These values, then, are said to "estimate" the relative degree of toxicity for a given compound.

Table 1 illustrates the wide range of doses which induce lethal effects in animals. As can be seen from the table, some chemicals cause death in microgram quantities and are consequently expressed as being extremely toxic. On the other hand, other chemicals may be relatively harmless following doses in excess of several grams. Over the years, a toxicity rating scale has been used to provide a qualitative or "ball-park" figure describing the severity of the expected toxicity of a compound. Table 2 shows

TABLE 1. *Approximate LD_{50} of a selected variety of chemical agents*

Agent	Animal	Route	LD_{50} (mg/kg)
Ethyl alcohol	Mouse	Oral	10,000
Sodium choloride	Mouse	i.p.	4,000
Ferrous sulfate	Rat	Oral	1,500
Morphine sulfate	Rat	Oral	900
Phenobarbital, sodium	Rat	Oral	150
DDT	Rat	Oral	100
Picrotoxin	Rat	s.c.	5
Strychnine sulfate	Rat	i.p.	2
Nicotine	Rat	i.v.	1
d-Tubocurarine	Rat	i.v.	0.5
Hemicholinium-3	Rat	i.v.	0.2
Tetrodotoxin	Rat	i.v.	0.10
Dioxin	Guinea pig	i.v.	0.001
Botulinus toxin	Rat	i.v.	0.00001

Intraperitoneal = i.p.; intravenous = i.v.; subcutaneous = s.c.
From ref. 7.

TABLE 2. *Toxicity rating chart*

Rating	Dose	Probable oral lethal dose for average 150-pound adult
Practically nontoxic	>15 g/kg	More than 1 quart
Slightly toxic	5–15 g/kg	Between pint and quart
Moderately toxic	0.5–5 g/kg	Between ounce and pint
Very toxic	50–500 mg/kg	Between teaspoonful and ounce
Extremely toxic	5–50 mg/kg	Between 7 drops and teaspoonful
Super toxic	<5 mg/kg	A taste (<7 drops)

From ref. 4.

such a typical rating scale which lists the categories of toxicity based on their probable oral lethal dose in humans. Another use of an LD_{50} determination is to compare it with the ED_{50}, or median dose of a chemical that is therapeutically effective in 50% of the subjects receiving it. From this comparison, a therapeutic index or "margin of safety" for the chemical can be established.

The therapeutic index (TI) is defined as the ratio of the LD_{50} to the ED_{50}. Figure 2 illustrates a hypothetical dose-response curve for the therapeutic effect and lethal effect of a given compound. Note that as the LD_{50} curve shifts to the left, the TI ratio becomes smaller and, thus, the compound has a reduced margin of safety (it is more toxic). An even more critical evaluation of a compound for its potential to produce toxicity relative to its margin of safety would be to calculate the ratio of the LD_1 to the ED_{99}.

With reference to Table 2, some compounds are considered relatively harmless because large quantities would need to be ingested prior to its toxic or lethal action. Table 3 shows that not all substances found around the home are toxic. These items are often involved in household poisonings and, unless massive quantities are ingested, there should be no serious toxic ef-

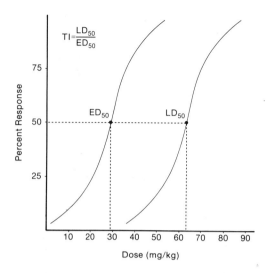

FIG. 2. A hypothetical dose response curve that illustrates the therapeutic effect (ED_{50}) and the lethal effect (LD_{50}) of a given chemical.

fects produced. Knowing when no antidotal treatment is needed is just as vital as knowing when treatment is required.

POISONING

Accidental and intentional poisonings are among the major causes of morbidity and mortality in the United States. The United States Consumer Product Safety Commission currently considers poisoning to be one of the leading causes of accidental death in children.

There is no way to accurately determine the exact extent of poisoning incidents. While it is reported that at least 5,000 to 10,000 Americans die from poisoning each year, there is currently no regulation that states these statistics must be gathered and documented. However, many people, including us, believe there is another group of victims, equal to in number or exceeding this 5,000 to 10,000 estimate, who die each year from unreported poisonings. These victims may have taken, for example, a medication which caused drowsiness while they were driving and caused a serious accident. The cause of death was reported as being an automobile accident, rather than as a poisoning event. Or, the victims may have been at work in a closed

area with a gasoline engine running and inhaled a large quantity of carbon monoxide. If they left the area and shortly thereafter collapsed of an apparent "heart attack," and their blood was never checked for carbon monoxide, then death may be reported as due to natural causes rather than to acute carbon monoxide poisoning.

Several million more people may be poisoned each year, but because of life-saving first aid measures that are quickly instituted, they survive the ordeal. Because of their survival, or because their poisoning was not especially remarkable, the event was never reported. Consequently, these people are also not accounted for in the total annual figure that lists poisoning incidence.

So it can be seen that an accurate estimation of the actual number of poisonings that occur each year is not available.

Causes of Poisoning

The leading single cause of all poisonings in the United States today is plants (Table 4). This should not be surprising in light of the popularity in cultivating them for both inside and outside the home. Furthermore, many of them bear fruit or berries that are just too attractive and enticing for inquisitive children. Few people who cultivate plants actually understand the potentially toxic effects which may occur following their ingestion. Therefore, they fail to warn children of the danger, and they take no precautionary measures to avoid the poisoning.

On the more positive side, however, most plant ingestions do not cause severe toxicity, and simple supportive and palliative measures are all that are usually necessary. There are exceptions, of course, and some plants are deadly if ingested. Plant poisoning is discussed later, in Chapter 12.

Approximately 40% of all serious intoxications are caused by a variety of household products. Soaps, cleaners, and detergents lead the list, with petroleum-based products (e.g., furniture polish, lighter fluid, gasoline, etc.) following close behind.

Drugs account for the next class of poisoning causes, with aspirin still constituting the major

TABLE 3. *Partial listing of nontoxic substances*[a]

Abrasives	Lubricant
Antacids	Lubricating oils
Antibiotics	Lysol® Brand disinfectant (not toilet bowl
Baby product cosmetics	cleaner)
Ballpoint pen inks	Magic Markers®
Bathtub floating toys	Makeup (eye, liquid facial)
Battery (dry cell) (1/5 MLD of mercuric	Matches
chloride)	Mineral oil
Bath oil (castor oil and perfume)	Motor oil
Bleach (less than 5% sodium hypochlorite)	Newspaper
Body conditioners	Paint (indoor or latex)
Bubble bath soaps	Pencil (lead-graphite, coloring)
Calamine lotion	Perfumes
Candles (beeswax or paraffin)	Petroleum jelly
Caps (toy pistol) (potassium chlorate)	Phenolphthalein laxatives (Ex-Lax®)
Chalk (calcium carbonate)	Plants (250,000 of 300,000 plants
Cigarettes or cigars (nicotine)	identified are nontoxic. If dangerous
Clay (modeling)	plant identified, induce vomiting)
Contraceptives	Play-Doh®
Corticosteroids	Polaroid® picture coating fluid
Cosmetics	Porous tip ink marking pens
Crayons (marked A.P., C.P.)	Prussian blue (Ferricyanide)
Dehumidifying packets (silica or charcoal)	Putty (Less than 2 oz)
Detergents (phosphate type, anionic)	Rouge
Deodorants	Rubber cement
Deodorizers (spray and refrigerator)	Sachets (essential oils, powder)
Elmer's Glue®	Shampoos
Etch-A-Sketch®	Shaving creams and lotions
Eye makeup	Shoe polish (most do not contain aniline
Fabric softeners	dyes)
Fertilizer (if no insecticides or herbicides	Silly Putty® (99% silicones)
added)	Soap and soap products
Fish bowl additives	Spackles
Glues and pastes	Spackling compound
Golf ball (core may cause mechanical	Suntan preparations
injury)	Sweetening agents (saccharin, cyclamate)
Greases	Teething rings (water sterility)
Hair products (dyes, sprays, tonics)	Thermometers (mercury)
Hand lotions and creams	Thyroid tablet 3 g
Hydrogen peroxide (medicinal 3%)	Toilet water
Incense	Tooth paste (with or without fluoride)
Indelible markers	Vaseline®
Ink (black, blue)	Vitamins (with or without fluoride)
Iodophil disinfectant	Water colors
Laxatives	Zinc oxide
Lipstick	Zirconium oxide

[a]In the event that large quantities of any of these substances are ingested, an authoritative reference source should be consulted.

share of all drug-related poisonings. While aspirin toxicity was a leading cause of poisoning by all means in children under 5 years of age for many years, its incidence has decreased significantly during recent years. This is largely a result of the Poison Prevention Packaging Act of 1970 which required safety closures on all commercial packages of aspirin-containing products. Regardless of adverse publicity to the contrary, most people do not mind receiving medicines and household products in safety closure containers (2).

Other commonly encountered drugs that reportedly are leading causes of poisoning include vitamins and minerals (particularly products containing vitamins A and D, and iron), sleep-

TABLE 4. *Major causes of poisoning (1978)*

Plants
Soaps, detergents, cleaners
Antihistamines, cold medications
Perfume, cologne, toilet water
Vitamins, minerals
Asprin
   Baby
   Adult
   Unspecified
Household disinfectants, deodorizers
Miscellaneous analgesics
Insecticides (excluding mothballs)
Miscellaneous internal medicines
Fingernail preparations
Miscellaneous external medicines
Liniments
Household bleach
Miscellaneous products
Cosmetic lotions, creams
Antiseptic medications
Psychopharmacologic agents
Cough medicines
Hormones
Glues, adhesives
Rodenticides
Internal antibiotics
Corrosive acids, alkalies
Paint

Modified from National Clearinghouse for poison Control Centers (10).

ing medications, antihistamines and cold remedies, and sedative and antidepressant medications.

It is also known that proper management of the poisoned patient saves lives. It is estimated that over three-fourths of all calls to Poison Control Centers can be handled adequately over the telephone, if sufficient, accurate information is given (8). All that is required is reassurance, not treatment. Since health professionals are readily accessible to most people, it is extremely important that they understand the basic principles of clinical toxicology, and understand how these principles apply to the poisoned patient.

Who Is Poisoned?

Statistics indicate that the majority of poisonings (approximately 75%) occur in children under the age of 5. Children over 5 years constitute the next group (approximately 15%), while adults comprise the remaining 10%. Although the number of poisonings in children under 5 is high, overall morbidity and mortality are remarkably low, except for certain classes of poisons which are invariably fatal (8).

The reasons why children under 5 years constitute the largest poisoning group are many and varied. No study of the basic principles of toxicology can be complete without mentioning what some of those causes are.

For example, a toddler's immediate environment includes all of those areas around the home about which adults are generally not concerned. Consequently, adults take few precautions to keep these areas secure and free from poisons. To illustrate, the area under the kitchen sink is out of immediate sight for most adults (Fig. 3). In order to view this area, an adult must stoop low, bend the knees, or actually sit on the floor. To a toddler, this area is in his direct line of sight and it affords him an entirely new world

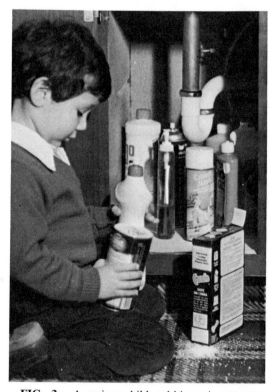

FIG. 3. A curious child and his environment.

to conquer. Another example is the mothballs that may have fallen from the closet shelf into a dark corner on the closet floor. They are probably never seen by an adult, but are quickly detected by an inquisitive toddler who believes they are candy to be devoured.

Children are also curious and investigative. A closed cabinet door, or even a high shelf, quickly becomes a major challenge to the child to see what's behind that door or on top of that shelf. A youngster may readily open the door or stack books or boxes on top of one another to get to the shelf. Many cases have been recorded where youngsters have built elaborate raised platforms to gain access to the top of the bathroom sink which then allow fairly easy access to the medicine cabinet. In many instances, these were constructed in only a few minutes while the parent was out of sight.

Many household products are marketed in attractive packages or contain enchanting labels that are intended to catch the eye of potential purchasers. However, these same labels that depict pictures of merry spring flowers, dancing maidens, musical notes, or citrus fruits also readily catch the roving eye and inquisitiveness of a young child. The bright red berries on the evergreen shrubbery outside the house may appear to be the same as the red berries in last night's dessert, and into the mouth they go.

The natural tendency of most children is to place anything and everything into the mouth. The fact that it may bear no resemblance to food, and perhaps doesn't even taste good, is purely coincidental to a youngster.

A young child actually does not distinguish between good versus bad tastes. Every parent is aware that young children will often readily accept and consume foods at the dinner table without thinking about the taste or appearance, until older brother or sister "reminds" them that they are not supposed to like the taste of certain vegetables and other foods. Thus, taste discrimination is a trait that is learned later. For example, a mothball, which an adult would immediately spit out, may remain for a long time in a child's mouth, sufficient to allow a significant amount of the chemical to be absorbed.

Parents often foster a poisoning because they take medication in the presence of their children. The old adage of "If I see it, I can do it" is especially prevalent in young children. Other times, parents administer candy-flavored medications or multiple vitamin products to children enticing them to readily take the product because of its "delicious candy" flavor. Youngsters who cannot distinguish between right and wrong, and who find this same bottle or a different container or a parent's prenatal vitamins or iron tablets (Fig. 4) unattended later on, may swallow a lethal dose, simply because they were told it was candy and tastes good.

McCormick et al. (9) present an interesting summary of poisonings of infants during diaper changing. Of 138 cases of poisoning that occurred during this procedure, 19% of the infants were directly given the poisonous material to keep them occupied. The authors admitted this number was probably even greater than the number that was reported.

A brief look around most homes should convince anyone that poisons are often left in easy viewing and, thus, are readily accessible to the unsuspecting. For example, count the number of unlabeled containers around the home that are filled with some liquid or solid substance. Also, look where these items, or even other items that do have appropriate labels, are stored. They are often found in unlocked cabinets, suit-

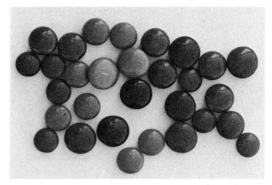

FIG. 4. Iron and vitamin tablets appear much the same as pieces of candy. Can you distinguish between them?

cases, on open shelves, in the bathroom corner, under the kitchen or bathroom sink, on the bedroom dresser or window ledge, on the workbench, etc. Too often an item that is normally kept in a secured area will be removed from that area for use, and then will remain within easy reach of some toddler's investigative fingers. It may even remain there for many days, weeks, or months until the user gets around to putting it away. Needless to say, poisoning takes only moments to happen.

Poisonings also occur because of the public's general unconcern or apathetic denial that a potential problem always exists. For example, cleaning aids, paint strippers and thinners, and other highly noxious products are used in nonvented areas. People work on an automobile, motorcycle, lawnmower, or other combustion engine left running in a closed garage, even though children are taught in grade school that this should not be done.

New products that may have been tested for their acute toxic potential are continually being introduced on the market. However, frequently, this toxic potential has not been tested over a period of time, or it has not been tested in persons of various ages, those with certain diseases, or when various diets are consumed. Also, many of these new products are extremely powerful, and the user may recall an older product that was similar but not exactly the same as the new product. If he uses it in the same manner as the older version, toxicity may occur.

Likewise, there is a wide variety of products on the market that exist in a concentrate form. One Poison Control Center reports it has observed severe burns occurring with alkali products whose pH was stated on the label as being "slightly alkaline" and, thus, seemingly safe on skin. However, this pH value referred to the diluted substance and not to the concentrate, whose pH in reality was in the dangerously caustic range.

Products often change their formulations. A toilet bowl cleaner which at one time may have been highly alkaline is now an acid-based product, and the switch in ingredients was made without apparent fanfare. An individual familiar with the older alkaline product may not even consider that the new product is completely different, especially since the name has not changed.

A common problem in acute poisonings occurs because the victim may not give the product's complete name. Therefore, the name is not descriptive of the constituents. For example, Clorox® is the name of a bleaching product that contains sodium hypochlorite. Clorox-2®, on the other hand, contains sodium perborate which must be antidoted differently than sodium hypochlorite. Drano® granules are sodium hydroxide, an alkali, and Drano® liquid drain cleaner is 1,1,1-trichloroethane, a moderately toxic hydrocarbon. So an important principle to remember is always make sure that the product name the victim states is actually descriptive of the ingredients.

A still more disturbing cause of poisoning exists because some products contain inaccurate or inappropriate antidoting information. Until recently, a salt solution to induce vomiting was considered appropriate to use for instances where emesis was indicated. However, it is now recognized that salt solutions may be more toxic than the actual poisoning event per se, and they have been the actual cause of some deaths (see Chapter 3). While labels on newly manufactured products no longer state that if the product is accidently swallowed, emesis should be induced with salt solution, many containers of these same products that were purchased 5 or 10 or even more years ago still exist around the home. The parent who is instructed by one of these older labels to administer a salt solution may be subjecting a poisoned victim to even more serious intoxication.

Consider another example of erroneous information (1). In this instance, a toddler swallowed a quantity of lye. First aid information on the label instructed that in case of ingestion, vinegar should be administered as an antidote. Vinegar was therefore given to the child with disastrous results. The mild acid actually increased the toxic effects of the lye due to an explosive exothermic (heat release) reaction which caused intense gastrointestinal damage that might not have occurred had the acid not been given.

While no one knows the exact extent of such inaccurate label information, it is thought to be extensive.

Where Poisonings Occur

Poisonings may occur anywhere, including around the home or workplace, at school, or on the road, and by any route of exposure. At home, most poisonings happen in the kitchen, followed by the bathroom, the bedroom, then all other sites together. It is not uncommon to hear a mother explain how her youngster got into some household cleaning agent found under the kitchen sink, or into a toilet cleaning aid, container of medicine from the bathroom, a medicine bottle, or cosmetic package in the bedroom. Likewise, reports are numerous which describe a person drinking a liquid from a soda bottle found in the garage that was apparently believed to be a palatable beverage but was subsequently shown to be gasoline, antifreeze, insecticide, or paint thinner. Even in the field, herbicides and insecticides serve as constant sources of poisoning through skin contact. The literature also abounds with reports of persons being intoxicated because they drank water which was transported in containers previously filled with insecticides or herbicides. Most accidental and suicidal poisonings occur through oral ingestion, while most industrial and agricultural toxicities follow pulmonary or dermal exposure (6).

Occasionally a farmer who is cleaning his liquid manure tanks is exposed to their toxic fumes (hydrogen sulfide), collapses, and dies after inhaling only a few breaths.

Another form of poisoning around the house can occur to anyone, but is especially prevalent to members of rural families during times of fertilizing the fields. In such incidences, application of liquid ammonia to the fields readily produces a cloud of ammonia gas which, if it carries across the field onto an adjoining plot where people are enjoying the evening on the patio, causes severe coughing, respiratory distress, and even death if enough is encountered.

At the place of employment, literally thousands of chemicals are present which may be accidentally ingested through contamination of food or water, or absorbed through the skin. Cases are documented whereby factory workers have taken certain chemicals home, apparently thinking they were nontoxic, but when used at home they caused serious toxicity.

In one instance, a family of three died when each of them ingested soup that had been seasoned with a lethal quantity of sodium nitrite. This was thought to have been placed in the salt container by a nonsuspecting father who brought it from his place of employment, apparently thinking it was table salt, sodium chloride.

An individual working in a ditch at a construction site around a busy highway, or in a tunnel, may become increasingly dizzy, lethargic, and ultimately unconscious, if the area where he is working becomes saturated with carbon monoxide from local traffic. Such poisoning encounters are fairly common around busy thoroughfares.

Schoolchildren, through negligence or perhaps even by mischievous intent, sometimes become careless with various chemicals from the chemistry laboratory, and these ultimately lead to some toxic episode. The fascination for metallic mercury has caused numerous reported toxicities, not through swallowing it, but by chronic inhalation of its vapors after being spilled on a living room carpet and dispersed into small globules with the vacuum cleaner.

Another example of reported unexpected toxic exposures resulted from aniline-containing products. These dyes are easily absorbed through the skin to cause methemoglobinemia. The route of exposure in these reports was from clothing stamped with laundry ink containing an aniline dye.

So it is easy to see that the potential for poisoning exists everywhere. Poisoning may result from chemicals in the air or water, from food because of residues or contamination, from medicines, or from other chemicals or poisonous products that are accidentally ingested.

When any one product or substance ingested by itself is not toxic per se, a combination of two or more different chemicals may be. For instance, we are all familiar with pharmacological examples of two drugs that, by themselves, at a particular dose, are not toxic. However, when they are combined, a serious toxicity occurs. Or, as will be described in Chapter 11, when chlorine bleach and a household cleaning product are mixed together, neither of which alone causes pulmonary irritation, they can produce a noxious gas which may cause serious toxic problems.

It is important to remember that the exact site of poisoning is not immediately necessary to antidoting the victim. It makes no difference whether the victim was intoxicated on the patio or in the bedroom. The problem exists and the victim's serious symptoms must be relieved as quickly as possible. On the other hand, knowing where poisonings occur is important because once the patient's immediate toxic symptoms are under control, this knowledge may help identify the specific cause in those cases where it is unknown. Then more specific antidotal measures can be instituted. Secondly, locating the site of poisoning will result in residues of the substance being removed or secured to keep others from ingesting it.

Knowing the major site of poisoning is also important for another, although frequently overlooked, consideration. During recent years a strong emphasis by the news media and health professions has been placed upon National Poison Prevention Week. The third week of March is set aside each year to make the American public more aware of the great potential and rapidity of poisoning around the home. People are advised to discard all unused chemicals and medications, and to move all potentially toxic substances out of the reach of children.

However, the "real world" situation is that many people can only be expected to do so much before they lose enthusiasm for the project. Thus, to assure the greatest public benefit will be derived from the least amount of effort, people should be advised to start this cleanup process at those sites around the home where the most significant problems exist. In other words, if an individual only secures, from a toxic substance standpoint, the kitchen and bathroom areas, then over 60% of all accidental

poisonings can, in theory, be prevented. If the bedroom is added, an additional 12%, or almost three-fourths of all accidental poisonings, may be prevented.

Does Poisoning Really Ever End?

Earlier in this chapter we posed the question, "When does toxicity end?" The answer may well be that it never ends. The possibility for toxic reactions to chemicals will always exist. However, their incidence, as just stated, can be reduced.

No health professional will be able to remove all toxic substances from the home and environment of the public he or she serves. This must be done at the home level. However, the public can be made aware of the problem and taught what should be done. This, then, is one of the basic principles of clinical toxicology. In other words, if poisoning is to be prevented or reduced in its intensity, the public must be made aware of the danger of chemicals.

So a fitting way to end this introductory chapter is to suggest specific means which will assure that the public is made aware of poison prevention techniques and will work toward reducing the chances for accidental poisoning. Teaching poison prevention awareness is every health practitioner's responsibility.

Make note of the points outlined in Table 5. Duplicate them into handout form and distribute them to all parents of small children. Better yet, mention the points whenever appropriate to any adult and urge that the points be taken seriously. Offer to speak about poison prevention topics to local service or PTA groups. Prepare slide shows for grade school children that depict the evils of poisons. Offer your time and talents to local news media as a source of information. Prepare press releases and radio spot announcements. The reception you will receive from both the media and public will be surprising.

Also, deterring symbols, such as *Mr. Yuk,* should be placed on containers which are toxic, and children should be instructed not to go near these items. Mr. Yuk and other symbols of poi-

TABLE 5. *Useful tips on reducing the incidence of poisoning*

Store all medication in a locked cabinet, out of the reach of children. Replace them immediately after use. Use child-resistant containers. Periodically check and discard medications no longer used. Flush them down the toilet, rinse containers, and discard.

Discard household cleaning aids or other products that are no longer being used. Flush them down the toilet, rinse containers well, and discard.

Store toxic household and garden products in cabinets fitted with safety latches and/or locks. When in use, always make sure an adult is present and that the product is put away immediately after use.

Work with household chemicals in a well ventilated area; do not mix chemicals (e.g., bleach and toilet bowl cleaner) unless specifically directed to do so.

Keep all items in their original containers. Never store toxic substances such as gasoline or insecticides in soda bottles or cups, or in any other unmarked or unapproved container. Use child-resistant containers and keep the caps securely shut between uses.

Never equate medicines with candy when administering drugs to children.

Never take medicines in front of small children, or joke, or make light of taking any medication, to a child.

Never take medicines in the dark or if you are not fully awake. If you normally wear glasses, put them on before taking the medication.

Keep poisonous plants away from children or others likely to ingest them. There is no reason, for example, to cultivate castor bushes that have deadly and enticing castor beans around a household with small children.

Educate children about the dangers of poisons in the home.

Use adhesive stickers showing Mr. Yuk, or similar characters, to help children identify dangerous substances.

In older houses, check for peeling paint or loose plaster, both of which can be a significant source of lead poisoning.

Never run fuel-consuming engines, kerosene heaters, etc. in a poorly ventilated area.

Formulate and rehearse a plan of action in case a poisoning should occur. Right now, look up important phone numbers (doctor, pharmacist, emergency rescue squad, etc.) and record these by the phone.

Make sure an up-to-date antidote chart is available. If in doubt about the validity of the one you have, bring it to a pharmacist or physician to check.

Stock emergency antidotes (activated charcoal and syrup of ipecac) and know how to use them.

soning (Fig. 5) have been developed to replace the older "skull and crossbones" reference. The public has become calloused to this symbol because it has been used indiscriminately, and, also, children might associate those items bearing the skull and crossbones with pirates and adventure.

Remember that Poison Prevention Week comes only once a year, but the message should be extended through the other 51 weeks.

SUMMARY

We must have a firm grasp on the fundamental elements of toxicology before specific events make sense. Thus, a few minutes spent reviewing these important points, by rereading this chapter, will be to our benefit.

If you have not already done so, read the book's preface at this time. It presents the philosophy of why this textbook was written. By understanding this, you'll have a better understanding of how to approach succeeding chapters.

Case Study

CASE STUDY: POISONING BY RAT POISON

History

A 24-month-old girl was hospitalized after her mother found her vomiting nearby an empty container of rat poison. The child had found the package in a low-lying cabinet, and emptied it into her cereal which she then ate. It was not packaged in a child-resistant container. The substance resembled cereal and smelled like peanuts, so the reason for the error was obvious.

The victim was treated with syrup of ipecac and a cathartic, and held for 2 days for observation during which time she received a vitamin supplement as her only other medication. She was released at the end of the second day, completely normal.

It should be noted that manufacturing of the product had been discontinued approximately 2 years before. The reason for this was because of the close visual similarity between the product and food, and

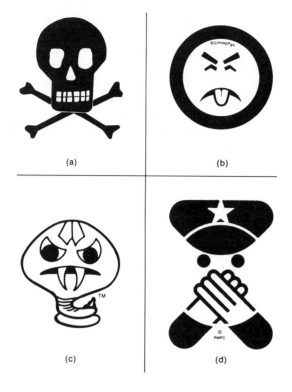

(a)

(b)

(c)

(d)

FIG. 5. Poison prevention symbols. **(a)** Traditional skull and crossbones; **(b)** Mr. Yuk; **(c)** SIOP; and **(d)** Officer Ugg.

because numerous poisonings with the same product had been reported in previous years. No packages were recalled from retail shelves, and the item may still be found.

Here we have a classical example that well illustrates many of the principles discussed in the text. The package of rat poison was found in a location generally unaccessible to adults, but easily noticed by the child. The product itself looked and smelled good, and it was apparently not repulsive to the taste. It was not packaged to prevent a child from getting into it and had no graphic poison identification on the label. Manufacture had long before been discontinued, although the product remained available for sale. Furthermore, although a poisoning occurred, the victim was not seriously harmed. (See ref. 12.)

Discussion

1. Outline the specific steps that could have been undertaken to prevent this poisoning. How should the child's parents guard against its recurrence?

2. What kinds of questions should you ask the parents if they were to call you for advice?

Review Questions

1. Discuss the probable origin of the term "toxicology," and what does it encompass?

2. Explain why M. J. B. Orfila is known today as the father of toxicology.

3. LD_{50} values are universally determined by all toxicologists using a standardized experimental protocol.
   A. True
   B. False

4. When we say its LD_{50} curve shifts to the left, how does this affect the therapeutic index for a drug?

5. Cite the figure usually presented that represents the number of people who die each year in the United States from poisoning. Why is this figure probably too low?

6. The majority of all poisonings occur in people of which of the following age groups?
   A. Under the age of 5 years
   B. 5–11 years
   C. 12–20 years
   D. 20 years and older

7. Explain why the individual depicted in Fig. 3 is especially vulnerable to accidental poisoning.

8. Cite ten important steps that may be taken to reduce the incidence of poisoning around the home.

9. Why is it important for consumers to know where most household poisonings occur?

10. A farmer who has been seriously intoxicated by fumes from a liquid manure tank is most likely suffering from poisoning by:
    A. Methane gas
    B. Ammonia gas
    C. Carbon monoxide
    D. Hydrogen sulfide

11. A period is set aside each year to be known as Poison Prevention Week. When does this occur?

12. List approximate quantities of a poison required by oral administration to be lethal in an average weight (150-pound) adult if the substance is labeled as shown:
    A. Practically nontoxic
    B. Moderately toxic
    C. Super toxic

13. List as many substances as you can that are commonly found around the home, which are considered to be nontoxic when ingested in normal quantities.

14. Which of the following toxicology subdisciplines is most closely associated with the medicolegal aspects of the toxic effects of chemicals on humans?
    A. Occupational toxicology
    B. Environmental toxicology
    C. Forensic toxicology
    D. Veterinary toxicology

15. Define the meaning of the term poison. What is meant by the statement that "all chemicals must be assumed to be toxic"?

16. What is an LD_{50} value? How does it relate to human toxicity?

17. Which of the following is the leading cause of all reported poisonings in the United States?
    A. Plants
    B. Soaps, cleaners
    C. Petroleum products
    D. Aspirin

18. Most plant ingestions do not cause severe toxicity problems.
    A. True
    B. False

19. A mother has phoned you to state that her young son has just swallowed some Clorox®. What is one of the first points you must clarify before antidotal therapy can proceed?

20. Newly manufactured products should no longer state on their label that salt solution should be used to induce emesis.
    A. True
    B. False

21. Vinegar is an appropriate antidote to administer to a person who has swallowed lye.
    A. True
    B. False

22. Most household poisonings occur at which of the following sites?
    A. Kitchen
    B. Bedroom
    C. Bathroom
    D. Garage

References

1. Anon (1977): Home-poison menace: inaccurate first-aid labels. *Medical World News*, March 21.
2. Biberdorf, R. L., and Forbes, D. S. (1977): Child-resistant medicine containers—Public use, preference and storage. *J. Am. Pharm. Assoc.*, 17:170–172.
3. Casarett, L. J., and Bruce, M. C. (1980): Origin and scope of toxicology. In: *Toxicology—The Basic Science of Poisons*, 2nd ed., edited by J. Doull, C. D. Klaassen, and M. O. Amdur, pp. 3–10. Macmillan, New York.
4. Gosselin, R. E., Hodge, H. C., Smith, R. P., and Gleason, M. N. (1976): *Clinical Toxicology of Commercial Products*, 4th ed. Williams & Wilkins, Baltimore.
5. Holmstedt, B., and Liljestrand, G. (editors) (1981): *Readings in Pharmacology*. Raven Press, New York.
6. Klaassen, C. D., and Doull, J. (1980): Evaluation of safety: Toxicologic evaluation. In: *Toxicology—The Basic Science of Poisons*, 2nd ed., edited by J. Doull, C. D. Klaassen, and M. O. Amdur, pp. 11–27. Macmillan, New York.
7. Loomis, T. A. (1978): *Essentials of Toxicology*, 3rd ed., Lea & Febiger, Philadelphia.
8. Lovejoy, F. H., and Berenberg, W. (1978): Poisoning in children under age 5. *Postgrad. Med.*, 63:79–89.

9. McCormick, M. A., Lacouture, P. G., Gandreault, P., and Lovejoy, F. H. (1982): Hazards associated with diaper changing. *JAMA*, 248:2159–2160.

10. National Clearinghouse for Poison Control Centers. (1980): Tabulations of 1978 case reports. *U.S. Dept. Health and Human Services, Rockville, Maryland*, 24:3.

11. Orfila, M. J. B. (1815): *Traite des poisons tires min-eral, vegetal et animal on toxicologie generale sous le rapports de la pathologie et de la medicine legale.* Crochard, Paris.

12. Schum, T. R., and Lachman, B. S. (1982): Effect of packaging and appearance on childhood poisoning. *Clin. Pediatr.*, 21:282–285.

13. Sonnedecker, G. (1963): *History of Pharmacy*. J.B. Lippincott, Philadelphia.

Factors That Influence Toxicity

2

SIGNIFICANCE

Poisonings do not always follow the "textbook" descriptions commonly listed for them. Signs and symptoms that are often stated as being pathognomonic (characteristic) for a particular toxic episode may or may not be evident with each case of poisoning. Poisoning victims may even display a behavior that is totally unexpected, and largely unpredictable.

It should be evident, then, that an experimentally determined acute oral toxicity expression, such as an LD_{50} value, is not an absolute description of the compounds' toxicity in all individuals. It neither assesses the inherent capacity of the compound to produce injury, nor reflects the victim's ability to respond in a manner other than predicted.

An extremely important principle always to bear in mind when evaluating a victim's response to a toxic chemical is that there are numerous factors which may modify the patient's responses to the toxic agent. Frequently the physician is faced with a bewildering situation. He strongly suspects the person has been subjected to an otherwise toxic exposure of some substance and may even await onset of certain symptoms, but the victim is not displaying what is expected. Or, it may be a situation where an ordinarily subtoxic dose of some chemical has produced poisoning symptoms that are quantitatively far beyond expectation. Perhaps much of the controversy associated with accurate interpretation of results or assessment of a patient's symptoms results from our failure to recognize the existence or importance of certain basic factors that may modify (increase or decrease) an individual's response to exposure by a chemical agent. Medical personnel should always keep these factors in mind during patient assessment. Realizing that these factors exist and are important to the patient is basic to our fundamental understanding of poisoning and the principles of clinical toxicology.

The factors (principles) that influence toxicity are essentially the same as those which determine a drug's pharmacological action. These are the factors that are studied early in pharmacology. However, we need to review these basic factors now, and briefly illustrate their importance in altering a toxic response. The following discussion is not meant to be a complete treatise on all the factors, but serves to illustrate the importance of assessing the poisoned patient in a holistic fashion.

COMPOSITION OF THE TOXIC AGENT

When referring to a toxic episode, a basic fallacy is the view that the responsible poison is a pure substance. This implies that there are no contaminants present, the vehicle and various adjuvants and formulation ingredients are innocuous, the victim has not taken any drugs previously, and there is no batch-to-batch variation in the product. These criteria are met in laboratory experimentation, but are rare in the "real world" of poisoning. We must always consider the possibility that the toxic episode may be the result of one or more toxic agents, including the vehicle. We have once again learned such a lesson in recent years about the importance of contaminants. Because of the presence of the toxic impurity, dioxin, in the herbicide, 2,4,5-T, severe toxic problems have occurred (see Chapter 9).

The physicochemical composition of the toxicant can sometimes be helpful in predicting the risk involved in exposure to a particular compound. In general, solids are less easily swallowed than liquids, and bulky, low-density solids are more difficult to consume than light, more fluffy compounds, especially for a small child. Thus, poisoning by these forms is less likely to occur than with liquids and small-size particles. The particulate size of the toxic agent is especially important in exposure by inhalation. Only particles having a small diameter (1 µm or less) will effectively reach the alveoli and be available for pulmonary absorption. Larger particles may, of course, be deposited on the walls of the throat and trachea to produce irritation to those tissues.

The pH of the compound is another factor which is definitely a predictor of its toxicity. If the chemical is a strong acid or base, obvious deleterious effects will occur with even a limited exposure to the compound, whereas ingestion of mildly acidic or alkaline substances may cause little more than localized gastric irritation.

Another factor which can modify the toxicity of an agent is its stability. Are breakdown products formed on storage? Will it remain active in a definite concentration? When added to water, does it change its chemical composition? These are important questions that need to be answered when establishing the toxicity potential of a compound.

Sometimes a compound, which was a pure chemical when packaged, may have undergone a chemical change to produce an entirely different species capable of causing toxicity symptoms which are unrelated to those expected from the original chemical. One such example is paraldehyde. This is a liquid sedative-hypnotic that produces, in overdose, its expected side effect of central nervous system (CNS) depression. However, paraldehyde that has been exposed to light and air may partially decompose to acetaldehyde. When acetaldehyde is ingested, nausea, severe reddening of the skin, coughing, and pulmonary edema are characteristically noted. Thus, a patient who ingested a large quantity of this impure paraldehyde solution and then displayed the latter symptoms could theoretically be described as having been poisoned by acetaldehyde, rather than by paraldehyde.

Suppose a caller explains that a victim has swallowed a particular substance identified by the label as an insecticide. The victim's parent reads the name of the insecticide from the container's label and describes the victim's behavior. You realize that the displayed symptoms do not match those expected from the particular insecticidal product. What is wrong?

The most obvious solution may be that the bottle contained a different substance than the label stated, or, possibly, an insignificant amount was ingested so that onset of expected symptoms may be delayed or may not even occur. Alternatively, the caller may have picked up the wrong container thinking that it was the one from which the ingestion occurred. In reality, the victim may have ingested an entirely different substance than that suspected by caller. But each poisoning incidence must be assessed by carefully examining all the facts rather than simply making an assumption and then proceeding with treatment; what actually happened in this example was that the puzzling symptoms were caused by some component of the product other than the primary labeled ingredient. In this case, the victim exhibited symptoms of nausea, coughing and gagging, and slight CNS depression from a petroleum distillate that served as the solvent for pyrethrins, the active insecticidal ingredient. The product was a pediculicide intended to kill head and body lice. Pyrethrins alone are not significantly toxic to people. Symptoms in this case were descriptive of the solvent, rather than of the pyrethrins. Had emergency personnel thought that the victim's symptoms would quickly dissipate because of the relatively nontoxic nature of the insecticide, and not have assessed the victim for "solvent" toxicity, a disastrous outcome may have resulted.

The first rule in identification of a potentially toxic substance is to check everything on the label to determine which substances in the product are potentially toxic, and which are probably not toxic. Additionally, after other factors have been quickly ruled out and the cause of poisoning is still unknown, an analytical as-

sessment of the product's composition should be determined, if possible, to ascertain whether it has undergone possible decomposition or alteration in contents to form a completely different chemical.

DOSE AND CONCENTRATION

One of the major factors influencing the toxic effect of a chemical is the dose or concentration. Remember, anything can be toxic if enough is taken (and, conversely, even the most toxic of substances may not be harmful when low concentrations are taken). The intravenous LD_{50} of distilled water in the mouse is 44 ml/kg, and for isotonic saline, 68 ml/kg (1). In these examples, it is obvious that both distilled water and isotonic saline are not generally considered toxic, but at a high enough volume or dose, their toxicity becomes evident.

Doses are normally calculated according to a person's weight, and larger doses usually imply a greater chance for a toxic response to occur. When a child accidentally ingests adult strength aspirin tablets (325 mg), as opposed to flavored baby aspirin tablets (81 mg), there is a greater risk for toxicity. It will obviously take fewer adult strength aspirin to produce significant toxicity (see Chapter 14).

With ingestion of a diluted solution of a potentially toxic compound, the chances for toxic effects to occur are greater than if the same quantity of substance was ingested in concentrated form. Diluted forms are more quickly absorbed and available to susceptible tissues. On the other hand, if the substance is an irritant, a diluted form may cause fewer toxic signs and symptoms (1).

ROUTES OF ADMINISTRATION

The manner by which a potentially toxic substance is introduced into the body can influence the time of onset, intensity, and duration of the toxic effects. The route of administration may also predict the degree of toxicity and possibly the target systems which will most readily be affected. A chemical injected by the intravenous route would be expected to be most toxic.

Administered by other routes, the approximate descending order of toxicity would be inhalation → intraperitoneal→ subcutaneous→ intramuscular→ intradermal→ oral→ topical (13). Of course, not all of these routes are important in clinical toxicology. However, it is not uncommon for poisoning to occur by subcutaneous or intradermal injection when an injected substance, intended for the intravenous route, was inadvertently injected outside the vein (18).

Oral

Most acute toxic episodes result from accidental or intentional ingestion of a toxic agent. The basic pharmacokinetic parameters governing absorption of drugs apply to toxic ingestions. We should remember that there is the potential for a compound to be absorbed throughout the gastrointestinal tract, including the buccal cavity and rectum. Absorption is dependent on the amount of nonionized form available. Gastric absorption is usually limited, but intestinal absorption is extensive because of its large surface area.

There are several important factors which may significantly modify the absorption of drugs and chemicals following oral administration.

First, a major consideration in the rate of absorption following ingestion is that the chemical must be dissolved. This is not a major concern with liquids, but for solid dosage forms, absorption is dependent on the dissolution rate. This also poses a concern for treatment of a poisoned patient. Many antidoting protocols suggest that ingested poisons should first be diluted and we generally adhere to this belief. There may be cases, however, where dilution would cause added adverse effects for the poisoned patient, by increasing the rate of absorption and production of heat. This will be discussed further in Chapters 3 and 8.

Another problem experienced with ingestion of large quantities of solid dosage forms is that they may clump together (form concretions) in the stomach. These may be difficult to remove by emesis or lavage. Lavaging until the return solution is clear may give the physician a false sense of security. It may be assumed that all of the stomach contents were removed (including the solid dosage form) but, in fact, the particles were too large to fit through the opening of the lavage tube. This mass of tablets or capsules may now behave more like a repository sustained-release dosage form.

The presence and type of food in the stomach can modify absorption of a compound. A meal rich in protein or fat usually delays absorption. Carbonated beverages increase the rate of intestinal absorption by increasing gastric emptying time, with evolution of carbon dioxide. Ingestion of a concentrated chemical frequently causes a decrease in absorption because of gastric irritation and constriction of the pyloric sphincter.

On the positive side, the oral route of intoxication may provide the body with a chance to readily metabolize (and, it is hoped, detoxify!) the ingested toxicant. The portal circulation transports all chemical substances absorbed from the gastrointestinal tract directly to the liver, the major organ of detoxification (13). This is especially beneficial for those compounds which undergo a significant first-pass effect. At the same time, some compounds (e.g., acetaminophen, carbon tetrachloride) are actually activated by the liver's enzymes to a more toxic form.

Inhalation

The lung is a large target organ that is constantly undergoing all sorts of insults from air pollutants, dusts, fibers, and other irritants. Serious toxic effects may follow from pulmonary absorption of vapors and aerosols. The pulmonary route can greatly accentuate the expected onset of toxicity for a given compound because of the lung's rich blood supply with its close proximity to alveolar air (10 μm) and the large surface area (50–100 m^2) of the alveoli. Toxicants that are absorbed by the lung fall into two categories: vapors and aerosols.

Vapors of toxicological significance consist of gases such as carbon monoxide, hydrogen sulfide, sulfur oxides, and nitrogen oxides. Vapor fumes from volatile liquids include chloroform, benzene, carbon tetrachloride; and fumes from solids include mercury vapor and several others. Transport of vapors across the alveolar membrane occurs by simple diffusion. The blood concentration of toxic chemical will depend on its solubility in blood, since blood equilibrates with alveolar gases almost instantaneously. In the case of hydrogen sulfide, a few inhalations of high concentrations of the gas may be all that is necessary to cause death.

Since aerosols are suspensions of particulate matter, the chief limiting factor in determining pulmonary absorption is the size of the particle. As stated earlier, only particles with a mean aerodynamic diameter of 1 μm or less will be transported into the alveolar region to be available for absorption into the bloodstream. Pulmonary absorption of soluble particles can occur by either the lipid-soluble diffusion or water-soluble filtration process.

Dermal Penetration

Percutaneous absorption involves the transport of a compound through the skin's various layers into the systemic circulation. Entry through sebaceous or sweat glands, or through hair follicles is another, although relatively uncommon, means. Skin is the most readily accessible organ to all forms of foreign chemicals. However, it is also an efficient barrier to most environmental toxins. Penetration by a chemical is time-dependent and a function of its lipid solubility and concentration gradient.

Most toxic skin exposures occur accidentally. The degree of toxicity is influenced by the compound involved and the condition of the skin. For example, cuts or abrasions on the skin's surface will allow the toxic agent to bypass the first layers of defense—the keratin and epidermis. They permit substances, that would generally not penetrate the epidermis, to easily pass into the deeper strata and into the circulatory system.

Industrial accidents involving the handling of extremely toxic solvents often occur. If a worker is heavily clothed and comes in contact with a chemical, the clothing may keep the toxic chemical localized to the area and extend the contact time with the skin. The type of chemical is also an important factor, because corrosive acids and alkali will initially increase the permeability by their destruction of the stratum corneum (see Chapter 8).

METABOLISM OF THE TOXIC AGENT

The metabolism of a toxic compound is generally recognized as the primary mechanism for its detoxification. Usually a toxic agent is metabolized to a more polar (less toxic) compound which is then readily excreted by the kidney. Unfortunately, this is not always the situation. Some chemicals are metabolized to compounds that are equally as active or sometimes even more active. Methanol, for example, must first be oxidized to its intermediate metabolites, formaldehyde and formic acid, to produce its most serious toxic symptoms, although methanol, per se, is a CNS depressant (Chapter 4). A partial list a chemicals known to be metabolized to more toxic compounds is presented in Table 1.

STATE OF HEALTH

As long as the patient's symptoms are managed and the toxic chemical undergoes typical

TABLE 1. *Representative examples of chemicals that are metabolized to more toxic substances*

Acetaminophen
Acetanilid
Aniline
Arsenicals, pentavalent
Carbon tetrachloride
Chloral hydrate
Codeine
Ethylene glycol
Heptachlor
Isopropanol
Methanol
2-Naphthylamine
Parathion
Pyridine
Schradan
Sulfanilamide
Tri-*o*-cresyl phosphate

metabolism to a nontoxic compound followed by excretion, the chances for survival are favorable. Most all descriptions of poisoning and patient prognoses are based on an otherwise healthy individual. However, the presence of hepatic or renal disease may significantly affect the pharmacokinetics of the toxic agent so that it becomes significantly more toxic. An example illustrated later in this chapter shows that infants who are deficient in certain hepatic enzymes react to some chemicals with severe toxicity. Although this is not a true analogy to a person with liver disease, the end result would be the same. Likewise, for persons with severe renal disease, certain drugs should be avoided in therapy (3). It stands to reason then that chemicals, in general, may be more toxic in such individuals.

Numerous other examples are also significant. Acidosis, from any cause, potentiates the action of tubocurarine and decreases the activity of insulin. Hypertensive patients may respond more intensely to chemicals that have sympathomimetic activity. Opiates and other chemicals that cause respiratory depression are more hazardous in persons with head injuries. Psychotomimetics may provoke recurrence of disease in patients with a past history of psychiatric disease. Most chemicals are passively absorbed across the mucosal surface of the small intestine and rely on physical contact with the mucosa for absorption. Disease states that cause diarrhea or constipation may decrease or increase the time of contact between chemical and absorptive sites and, thus, lower or enhance absorption. Stress-mediated changes in hormonal levels (e.g., hyperthyroidism) may alter the toxic effects of certain chemicals (4). The list of examples is lengthy.

AGE AND MATURITY

The patient's age must always be considered before the extent of toxic reactions can be fully assessed. Most anticipated toxic effects, as well as reported prognoses, are based on individuals who are *neither* too young nor too old. Unfortunately, not all victims of poisoning are of this ideal age. In fact, as we learned in Chapter 1, most accidental poisonings occur in persons of less than 5 years. Also, we are just beginning to understand the area of geriatric pharmacology and toxicology. Age as a factor relating to a difference in toxicity between infants and adults may be exemplified by considering the classic chloramphenicol-induced gray-baby syndrome.

In the early 1960s, it was still popular practice to administer the antibiotic, chloramphenicol, to premature infants as a prophylactic measure. It became apparent after several years of such therapy, that a numbr of infants receiving this antibiotic were being intoxicated with it. Within days of initiation of treatment, signs and symptoms of aplastic anemia appeared (5,11).

Chloramphenicol is normally excreted in adults largely as the glucuronide metabolite. No adult had ever before been reported to experience aplastic anemia from chloramphenicol, and it may have been assumed that children also form the glucuronide metabolite and readily excrete the drug. After considerable study, however, it was learned that infants were unable to metabolize chloramphenicol to its detoxified metabolite because their hepatic enzymes were not fully developed. Blood levels of the antibiotic increased to toxic levels, and only a few doses were sufficient to cause a potentially lethal effect. However, once an infant developed adequate liver microsomal enzymes, chloramphenicol would be metabolized normally. The incidence of aplastic anemia would then decrease proportionately. The problem was even further compounded by inadequate renal excretion of unconjugated drug (16).

In geriatric patients the toxic effects of an injected drug may be reduced because of a generalized physiological reduction of blood supply into tissues. Similarly, the toxic response from an orally ingested drug or chemical may also be reduced, because once absorbed less of the substance will be delivered to a particular tissue site. This entire process, in elderly people, may be complicated even more because of their having, in general, a greater incidence of debilitating diseases (e.g., hepatic, renal, and cardiovascular) which may further reduce their ability to detoxify, excrete, or distribute the drug or chemical.

Age-related differences in an individual's susceptibility to a drug or poison are not based solely on rates of metabolism, distribution, or excretion. Absorption may also be adversely affected or modified because of geriatric diets which may vary from those of younger adults.

NUTRITIONAL STATE AND DIETARY FACTORS

Certain nutritional factors such as the food or liquid contents of the stomach (e.g., acidic or alkaline, hot or cold, high-fat or lean, high or low volume, and viscosity) are extremely important to the absorption characteristics of many chemicals.

We know the importance of taking drugs on an empty stomach. In general, higher blood levels are achieved when drugs are taken on an empty stomach, than if similar doses of these same drugs are taken when food is in the stomach (8).

Certain foods may significantly increase or decrease drug absorption. A frequently stated example relates to the calcium in milk, which may bind to tetracycline, and thus reduce its absorption (6). Fatty foods, on the other hand, enhance griseofulvin absorption (7).

Certain foods may antagonize drug effects. For example, foods rich in pyridoxine may significantly lower the pharmacological action of levodopa (9).

Nutritional effects on absorption are not limited to drugs. For example, heavy metal absorption is influenced by diet. Calcium, iron, fats, and protein are all reported to enhance lead absorption (2). Deficiency of calcium, iron, or protein, on the other hand, enhances cadmium absorption.

Also, some foods can actually increase the toxicity of certain drugs by means other than influencing their absorption. An excellent example is those foods that are rich in the pressor amine, tyramine (Table 2). If one of these foods is ingested while an individual is taking a mono-

TABLE 2. *Foods containing large amounts of tyramine*

Aged cheese
Beer
Canned figs
Chianti wines
Chicken liver
Chocolate
Pickled herring
Raisins
Sherry
Sour cream
Soy sauce
Yeast extracts

amine oxidase inhibiting drug (e.g., pargyline, phenelzine), severe symptoms of hypertensive crisis and even death may occur. Tyramine in foods is ordinarily metabolized to a nontoxic substance by monoamine oxidase which is located within the cells lining the gastrointestinal tract. This occurs as tyramine enters these cells during absorption into the blood. Little or no tyramine is, therefore, absorbed. However, when monoamine oxidase enzyme is inhibited, tyramine is not metabolized and is absorbed into the blood where it causes its toxic pressor effect.

Individuals on a starvation diet, or those who have a low protein intake, may have lower-than-normal plasma levels of albumin (19). Consequently, this may leave a proportionately greater amount of an ingested drug in its free form that normally binds to albumin. Since it is the free form of a drug (versus that which is protein bound) which causes toxicity, the drug will be more toxic. Also, a low dietary protein intake may result in a decreased level of hepatic microsomal enzymes and, thus, the metabolic processes may proceed less readily.

GENETICS

A new word, *pharmacogenetics*, has entered the toxicologist's vocabulary in recent years. While frequently used interchangeably with the term idiosyncrasy, pharmacogenetics describes the differences in an individual's response to drugs and chemicals that are related to hereditary influences.

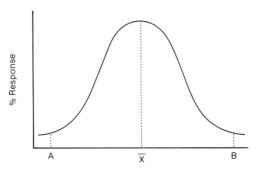

FIG. 1. A normal distribution curve.

It is commonly recognized that if a population of men is sampled and their body weights measured, the results would distribute graphically as shown in Fig. 1. The largest majority of men would weigh close to the arithmetic mean of the group. Additionally, a few would weigh much less (Fig. 1,A) while others would weigh much more (Fig. 1,B). The form of the graph would assume the shape of a normal distribution that is also characteristic of numerous other factors which can be measured within a population (e.g., height, blood pressure, intelligence, etc.). Each of these values is determined by a multiplicity of variables which are largely inherited.

However, occasionally a bimodal, or even trimodal curve (Fig. 2) results when some response is measured, and an entirely different variable then becomes important to our understanding of toxicology.

To illustrate the importance of pharmacogenetics as it relates to drug toxicity, consider the drug succinylcholine. This depolarizing skeletal muscle relaxant drug is given by infusion during surgery to permit procedures at a lighter stage

of general anesthesia than would be necessary without it. All skeletal muscle activity, including that of respiration, is depressed.

Ordinarily the biotransformation of succinylcholine proceeds as shown in Fig. 3. Most people quickly inactivate the drug by hydrolysis to its first inactive metabolite, succinylmonocholine. This occurs via the plasma enzyme, pseudocholinesterase (10). Thus, the initial step proceeds quickly, and within minutes the drug's activity is lost. So, once intravenous infusion is halted, skeletal muscle tone begins to increase and the patient's normal respiration is restored. Metabolism is later completed by liver enzymes, resulting in succinic acid and choline, but this step takes more time.

The problem arises because some people exhibit an unusual susceptibility to succinylcholine (10). They possess an atypical pseudocholinesterase and, consequently, cannot undergo the initial detoxifying step that normally occurs in the same time frame. Metabolism of succinylcholine in these individuals is slower. Thus the individual receiving succinylcholine experiences prolonged apnea and skeletal muscle relaxation that may last for several hours after discontinuation of infusion.

Figure 4 illustrates the rate of hydrolysis of succinylcholine by plasma containing normal pseudocholinesterase versus plasma with the atypical enzyme. It can readily be seen that the atypical enzyme hydrolyzes succinylcholine at a greatly reduced rate. This medical problem has been carefully investigated and results of numerous studies have shown that one person in about 2,000 possesses the atypical enzyme and genetic background that favors this prolonged action to succinylcholine.

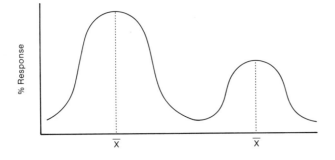

FIG. 2. A bimodal distribution curve showing two population groups.

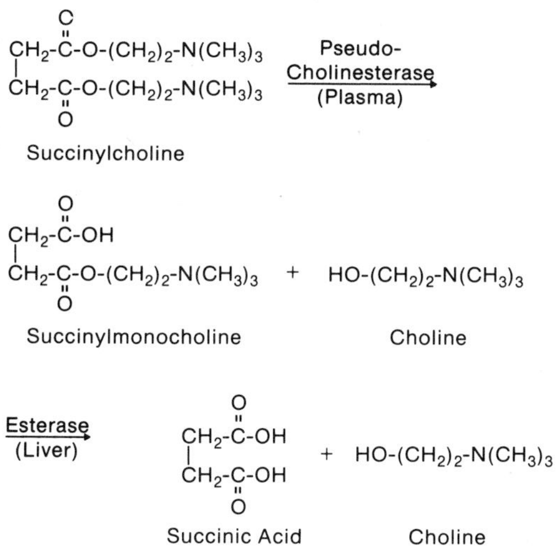

$$CH_2\text{-}\overset{\overset{\displaystyle O}{\|}}{C}\text{-}O\text{-}(CH_2)_2\text{-}N(CH_3)_3$$
$$CH_2\text{-}\underset{\underset{\displaystyle O}{\|}}{C}\text{-}O\text{-}(CH_2)_2\text{-}N(CH_3)_3$$

$\xrightarrow{\text{Pseudo-Cholinesterase (Plasma)}}$

Succinylcholine

$$CH_2\text{-}\overset{\overset{\displaystyle O}{\|}}{C}\text{-}OH$$
$$CH_2\text{-}\underset{\underset{\displaystyle O}{\|}}{C}\text{-}O\text{-}(CH_2)_2\text{-}N(CH_3)_3 \quad + \quad HO\text{-}(CH_2)_2\text{-}N(CH_3)_3$$

Succinylmonocholine   Choline

$\xrightarrow{\text{Esterase (Liver)}}$
$$CH_2\text{-}\overset{\overset{\displaystyle O}{\|}}{C}\text{-}OH$$
$$CH_2\text{-}\underset{\underset{\displaystyle O}{\|}}{C}\text{-}OH \quad + \quad HO\text{-}(CH_2)_2\text{-}N(CH_3)_3$$

Succinic Acid   Choline

FIG. 3. Biochemical transformation of succinyl-choline.

Most genetically-controlled differences in a person's response to drugs and chemicals are due to differences in rates of metabolism. However, the same consideration should be extended to variations in absorption, distribution, and excretion. A partial list of important genetically-controlled conditions in which individuals display altered responses to drugs and chemicals is presented in Table 3.

SEX

Toxicologists are only beginning to understand the differences between drug and chemical responses in males and females. While significant quantitative differences in pharmacological responses have been experimentally shown in animals to occur to a variety of drugs and chemicals (6), such a definitive statement on the expected toxicity of drugs and chemicals cannot be stated at this time.

For example, some studies report that a sex-related difference exists for absorption of erythromycin, resulting in less of the drug being absorbed by women, following oral administration (14,15). Females have also been reported in one study to have lower serum phenytoin levels than men, because of their increased metabolism rate (17). While the pharmacological activity and onset, as well as severity of adverse reactions (e.g., nausea, vomiting, etc.) for these drugs may differ among the sexes, there is still no definitive evidence that an acute toxic dose of either of them will produce significantly different toxic manifestations between men and women.

It should also be pointed out that most studies which report sex-related differences in drug action are conducted with pharmacologic, rather than toxic, doses of the drug.

Several other important considerations do need to be considered. For example, men traditionally weigh more than women. Therefore, a dose of a chemical in a male would be expected to produce lower blood and tissue levels than the same dose taken by a female, simply because of the male's larger blood volume and greater tissue mass which dilute the chemical. Additionally, differences in quantities of muscle mass and fat tissue may be important determinants for blood levels reached by certain drugs and chemicals. For substances that are injected intramuscularly, lower blood levels can be expected with those drugs in individuals (usually

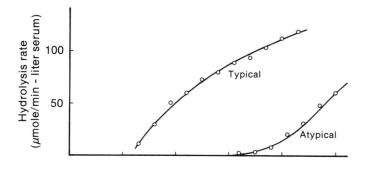

FIG. 4. Rate of hydrolysis of succinylcholine in the presence and absence of the normal enzyme. (From ref. 12.)

TABLE 3. *Examples of pharmacogenetic-related differences in response to selected drugs*

Genetic abnormality	Drug/chemical	Response
Atypical pseudocholinesterase	Succinylcholine	Prolonged skeletal muscle relaxation; apnea
Deficient NADH methemoglobin reductase	Nitrates Chlorates Oxidizing agents	Abnormally high and prolonged methemoglobin levels
Deficient hepatic acetyl transferase	Isoniazid Hydralazine Phenelzine	Enhanced toxicity, qualitatively and quantitatively
Deficient glucose-6-phosphate dehydrogenase	Acetylsalicylic acid Primaquine Quinine Nitrofurantoin Naphthalene Fava beans	Hemolytic anemia
Abnormally sensitive δ-amino-levulinic acid synthetase	Barbiturates	Hepatic porphyria
Presence of atropine esterase (rabbits)	Atropine	Atropine resistance
Increased hepatic enzymes	Warfarin	Warfarin resistance

men) with a greater muscle mass. Also, drugs with a high lipid coefficient that normally partition into fat may produce different toxicological responses in different sexes, based on the individual's ratio of body fat/total weight. Admittedly, many of these factors are of more theoretical interest and experimental significance than of clinical importance. However, they illustrate the extent of variability that a chemical may produce in different people.

At present, there is little clinical information concerning differences in toxic reactions between the genders. While quantitative differences may occur, qualitative differences probably do not. An acute toxicity response should be managed in a similar manner for both men and women, depending on severity of symptoms.

ENVIRONMENTAL FACTORS

Temperature

The response of a biological system to a toxic agent decreases as the environmental temperature is lowered, but the duration of the overall response may be prolonged. The reasons for these apparent discrepancies are related, first, to a decreased rate of absorption occurring in the colder environment; and, second, discrepancies occur because once the drug or chemical is absorbed, its effects may be prolonged owing to a lowered rate of metabolic degradation and excretion.

Additionally, some drugs are more toxic in certain environmental temperatures than in others. For example, atropine-like compounds may produce significantly greater toxicity in a warm environment than in a colder one. Because anticholinergic agents inhibit sweating, the body temperature becomes elevated because the absence of perspiration prevents cooling of the body; so the toxic effects are from hyperthermia.

Alternatively, drugs such as reserpine and chlorpromazine that suppress the body's thermal regulatory center may be more toxic at certain temperatures. Such drugs permit the body temperature to assume that of the environment. Therefore, an individual's body temperature tends to rise in a warmer climate and decrease in a colder climate.

In either instance, the factor to be clearly concerned with is temperature; perhaps hyperthermia in the first instance, and hypothermia or exposure at the lower temperature.

Occupation

Individuals working in industries where organic compounds such as chlorinated hydrocarbon pesticides or volatile substances are used may have an enhanced ability to metabolize drugs and chemicals. The reason for this is related to the chemical's presence in the environment, which may have enhanced the worker's liver microsomal enzyme activity. His expected reaction to a toxic dose of any subsequent chemical, normally detoxified by the liver microsomal system, would be less than normal. Of course, his reaction would be greater than normal for those substances listed in Table 1 that are metabolized to a more toxic form.

Living Conditions

The final factor we will consider is the living conditions to which a person is subjected. We should remember that the potential relevance of this factor is based on animal studies and its relation to humans can only be surmised. If clinically significant, the living conditions of an individual could be an extremely important factor to consider. We include it here to stress the importance of understanding all ramifications when attempting to interpret the events of a poisoning. The amphetamine-aggregation toxicity test can be used to illustrate this factor.

The LD_{50} value for amphetamine is determined for mice placed singly in a container. As the number of animals that are placed in the container increases, the LD_{50} decreases (i.e., the drug becomes more toxic). There seems to be a crowding factor related to living conditions that significantly affects the toxic dose of amphetamine.

More work is needed to ascertain if this response is significant in humans, and, if so, for what chemicals. If it does hold for people, it may at least partially explain differences in toxicity of a chemical in people of rural areas versus people living in crowded urban settings. At present, we should consider that factors such as crowding in living conditions, noise, and social pressures are important areas for research, but difficult to quantify.

SUMMARY

Our understanding of the factors that may modify chemical activity in the body will be enhanced if we realize that most of these factors are based on important pharmacological principles and common sense. Any individual factor discussed in this chapter is not more important than the others. Indeed, we included the ones in this chapter simply to illustrate the importance of the topic in general, rather than to specify these as being more relevant than the ones not listed.

As we will see again and again throughout this book, victims of poisoning frequently respond in an unpredictable manner. Understanding why their responses may vary from the "normal" will greatly aid our understanding of how to best manage the patient.

Review Questions

1. Discuss the meaning and the relevance of the term pathognomonic when it refers to symptoms relating to a poison.

2. How do the factors that influence toxicity which are discussed in this chapter compare or contrast to means for influencing a pharmacological (beneficial) response?

3. Discuss how chloramphenicol induces fatal aplastic anemia in neonates. Why is this not a clinical problem in adults?

4. Geriatrics frequently show a different response to a toxic chemical than younger adults. Cite the various factors that influence this difference in response.

5. Which of the following is a true statement?
   A. In general, chemicals are absorbed more rapidly when food is present in the stomach

B. Foods rich in ascorbic acid may significantly reduce the pharmacological effect of levodopa

C. Calcium, iron, and fat all enhance lead absorption

D. Tyramine-containing foods may induce a hypotensive crisis

6. A patient with a deficiency of the hepatic enzyme acetyl transferase should receive which of the following substances with extreme caution?
   A. Atropine
   B. Succinylcholine
   C. Nitrate
   D. Isoniazid

7. A deficiency of methemoglobin reductase will most likely cause an adverse reaction if which of the following is ingested?
   A. Atropine
   B. Succinylcholine
   C. Nitrate
   D. Isoniazid

8. The protein composition of a diet may affect an individual's response to a subsequently encountered poison. State several means by which this occurs.

9. The term pharmacogenetics may be a more accurate description of what other word in common use in pharmacology and toxicology?

10. Succinylcholine is initially detoxified by enzymes found in the:
    A. Lung
    B. Plasma
    C. Liver
    D. Kidney

11. Most poisons are pure substances.
    A. True
    B. False

12. Dioxin is a toxic contaminant of what herbicide?

13. How important is a product's vehicle or solvent to the product's overall toxicity potential?

14. Rank order each of the following routes of exposure according to approximate descending order of toxicity: oral, intraperitoneal, inhalation, intradermal, topical, intramuscular, subcutaneous, intravenous.

15. Why is knowing the route of administration of a toxic substance important? Cite as many reasons as you can.

16. Atropine toxicity may be influenced by the environmental temperature. It is reported to be more toxic at which of the following climates?
    A. Hot environment
    B. Cold environment

17. Inhaled particles must be smaller than a particular size in order to reach the alveoli. What is this critical size?

18. Cite the expected toxic response from an overdose of paraldehyde. When effects other than those you listed occur, what are the probable reasons for their occurrence?

19. Assume that an individual has ingested a pediculicide product containing the insecticide, pyrethrins. Explain how a toxic reaction from this product would most likely occur.

20. Hepatic porphyria results from barbiturate administration to a person who has:
    A. Atypical pseudocholinesterase
    B. Deficient glucose-6-phosphate-dehydrogenase
    C. Deficient hepatic acetyl transferase
    D. Sensitive δ-aminolevulinic acid synthetase

21. Concentrated forms of most chemicals are more quickly absorbed than diluted forms.
    A. True
    B. False

22. Which of the following is a toxic gas (as opposed to a vapor fume)?
    A. Carbon tetrachloride
    B. Nitrogen oxide
    C. Volatilized mercury
    D. Benzene

23. Discuss why the most significant toxic response from ingested methanol may be delayed for many hours after ingestion.

24. An orally ingested chemical will be absorbed in its:
    A. Ionized form
    B. Nonionized form

25. What does it mean when an ingested solid dosage form forms a concretion? What is the limi-

tation to using a gastric lavage tube to remove these poisons?

26. Carbonated beverages increase gastric emptying time.
    A. True
    B. False

27. All of the following substances are metabolized to more toxic compounds *except*:
    A. Acetaminophen
    B. Carbon tetrachloride
    C. Phenytoin
    D. Parathion

28. Acidosis potentiates the activity of insulin.
    A. True
    B. False

29. Discuss the route a chemical takes, once it is absorbed from the gastrointestinal tract, to get to the liver, its site of detoxification.

30. Inhaled poisons may be severely toxic because of the large surface area of the alveoli, which places the substance in close contact to a large amount of blood. What is the approximate size of this surface area?

References

1. Balazs, T. (1970): Measurement of acute toxicity. In: *Methods in Toxicology*, edited by G. E. Paget, pp. 10–15. F. A. Davis, Philadelphia.
2. Barltrop, D., and Khoo, H. E. (1975): The influence of nutritional factors on lead absorption. *Postgrad. Med. J.*, 51:795–800.
3. Bennett, W. M., Singer, I., and Coggins, C. J. (1974): A guide to drug therapy in renal failure. *JAMA*, 230:1544–1553.
4. Boyd, E. M. (1972): *Predictive Toxicometrics*. Scientechnia Ltd., Bristol, England.
5. Burns, L. E., Hoggman, J. E., and Cass, A. B. (1958): Fatal circulatory collapse in premature infants receiving chloramphenicol. *N. Engl. J. Med.*, 261:1318–1321.
6. Chin, T. F., and Lach, J. L. (1975): Drug diffusion and bioavailability: Tetracycline metallic chelation. *Am. J. Hosp. Pharm.*, 32:625–627.
7. Crounse, R. G. (1961): Human pharmacology of griseofulvin: The effect of fat intake on gastrointestinal absorption. *J. Invest. Dermatol.*, 37:529–533.
8. Doull, J. (1980): Factors influencing toxicology. In: *Toxicology—The Basic Science of Poisons*, 2nd ed., edited by J. Doull, C. D. Klaassen, and M. O. Amdur, pp. 70–83. Macmillan, New York.
9. Gillespie, N. Ĝ., Mena, I., Cotzias, G. C., and Bell, M. A. (1973): Diets affecting treatment of parkinsonism with levodopa. *J. Am. Diet. Assoc.*, 62:525–528.
10. Goldstein, A., Aronow, L., and Kalman, S. M. (1974): *Principles of Drug Action*, 2nd ed. Harper & Row, New York.
11. Iossifides, I. A., Smith, I., and Keitel, H. G. (1963): Chloramphenicol-bilirubin interaction in premature babies. *J. Pediatr.*, 62:735–741.
12. Kalow, W. (1962): *Pharmacogenetics: Heredity and the Response to Drugs*. W. B. Saunders, Co., Philadelphia.
13. Klaassen, C. D., and Doull, J. (1980): Evaluation of safety: Toxicologic evaluation. In: *Toxicology—The Basic Science of Poisons*, 2nd ed., edited by J. Doull, C. D. Klaassen, and M. O. Amdur, pp. 11–27. Macmillan, New York.
14. Lake, B., And Besll, S. M. (1969): Variations in absorption of erythromycin. *Med. J. Aust.*, 1:449–450.
15. Philipson, A., Sabath, L. D., and Charles, D. (1976): Erythromycin and clindamycin absorption and elimination in pregnant women. *Clin. Pharmacol. Ther.*, 19:63–77.
16. Sande, M. A., and Mandell, G. L. (1980): Antimicrobial agents—Tetracycline and chloramphenicol. In: *The Pharmacological Basis of Therpeutics*, edited by A. G. Gilman, L. S. Goodman, and A. Gilman, pp. 1181–1189. Macmillan, New York.
17. Sherwin, A. L. (1974): Effects of age, sex, obesity and pregnancy on plasma diphenylhydantoin levels. *Epilepsia*, 15:507.
18. Teitelbaum, D. T., and Ott, J. E. (1969): Elemental mercury self-poisoning. *Clin. Toxicol.*, 2:243–248.
19. Welling, P. G. (1977): Influence of food and diet on gastrointestinal drug absorption: A review. *J. Pharmacokinet. Biopharm.*, 5:291–334.

Principles in Management of the Poisoned Patient

3

One of the most important aspects in managing a poisoning or toxic exposure is knowing what to do, and in what order to do it! As we shall see later in this chapter, knowing "what to do" involves much more than routinely providing victims of poisoning with an agent to reduce absorption of the poison or nullify its effects. Rather, there are established rules for antidoting poisons that include general and specific principles designed to keep the individual alive, or at least to prevent more serious damage from occurring.

Throughout history, numerous methods have been advocated for antidoting the toxic effects of chemicals. These have ranged from carrying talismans (charms) and chanting prayers, to making incisions in the body, or to blood-letting with leeches. We must wonder if many victims undergoing these primitive treatments would have been better off taking their chances with the poison rather than subjecting themselves to these so-called antidotal measures. Even the immortal Orfila once advised the use of antidotes which, although in his time were considered efficacious, now are known to have little, if any, value, or, in some cases, even to be toxic in their own right.

The art of toxicology has developed today to unprecedented stature. Analytical methods are now available that permit detection of quantities of a poison in blood, urine, and other body fluids in the nanogram range (10^{-9} g) and less. Poisonous substances in air samples can be detected in quantities of parts per billion or less. We would like for emergency antidotal treatment methods to evolve similarly, but this has not occurred. Many commonly recommended procedures for antidoting a poison still remain at their formative stages; they are perhaps best described as crude.

For example, the two agents most commonly recommended to treat a wide variety of poisonings in people of almost all ages include activated charcoal, a residue of burnt wood, and syrup of ipecac, derived from a crude plant. Crude they are, perhaps, but if we examine the data that depict outcomes of poisoning when one of these substances is used versus when it is not used, it readily can be seen that somebody must be doing something right! Of course it must be realized that many of these poisonings may not have been sufficiently serious to warrant antidotal therapy. So it is possible that the figures infer a positive benefit that really does not exist. Still, they may reflect the truth, and this is the premise we will follow throughout this book.

Successful antidoting of a poisoned victim involves following a general outline as depicted in Fig. 1. Overriding all other considerations must be the fact that the *patient* is first treated, followed, second, by the poison. In other words, it is of little value to attempt to remove a chemical from the victim's stomach if he has stopped breathing or his heart is fibrillating. Therefore, always assess the patient's condition *first*, then decide what must be done and in what order. Once the victim is stabilized, and only then, try to identify the poison, the quantity involved, and how much time has elapsed since exposure. Then proceed with antidoting the poison.

NONSPECIFIC ANTIDOTES

Certain generalized procedures exist for antidoting most poisons. For example, most ingested substances may be successfully removed by emesis or be adsorbed onto activated charcoal. Most inhaled poisons are treated with oxygen therapy. Most skin contamination is successfully managed by washing with soap and water. Thus, contrary to popular belief, antidoting poisoning is not an unapproachable activity requiring an infinite stock of specific antidotal substances. Antidoting is, by and large, nonspecific.

Throughout this book, poisoning is discussed and specific antidoting methods are mentioned when these are appropriate. As a general rule, the nonspecific measures to be used for a particular toxic emergency (e.g., emesis, adsorption, etc.) are not mentioned. It will be assumed that all emergency measures have been initiated first. The same holds true for supportive therapy. These are, of course, first-line procedures and, when appropriate, are to be instituted.

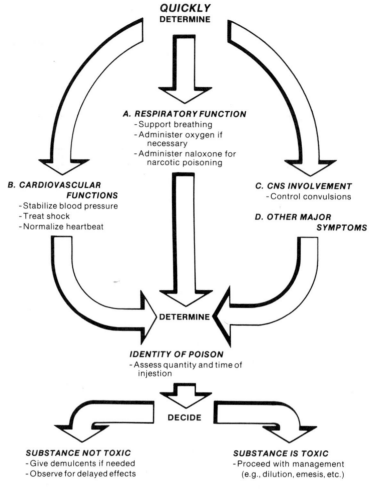

FIG. 1. The flow chart illustrates the steps involved in assessment and management of a poisoned patient.

SHOULD ANTIDOTING BE INSTITUTED?

One of the first questions that must be answered when a poisoning ingestion is suspected is whether the victim is actually a candidate for antidotal therapy! This question has no absolute answer although certain principles hold true for some poisonings.

When poisoning is suspected, but not known for sure, and if the suspected poison is known to be extremely toxic, then antidotal therapy should be initiated without further delay. There are numerous poisons that do not cause symptoms until many hours after exposure. When

the ingested quantity of a poison is unknown, it should be assumed that it is sufficient to cause serious problems.

If a victim is known to have previously swallowed a poison (e.g., a toxic amount of aspirin tablets) but still has not displayed symptoms, antidotal therapy should be initiated. Sometimes people are reluctant to administer an emetic an hour or more after a poisonous substance was swallowed, thinking it is too late for the emetic to be effective. There are many cases on record, however, where 8 to 12 or more hours after ingestion a victim has been made to vomit large clumps of poison (e.g., a bolus of aspirin tablets not yet dissolved). Similarly, as will be stated later, activated charcoal may be an effective adsorbent many hours after the poisoning, and long after the poison has left the stomach. This is particularly true for those toxic substances which undergo excretion by the enterohepatic circulation. Activated charcoal given over a period of hours can effectively reduce the blood concentration of these agents by decreasing their absorption.

Above all, no poisoning event, confirmed or suspected, should be brushed aside as unimportant. All patients deserve an accurate assessment and must receive therapy when appropriate.

CLINICAL EVALUATION

A victim of poisoning must be carefully evaluated for extent of poisoning before definitive therapy can begin (Fig. 1). This task is frequently difficult because the poisoned individual may be unconscious, unresponsive, or confused. The victim may present with a variety of signs and symptoms which are sometimes associated with a specific class of drugs (Table 1). An accurate history of the patient may be difficult or even impossible to obtain, or symptoms may suggest one cause of poisoning with a probable prognosis, but the circumstances of the poisoning strongly indicate an entirely different cause. As a result, the emergency personnel must make quick decisions on what to do and where to start in treating this poisoned patient. The following steps should be followed in the approximate order indicated.

Assess cardiorespiratory functions: If breathing is seriously affected, make sure oxygen is available and resuscitate if necessary. When administering oxygen, remember that respiration is depressed as oxygen content of the blood increases, and is increased as carbon dioxide levels increase. So, for poisoning by a respiratory depressant, the patient must be carefully observed during oxygen therapy.

Assessment of neurologic function is extremely important in the clinical evaluation of the poisoned patient. The stages of CNS depression and excitation are listed in Table 2. This classification of neurologic stability is often used in the initial assessment of the poisoned patient, as well as in the evaluation of the progress of treatment.

Often the characteristic clinical manifestation of the poisons listed in Table 1 can lend support to an accurate diagnosis of a poisoning, especially if it is of unknown origin. However, one must be cautioned *not* to expect to determine an unknown toxic ingestion just by following this chart!

Once the poisoned patient has been stabilized, or is at least out of immediate danger, additional steps can be taken to remove the poison, prevent or delay its absorption, and enhance its excretion.

Another point to stress which will aid in the clinical evaluation of the poisoned patient is the use of a toxicological analysis of blood, urine, and vomitus. There are several qualitative and quantitative methods available which can quickly identify the presence of a toxic substance. The results of these tests can be used to aid in the diagnosis of the poisoned patient, evaluate the progress of treatment, and predict outcomes of treatment.

DILUTION OF THE POISON

The initial procedure generally recommended whenever ingestion of a poison is suspected is to dilute it (44). Water is the best and, indeed, the only fluid that should be used when identity of the poison is unknown. Water is available in most homes, even if its supply has been cut off (e.g., in the refrigerator). A rule of thumb often stated in the literature is to administer 1 to 2 cupfuls to a child and 2 to 3 cupfuls to an adult. A better rule is to offer the victim a quantity that can be comfortably swallowed. Never force fluids beyond the point of comfortable ingestion. Excessive liquid may distend the stomach wall to cause premature relaxation of the pyloric sphincter, with subsequent emptying of the gastric contents into the duodenum. Once this occurs, it becomes much more difficult to remove the poison before it is absorbed.

TABLE 1. *Characteristic manifestations of poisoning*

Signs or symptoms	May be caused by:
Ataxia	Alcohol, barbiturates, bromides, phenytoin, hallucinogens, heavy metals, solvents (organic)
Breath odor	Alcohol: ethyl alcohol Garlic: arsenic, organophosphates, phosphorus Bitter almonds: cyanides Acetone: isopropanol, nail polish remover, salicylates Pungent: ethyl chlorvinyl Violets: turpentine Wintergreen: methyl salicylate Pearlike: chloral hydrate Others (characteristic): ammonia, gasoline, kerosene, petroleum distillates, phenol
Coma; drowsiness	Alcohol, antihistamines, antipsychotics, antidepressants, barbiturates and other sedatives, narcotics, salicylates
Fasciculations; convulsions[a]	Alcohol, amphetamines, antihistamines, barbiturate withdrawal, chlorinated hydrocarbons, cyanide, isoniazid, lead, organophosphate insecticides, methaqualone, plants (some), salicylates, strychnine, tricyclic antidepressants, phenothiazines
Gastrointestinal	
Emesis (frequently bloody)	Boric acid, caffeine, corrosives, heavy metals, phenol, salicylates, theophylline
Abdominal colic	Arsenic, heavy metals, lead, organophosphates, mushrooms, narcotic withdrawal
Diarrhea	Arsenic, boric acid, iron, mushrooms, organophosphates
Constipation	Lead, narcotics
Heart rate	
Bradycardia	Digitalis, narcotics, sedatives
Tachycardia	Alcohol, amphetamines, atropine, salicylates
Mouth	
Dry	Amphetamine, atropine, antihistamines, narcotics
Salivation	Mushrooms, organophosphates, mercury, arsenic, corrosives, strychnine
Gum discoloration	Lead and other heavy metals
Paralysis	Botulism, heavy metals
Pupils	
Miosis	Mushrooms (muscarinic type), narcotics, organophosphates
Mydriasis[b]	Amphetamine, antihistamines, atropine, barbiturate (coma), cocaine, glutethimide, LSD, methanol, opiate withdrawal, tricyclic antidepressants
Nystagmus	Barbiturates, phenytoin, sedatives
Vision disturbance	Botulism, methanol, organophosphates
Hallucinations	Alcohol, cocaine, LSD, mescaline, PCP
Respiration	
Rapid rate	Amphetamines, barbiturates (early), methanol, petroleum distillates, salicylates
Slow rate	Alcohol, barbiturates (late), narcotics
Paralysis	Botulism, organophosphates
Wheezing; pulmonary edema	Narcotics, organophosphates, petroleum distillates
Skin	
Cyanosis	Nitrites, strychnine, carbon monoxide
Red, flushed	Alcohol, antihistamines, atropine, carbon monoxide, boric acid, cyanide
Purpura	Salicylates, snake and spider bites
Jaundice	Acetaminophen (delayed), arsenic, carbon tetrachloride, castor bean, mushroom (delayed)
Sweating	Amphetamine, barbiturate, cocaine, LSD, mushrooms, organophosphates
Needle marks	Amphetamine, narcotics, PCP
Bullae	Barbiturates, carbon monoxide

[a]May be caused by any substance which causes hypoxia.
[b]May indicate severe stage of narcotic poisoning, caused by hypoxia.
From ref. 39.

TABLE 2. *Neurologic status*

CNS depression or excitation	Symptoms
Depression	
Stage 0	Asleep; drowsy, but accountable; responds to verbal commands
Stage 1	Corneal, gag, and deep tendon reflexes present; responds to pain
Stage 2	Deep tendon reflexes present; gag reflex present; no response to pain
Stage 3	Deep tendon reflexes absent; no response to pain; may have decorticate or decerebrate rigidity
Stage 4	Stage 3 symptoms plus cardiovascular and respiratory compromise; convulsions may be present
Excitation	
Stage 1	Restlessness; insomnia; tachycardia; flushed face; mydriasis
Stage 2	Stage 1 symptoms plus convulsions and mild pyrexia
Stage 3	Arrhythmia; delirium and mania; hypertension; hyperpyrexia
Stage 4	Stage 3 symptoms plus convulsions and/or coma

From ref. 45.

Water is given to accomplish at least two functions. First, it reduces gastric irritation that many ingested poisons cause. Second, and even more important, it adds bulk to the stomach that will be needed later for emesis. Emesis can only be successful if there is fluid or similar bulk present in the stomach to mix with the poison and provide a vehicle for its expulsion.

Under no circumstance should any liquid other than water be given unless it is specifically indicated. A child may refuse to drink water and insist on a carbonated beverage to which an unsuspecting parent complies. These release a large volume of carbon dioxide gas within the stomach to cause its distention, with possible resultant premature opening of the pyloric sphincter. Additionally, if the ingested poison were corrosive, the gas may potentiate perforation of the gastric lining, or force the substance into the esophagus where it could induce further corrosive damage.

Milk contains an absorbable fat that readily mixes with a wide variety of lipid substances. If it is given when such a poison has been swallowed, both substances may be absorbed into the body. More serious toxicity may result than would otherwise have been expected. Also, milk has been shown to delay the onset of emetic action of syrup of ipecac. Figure 2 summarizes the results of a study that illustrates this point (50). Ten subjects received ipecac syrup with either water or milk. The trials were separated by one week. Given with water, the mean time to onset of emesis was 24 min; with milk it increased to 35 min. The difference was statistically significant (i.e., milk did indeed delay onset of action).

One question that frequently emerges is whether acidic or alkaline substances should be "neutralized" by administering an acidic or alkaline fluid. In no instance should this be attempted. The heat released by exothermic reaction when acid mixes with base may cause irreversible tissue damage. Also, to be practical, it is not possible to effectively neutralize

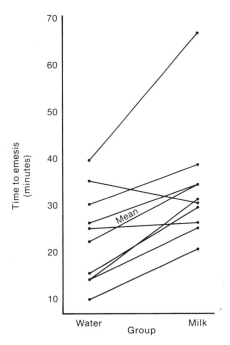

FIG. 2. Delayed onset of ipecac when taken with milk compared to water. (From ref. 50.)

strongly acidic or alkaline substances with another product (having an opposite pH) that is commonly found around the home or even in a hospital emergency room.

Whether ingested poisons should or should not be diluted is still being debated by some authorities. Not all of them place high priority on the importance of dilution of an ingested poison (16,30). One of the basic adages of pharmacology is that chemicals are more readily absorbed into the blood when they are diluted. Also, as we shall see in Chapter 8, dilution of strong acids or bases may cause more problems than benefits. Whereas dilution followed by emesis (when appropriate) seems to offer certain advantages, the American Association of Poison Control Centers has recently stated that oral dilution generally should not be used (28).

EMESIS

General Considerations

For many years emesis has been a mainstay for treating poison ingestions. Drugs (emetics) have been used for this purpose since earliest recorded history, and indeed some of these are still being used today. Even ipecac has been in use for several hundred years.

Chemically induced emesis is generally accepted as the first-line procedure for antidoting poisons because it can be easily accomplished by most persons at home. However, in recent years many of the common techniques and drugs recommended for inducing emesis have been shown to be ineffective, and in some instances dangerous. Thus, emetics, as a means to reduce the amount of poison available for absorption, are being seriously questioned for their overall value in treating poisoning. Nevertheless, they still occupy an important position in antidoting many poisons.

Certain precautions (Table 3) are valid for all emetics and should be remembered whenever their use is contemplated. If the victim is unconscious, the danger exists that vomitus may be aspirated into the lungs and cause chemical pneumonia. If the poison is a convulsant, forced emesis may precipitate convulsions.

TABLE 3. *Conditions in which emesis should not be attempted*[a]

Do not induce vomiting if the poison is a:
convulsant
hydrocarbon
corrosive acid or caustic alkali

Do not induce vomiting if the patient:
is unconscious or comatose
has severe cardiovascular disease or emphysema, or extremely weakened blood vessels
is under 6 months of age

[a]Emesis may be induced under certain circumstances; see Chapter 7.

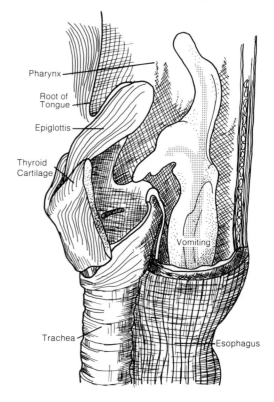

FIG. 3. Graphic representation illustrating the manner in which vomitus can easily be aspirated into the trachea.

For petroleum or pine distillates, special care is needed when dealing with acute ingestions. Because of their low surface tension and viscosity, these substances are readily aspirated into the lungs during emesis (Fig. 3) and may cause chemical pneumonitis. The presence of one of these substances in the esophagus, close to the trachea, is cause for alarm as it is initially swallowed. To subject the victim to increased exposure time during vomiting increases the chance for aspiration even more. It is true that some controversy exists on the proper emergency care concerning the use of emesis when one of these substances has been swallowed. However, as will be explained in Chapter 7, this procedure should only be performed by qualified medical personnel and only in an appropriate medical setting.

If the poison is a corrosive acid or alkali, emesis should be avoided because it may incite further damage to the esophagus as the substance is brought up. The tissue damage induced by these substances is related, in part, to the contact time between poison and tissue.

Children under 6 months of age should not receive syrup of ipecac. Their gag reflex is poorly developed and emetics may cause choking with aspiration. For children under 6 months, lavage is preferred.

Emetics should be used with care in persons with severe cardiovascular disease, aneurysms, severe emphysema, or other conditions where the blood vessels are weakened.

Frequently overlooked in the directions for administering emetics is an additional precaution. Vomiting should only be undertaken if there is sufficient bulk (e.g., fluid) in the stomach to serve as a carrier for the ingested poison. Frequently the quantity of poison swallowed may be too small to be expelled on its own. Thus, as stated earlier, water should be given prior to, or along with, an emetic.

SYRUP OF IPECAC

Use of ipecac dates back several centuries when it was first mentioned in the *Natural History of Brazil* [1648]. Ipecac root was brought to Europe in 1672 as a "cure" for dysentery. However, its popularity was limited because the excessive doses usually recommended caused many undesirable effects. But these problems were worked out and ipecac was recommended to treat a wide variety of conditions.

As recently as 1965, syrup of ipecac was listed by several references as an alternative to sodium chloride, powdered mustard, or mechanical stimulation of the pharynx as a method to induce vomiting. Its action was described as being generally slow, with vomiting occurring after 30 to 60 min. It was also considered to be toxic if too much was given. Much of this toxicity was actually due to the fluid extract (which is 14 times more potent than the syrup). Most reference sources stated that other, more effective, methods should preferentially be used for inducing vomiting or antidoting poisons.

In 1964 the Food and Drug Administration required that ipecac be purchased only on prescription order. In late 1965, however, at the request of pharmaceutical and medical associations, this restriction was lifted and, now, sale of one ounce of ipecac syrup over-the-counter is permitted.

Ipecac causes emesis through both an early and late phase of vomiting (35). Early vomiting usually occurs within 30 min and is due to a direct stimulant action on the gastrointestinal tract. A later phase occurs after 30 min, resulting from direct stimulation of the medullary chemoreceptor trigger zone. Therefore, if vomiting does not occur within the first 15 to 20 min, the drug should not be discounted as ineffective. Vomiting may occur later through a different mechanism. On the other hand, many physicians recommend that a second dose be given 20 to 30 min following the first dose if vomiting has not yet occurred. No more than two doses of ipecac should be given to induce vomiting following an acute toxic ingestion.

The effectiveness of syrup of ipecac as an emetic has been variously reported as poor to excellent. Some studies indicate that a significant number of people will not vomit with the substance. However, most studies have definitely established that syrup of ipecac is an effective emetic, even for poisons that have antiemetic activity.

Manoguerra and Krenzelok (36) reported that 81% of 232 patients given a single dose of syrup of ipecac vomited; an additional 15% vomited when the dose was repeated. The average length of time from ipecac administration to vomiting was 24 min. Of 63 patients who swallowed drugs with antiemetic properties, 81% vomited after the first dose and an additional 14% required a second dose.

A practical way to look at the issue is to assume that even if a poisoned victim vomited only a portion (e.g., one-fourth or one-half) of the ingested substance, this could be a sufficient amount to change the prognosis from "critical" to a point where there is a greater chance for survival!

Toxicity of Ipecac

Generally, syrup of ipecac is safe and well tolerated by most persons. In reports summarizing studies of nearly 7,500 persons who received the emetic, no serious systemic toxicity was noted when it was used correctly.

A variety of toxicities to ipecac have been reported in other studies, however (Table 4) (35). The most frequently encountered and potentially serious toxic reaction is on the cardiovascular system. In these reports, ipecac was given usually to induce emesis following ingestion of drugs with potent antiemetic action. Manno and Manno (35) considered these intox-

TABLE 4. *Symptoms of ipecac toxicity*

Cardiovascular
ECG irregularities
Hypotension
Tachycardia or bradycardia
Gastrointestinal
Abdominal cramping
Diarrhea (severe)
Nausea and vomiting
Neuromuscular
Convulsions
Skeletal muscle weakness, aching, or stiffness
Tremor
Miscellaneous
Blood dyscrasias
Dehydration
Dyspnea
Fever
Hyponatremia
Shock

From ref. 35.

ications as senseless since, in their opinion, emetics should not be given for poisoning by antiemetics. Obviously, much discrepancy exists. However, toxicity is rarely seen in the dosage range used therapeutically or from one ounce of the syrup (the maximum amount most people have on hand at any one time). On the other hand, if syrup of ipecac does not produce emesis within 20 to 30 min of the second dose, some authorities suggest that it should be removed by gastric lavage. Again, this is a difficult concept to support since ipecac does produce a second-phase central action and if sufficient time is permitted to elapse, emesis should occur.

General Considerations for Using Syrup of Ipecac

The emetic can be safely given at home by parents, after receiving proper medical advice. Assuming that it may take approximately 20 to 30 min after administration before vomiting begins, much valuable time will be saved if people always have the antidote readily available. For example, emergency medical vehicles usually stock syrup of ipecac. If it takes 10 min for the vehicle to reach a home, plus another 20 to 30 min to induce vomiting, serious poisoning may occur within this period. Worse yet, if treatment is not instituted until the victim arrives at the hospital, even more valuable time will be lost. Therefore, parents of small children should be strongly urged to keep an ounce of ipecac syrup handy at all times.

There is another advantage to giving the antidote at home, followed by a ride to a hospital. The gentle jostling by riding in a vehicle (especially with the windows closed and heater on) may help promote more rapid emesis.

Another reason for quick use of syrup of ipecac in poisonings is that drug-induced emesis is generally less traumatic to the patient than gastric lavage. Insertion of a lavage tube is unpleasant to most people, especially children, and must only be undertaken by qualified personnel. Lavage is slow, relatively inefficient, and can cause complications of forcing material out of the stomach into the intestine where it cannot readily be recovered. Chemical emetics can also recover particles of material that are too large to pass through the opening of a lavage tube.

APOMORPHINE

Apomorphine is a morphine derivative that produces quick emetic action, usually within 1 to 3 min, through direct stimulation of the chemoreceptor trigger zone. This action is more pronounced than with syrup of ipecac and can usually be relied on to cause forced ejection of the stomach contents (15). It also has the advantage that it can be used along with orally administered activated charcoal, whereas syrup of ipecac must be given at least 30 min before activated charcoal.

The disadvantages of apomorphine are that it must be freshly prepared and given by injection, and it should only be administered by qualified medical personnel. Thus, it is not appropriate for home use.

Apomorphine also depresses the CNS. If the ingested poison is a respiratory depressant, apomorphine generally should not be used.

To overcome the effect of the protracted emetic action and respiratory sedative properties of apomorphine, some physicians advocate administering a narcotic antagonist, such as naloxone, shortly following the onset of emesis.

Although it is a narcotic, apomorphine is not a controlled substance. It was deleted from its original C-II status because there is little abuse potential. After all, who would willfully abuse a drug that causes vomiting? Also, when needed, it must be readily available without having to cut through bureaucratic red tape.

SOAP SOLUTION

When rapid emesis is indicated and syrup of ipecac is not available, one alternative is to administer a liquid detergent (29). Two to 3 tablespoonfuls should be mixed with 6 to 8 ounces of water and administered. Detergents are believed to produce emesis by direct stimulation of the gastrointestinal mucosa, thus their

action is rapid. In one study, the mean time to emesis was less than 10 min, compared to 15 to 20 min for syrup of ipecac (29). The solution is difficult to swallow, so this method usually has poor patient acceptance.

Persons being instructed to use liquid detergents should be cautioned *not* to use laundry detergents or electric dishwashing cleaning products. These are potentially corrosive and may cause injury.

MECHANICAL STIMULATION

When syrup of ipecac is not available, some recommend stimulating the back of the tongue or the pharynx. This involves placing the victim in a spanking position, and gently stroking the area with a blunt object such as a spoon or tongue depressor. Fingers are not advised since the victim may reflexly bite down as he is gagged, causing injury to the individual's finger.

The advantage of this procedure is its ready availability. Its major disadvantage is its lack of effectiveness: Gagging is not the same as vomiting. In a study of 30 poisoned children, only 2 children vomited following mechanical stimulation, and the volume was insignificant (2 ml and 4 ml, respectively). All victims had previously been given 6 to 8 ounces of fluid (21).

OUTMODED EMETICS

Numerous substances have been advocated over the years as emetics. *Potassium* and *antimony tartrate* (tartar emetic), *copper sulfate*, and *zinc sulfate* were once considered to be outstanding emetics. However, because of their erratic, slow action and possible toxicity if absorbed, they should no longer be recommended. *Mustard powder* mixed in water was formerly advocated. However, it is unreliable as an emetic, and few households actually have it available. It also produces an extremely gritty, bitter taste in the mouth; thus valuable minutes may be wasted in first trying to locate the powder and second, in trying to coax an unwilling child to ingest it. Therefore, mustard powder is no longer recommended as an emetic. Condiment (spice) mustard does not possess emetic value.

SALT SOLUTION

Problems with Salt

Whereas numerous reference books, first aid charts, and some package labels still advocate inducing vomiting with a salt solution, this measure is now considered to be potentially dangerous (9,24,42). To illustrate this change in thinking, several points must be considered.

Because of a variation in different household tablespoon measures, and because of the intense anxiety felt by a parent who is attempting to antidote a poisoned victim (usually a child) and who interprets the directions as meaning that "if one tablespoonful of salt is good, then two would be even better," extremely large, toxic doses are frequently given. Advice from doctors, pharmacists, and emergency room personnel has long been to administer "a strong salt solution" rather than specifying an actual quantity. In some reported cases, children have received more than 4 heaping tablespoonfuls of salt given repeatedly, two to three times.

Toxicity of Salt

When salt solution is administered and emesis does not occur, the salt is absorbed into the blood. As sodium levels rise, this increases the tonicity of extracellular fluid (blood). Intracellular fluids then move outward into the blood to dilute it, as is understood from the basic laws of osmosis. This results in crenation (shrinking) of these cells. At the same time, it also results in an increased intracranial pressure.

Whereas all cells of the body may be affected, the first to respond are those within the CNS. The shrunken cells cannot perform their normal activities. Thus, the combination of damaged brain cells with disturbed metabolic functions, along with distension of the intracranial blood vessels leads to severe intraventricular hemorrhage and thrombosis occurring throughout the brain. When this occurs, death is imminent.

ADSORBENTS

Another means to reduce absorption of an ingested poison is by use of an adsorbent. While several such substances, including kaolin, Fuller's earth, cholestyramine, pectin, and attapulgite are occasionally recommended as adsorbents, they are not acceptable as general antidotes (8,32). Only activated charcoal should be used for routine adsorption of gastrointestinal poisons. But we still should remember that because an adsorbent is not useful for routine antidoting purposes, this does not mean it is entirely without value. Fuller's earth, for example, has been shown to have a high affinity for the herbicide paraquat (10). Similar high affinities for specific adsorbents may ultimately be shown through continued research.

Activated Charcoal

Activated charcoal used to treat poisoning can be traced to the time of Hippocrates (31). From that point until the 19th century its use was widely recommended to treat a variety of common ills.

The first to specifically demonstrate activated charcoal's adsorbent activity and usefulness to reduce absorption of poisonous substances was a French chemist named Bertrand. He publicly demonstrated its efficacy in 1813 by swallowing 5 g of arsenic trioxide mixed with activated charcoal. He suffered no untoward symptoms of toxicity. A few years later, in 1831, a French pharmacist named Touery conducted an even more impressive demonstration than that of Bertrand. Touery swallowed ten times the lethal dose of strychnine which had been mixed with activated charcoal. He stood before members of the French Academy of Medicine for several hours waiting for symptoms of strychnine toxicity which he was confident would never occur. Luckily, he was correct! While this demonstration must have been dramatic at the time, there is little written evidence today to suggest that it made any significant impact on French medical practice. In fact, it would be another 5 years before the Academy formally mentioned it.

Through the first 30 or 40 years of the 20th century, activated charcoal did not receive high praises as an antidote. There were few studies conducted that demonstrated its absolute role in adsorbing poisons from the gastrointestinal tract. During this period also, it was common to mix activated charcoal with tannic acid and magnesium oxide to form the traditional "universal antidote" which, for so many years, dominated all other antidotes as being the "best method" for treating most cases of ingested poisons. By the mid-1960s, toxicologists had developed renewed interest in activated charcoal and began looking at it more seriously. It has been intently studied ever since.

There are many reasons we may speculate as to why activated charcoal was neglected until recently. Its physical characteristics make it undesirable to force upon a poisoned patient. Additionally, in some incidences the substance has been used indiscriminately, leading to numerous negative reports of its adsorptive value. Many of the earlier studies with activated charcoal were conducted with animals or *in vitro* models, and few attempts were made to correlate these findings with clinical efficacy. Many of the clinical studies that were conducted were not particularly useful since they analyzed extremely small doses of drugs or poisons that were far below those encountered in most actual poison situations. Many other studies employed doses of activated charcoal that were too small to show beneficial results.

Perhaps the greatest deterrent to the serious use of activated charcoal relates to the notoriety of the "universal antidote." This substance (1 part tannic acid, 1 part magnesium oxide, and 2 parts activated charcoal) was popularized years ago as a first choice antidote for emergency treatment of poisoning by a variety of substances. However, experimental evidence subsequently showed that it was not the effective measure for which it was originally promoted. No doubt numerous physicians and emergency room personnel may have automatically believed that its activated charcoal component, used alone, was likewise not effective.

We now know that the activated charcoal component of "universal antidote" adsorbs part of the magnesium oxide and/or tannic acid (22). This reduces its overall adsorptive property and,

therefore, its antidotal efficacy. Also, tannic acid may be absorbed into the blood and has been shown to be hepatotoxic in certain animal species (41). Thus, "universal antidote" is no longer recommended as an emergency antidote and, in fact, may be downright hazardous to use (3).

Activated charcoal is regarded today as one of the most important of the various substances available for removing ingested chemicals from the gastrointestinal tract. It is also used in hemoperfusion units for removing toxic substances from the blood. Whenever an emetic cannot be used, or following successful chemical induction of emesis, or when the patient is unconscious, activated charcoal may be given.

Activated charcoal reduces absorption of a wide variety of poisons but has little or no effect on others (Table 5). In the stomach and the intestine, poisons diffuse through the numerous pores on the charcoal surface and form tight chemical bonds. This charcoal-chemical complex then passes out of the body.

Activated charcoal possesses several important advantages over syrup of ipecac. For example, it is not contraindicated when poisoning was caused by any of the substances in Table 3. While it is not useful for the poisons listed in Table 5, it is quite effective for most other commonly encountered poisons. Its only restriction to administration is when there is an absence of bowel sounds.

Time Interval

For maximal antidoting effect, activated charcoal should be administered within 30 min of the poison ingestion. However, when used

TABLE 5. *Chemicals that are poorly or not adsorbed by activated charcoal*

Alkali
Boric acid
Cyanide
DDT
Iron salts
Malathion
Mineral acids
Water insoluble compounds

with drugs that slow gastric emptying (e.g., anticholinergics, sedatives, etc.) beneficial results have been obtained when the antidote was given 6 to 8 hr following poison ingestion. Following aspirin ingestion, a 9- to 10-hr interval between ingestion of drug and charcoal has still produced beneficial results.

Two studies illustrate that charcoal effectively reduces the quantity of various drugs and chemicals from the gastrointestinal tract. In the first instance (Fig. 4), subjects received a dose of phenobarbital alone, or with charcoal concurrently, or at various time intervals (40). Activated charcoal was effective even when administered 10 to 48 hr after drug ingestion (Fig. 4).

In the second instance (Fig. 5), volunteers took a dose of nortriptyline followed with a single dose of activated charcoal 30 min later, or multiple doses ranging over the next 6 hr (20). The results clearly indicate that repeated administration of the adsorbent significantly reduced absorption of nortriptyline more than did a single dose.

Burnt toast scrapings and crushed coal are unacceptable substitutes for activated charcoal. Commercial activated charcoal tablets and charcoal products intended for any purpose other than medicinal (e.g., water filtration, fish tanks, etc.) are not adsorptive to the same extent and, therefore, have no place in emergency antidoting procedures.

Dose

The usual recommended dose of activated charcoal is 50 to 60 g for an adult and 15 to 30 g for a child. Recent studies indicate that doses of activated charcoal approaching 100 to 120 g are more appropriate for adults. Experts generally agree that activated charcoal should be given in a relative dose ratio of at least 10:1, charcoal to drug. This ratio might be unrealistic in a child, however (Fig. 6). The important point to remember is that enough activated charcoal must be given to do its job, and there does not seem to be a dose which is too much.

While sometimes reported that food present in the stomach or intestine will reduce the adsorptive properties of activated charcoal, from a practical standpoint this effect is insignificant. However, some recommend that a higher dose be given when food is known to be in the stomach.

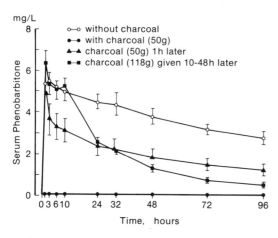

FIG. 4. Effect of activated charcoal on serum phenobarbitone (phenobarbital) concentration. Subjects received 200 mg phenobarbitone with or without activated charcoal. (From ref. 40.)

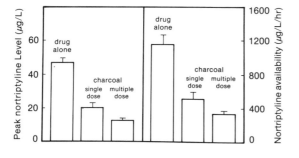

FIG. 5. Effect of activated charcoal on peak plasma nortriptyline levels and nortriptyline availability. (From ref. 20.)

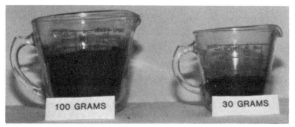

FIG. 6. Graphic illustration showing the bulkiness of 30 g and 100 g of activated charcoal.

Use with an Emetic

Activated charcoal should not be given within 30 min of syrup of ipecac unless the victim has already vomited (27). If both substances are to be administered, ipecac should precede the charcoal. This is important to remember because emetine and cephaeline, which comprise over 90% of the active emetic alkaloids of ipecac (19), are adsorbed onto the activated charcoal, negating their action.

Consideration should be given to combining activated charcoal with apomorphine if immediate emetic action is wanted. Decker and colleagues (23) have shown (Fig. 7) that administration of either activated charcoal or apomorphine alone decreases blood levels of

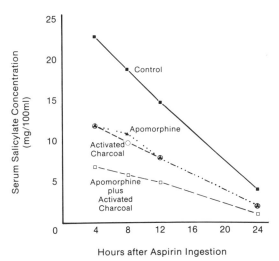

FIG. 7. The effect of activated charcoal and apomorphine, alone and in combination, on serum salicylate concentration. Subjects took a single oral dose of aspirin alone or in combination with one or more of the antidotes. (From ref. 23.)

salicylate. However, when both agents are given, blood levels are reduced even more.

Administration

Activated charcoal is unsightly, and readily adsorbs materials from the air and water when mixed and allowed to stand. Therefore, it should be added to sufficient water in a dark container (to keep youngsters from seeing it!) and used immediately. Several commercial products contain a premeasured quantity of the substance in a tightly closed, dark plastic bottle. Water is added to the powder, and following vigorous shaking the mixture is administered directly from its container.

The substance does leave a gritty sensation in the mouth, discolors the gums and mouth to some extent, and sticks to the throat. For these reasons, some medical practitioners argue that a child will refuse to drink it (5). However, the validity of this statement has been tested, and while some resistance may be met, it is accepted by most (14). Today, there are liquid activated charcoal preparations available which have met little resistance among children and are easily administered by nurses.

Various flavoring and thickening agents have been added in an attempt to increase palatability of an activated charcoal slurry (25,33,37,53). These include sodium algenate, carboxymethylcellulose, carageenin, bentonite, gelatin, ice cream and sherbet, jams and jellies, cocoa powder, fruit syrups, saccharin sodium, and sorbitol. Caution is advised before any such substances are added, however.

To illustrate, Levy et al. (33) demonstrated that aspirin adsorption onto activated charcoal was reduced by nearly 25% when melted ice cream was mixed with the charcoal.

CATHARTICS

Toxic substances may be effectively removed from the gastrointestinal tract with the use of a saline cathartic (Table 6). This reduces the contact time between the poison and the absorption sites and, in turn, reduces the potential for toxicity. However, the evacuation action of saline cathartics may require several hours for completion (17). Furthermore, addition of a saline cathartic to the regimen of a patient receiving activated charcoal does not enhance the effect of the charcoal alone (49).

Cathartics can usually be recommended for most intoxicated patients (28,43), although some authorities stress that this procedure is best left to the discretion of a physician or emergency room personnel.

Catharsis should not be attempted when the poison is strongly corrosive, as it may increase the extent of chemical injury. It should not be performed when the patient has electrolyte disturbance or an absence of bowel sounds. Aside from a few exceptions (i.e., castor oil for phenol intoxication, and mineral oil for fat-soluble vitamin overdoses) no other stimulant or lubricant cathartic should be recommended. Additionally, magnesium-containing cathartics should not be given to persons with compromised renal function because of the possibility of causing CNS depression due to accumulation of high concentrations of magnesium in the serum (13).

TABLE 6. *Cathartics used in poison treatment*

Cathartic	Dose (p.o.)	
	Child	Adult
Magnesium sulfate (Epsom salts)	0.25 g/kg	5–10 g
Magnesium citrate solution (citrate of magnesia)	150 ml	300 ml
Sodium sulfate	250 mg/kg	15 g
Sodium sulfate/sodium phosphate mixture (Fleet Phospho-Soda)	20 ml[a]	40 ml[a]

[a]Diluted with water.

Sodium-containing cathartics are, likewise, best avoided by persons with congestive heart failure or other conditions where fluid retention would pose a significant danger.

LAVAGE

Lavage (F. *laver* = to wash) is a process of washing out the stomach with various solutions, including water, saline, sodium bicarbonate, calcium salts, tannic acid, or potassium permanganate. It is sometimes indicated when the poison must be quickly removed from the stomach before emesis can be effective, or when emesis is contraindicated.

The patient is placed on the left lateral side to permit pooling of gastric contents (in this position the pylorus is pointed up) and reduce the chance for emptying into the small intestine. Also, the patient's head should be lower than the rest of the body. The largest tolerable catheter is inserted into the stomach. The mouth or nose can be utilized as a route of entry. When the nasal route is used, the size of the tube is limited, so this method is less useful for withdrawing large particles. Regardless of the route of entry, a syringe is then attached to the outer end of the catheter. The next step is to attempt to aspirate as much of the stomach contents as possible, then the lavaging solution is introduced into the stomach (50–100 ml aliquots for children and 200–300 ml aliquots for adults). Generally, 1 to 2 L are used, but there are occasions when more will be necessary (e.g., if large quantities of a toxic substance were ingested or if the person has recently swallowed large pieces of food). The consensus is to lavage until clear, that is, keep introducing lavage solution into the stomach and withdrawing it until the return solution is clear. Caution must be exercised with this action. There is always the possibility that even though the patient was lavaged until clear, there may still be some particles remaining in the stomach. This point will be illustrated in several of the case studies presented later in this book.

Lavage is not always considered to be a procedure of first choice for removing ingested poisons, and can be associated with numerous risks. For example, the tube may be accidentally inserted into the trachea. Improperly used, lavage may incite a greater risk for aspiration of solution. The tube may cause perforation of the stomach or hasten its emptying time into the intestine. If a cool lavaging solution is used too rapidly, the body temperature may be rapidly lowered. Some lavage solutions are toxic in their own right and if left in the stomach too long, or if incompletely removed, may cause more harm than good. Furthermore, recent studies have shown that lavage may not actually remove a significant amount of the poison (2,18). Lavage is also inappropriate for removing large clumps of solid substances since they usually will not fit through the tube opening.

FORCED DIURESIS

Forced diuresis is employed to help remove chemicals from the blood after they have been absorbed. It is useful when the compound or its active metabolite is eliminated in the urine and when diuresis enhances this excretion. The procedure is based on increasing the volume of flow of urine through the renal tubules so the chemical may be more quickly eliminated. The objective is to maintain a urine output of 300 to 500 ml/hr, or 8 to 14 L/day. While many diuretic agents have been recommended over the years, either mannitol or furosemide is generally used today. Mannitol increases urinary output through osmotic attraction. Furosemide reduces fluid reabsorption in the descending limb of Henle's loop.

Forced diuresis is beneficial for some, but not all, chemicals (Table 7) (13,51). Those chemicals which are not normally reabsorbed by the kidney will not be significantly lowered in concentration with forced diuresis. Thus, merely increasing the urinary flow is not a means to remove many chemicals from the blood.

Whenever the procedure is contemplated, the patient must first be assessed for renal function and urine flow, acid-base balance, and cardiopulmonary status. The central venous pressure must be constantly monitored to prevent fluid

TABLE 7. *Forced diuresis*

Substances removed by forced diuresis	
Amphetamine	Penicillin
Alcohol	Phencyclidine
Aniline	Quinine
Barbiturates, long-acting	Quinidine
	Salicylates
Bromides	Strychnine
Ethylene glycol	Sulfonamides
Isoniazid	
Lithium	

Substances not removed by forced diuresis	
Acetaminophen	Glutethimide
Barbiturates, short- and medium-acting	Methaqualone
	Phenothiazines
Ethchlorvynol	Tricyclic antidepressants

imbalances. Other inherent dangers from the procedure include water intoxication, cerebral and pulmonary edema, and fluid and electrolyte imbalance.

At best, forced diuresis may increase the excretion of a chemical twofold. A better procedure is to couple this with acidification or alkalinization of the urine so that ion-trapping is greater. Ascorbic acid or ammonium chloride will acidify the urine to an end point of 5.0, and sodium bicarbonate alone or with acetazolamide accomplishes alkalinization to a pH of 8.0. Acetazolamide must not be used alone since it causes a mild systemic acidosis, which may cause an unfavorable pH ratio between blood and tissues.

To illustrate, excretion of basic chemicals, such as quinine and quinidine, amphetamine, phencyclidine, strychnine, and phosphorus will be hastened when the urine is acidified. Phenobarbital excretion has been shown to increase sevenfold when forced alkaline diuresis is employed (47). Alkalinization with forced diuresis is also effective for such organic acids as salicylates, arsenic, isoniazid, lithium, meprobamate, and naphthalene.

DEMULCENTS

Occasionally all that is needed to treat a poisoning is a demulcent. Many plants and chemicals irritate the oral and gastric mucosa, but cause no serious toxicity. For these, ice cream, milk, or another soothing agent will reduce the irritation and help the victim feel better. Beaten egg whites (up to a dozen for an adult) have been given for corrosive intoxications. Egg white serves as a source of readily available protein that, in theory, helps keep the corrosive away from the gastric mucosa.

Demulcents are also of benefit when treatment is not needed, but it is obvious that the patient or parent of the patient demands that something be done. Thus, a demulcent frequently serves as important placebo or palliative therapy.

DECONTAMINATION

Numerous lipid-soluble chemicals can be absorbed through the skin and cause systemic symptoms of toxicity within minutes of absorption. It is, therefore, important that whenever the skin is contaminated that the poison be washed off at once. All contaminated clothing should be removed. The skin should be thoroughly flushed with water and washed with mild soap. Special care should be observed to avoid briskly rubbing the area, as this may promote absorption or cause abrasion which, in turn, may increase the absorption of many chemicals. Some authorities recommend that tincture of green soap (soft soap liniment, which contains 30% alcohol) be used to clean the area, as its alcohol content will readily solubilize some poisons. However, few homes have this substance readily available, and valuable time may be lost while trying to locate it. Ordinary soap is adequate for most routine procedures.

No creams or ointments should be placed over the contaminated area. These will need to be removed later before an attending physician can proceed with treatment. Also, occlusive products make decontamination more difficult.

The eye poses a special problem to spilled or splashed chemicals. Many substances are absorbed within minutes through the cornea, causing permanent damage to eye structures, including loss of eyesight. When contamination of the eye occurs, irrigation with warm water

must be immediately instituted and be continued for at least 15 to 20 min to dilute and remove the substance. Remove contact lenses, if present, and hold the head directly under a softly flowing stream from the tap or from a container. Medicine droppers or irrigation syringes are inadequate because they do not hold a sufficient reservoir of water. Immediately after irrigation, the patient should be taken to a physician for further care.

DIALYSIS AND HEMOPERFUSION

The following procedures are limited in scope and are not routinely performed for every toxic ingestion. However, they are now being employed more frequently as adjuncts to management of the severely intoxicated patient. The basic principles involved will add to our overall approach to the management of the poisoned patient.

One should be aware that for a comatose patient, the number and severity of complications that may develop increase with the length of time the patient remains in a coma (7,10). It is, therefore, desirable to reduce this time period by any means available. Still, it must always be remembered that even though the concentration of the poison in the blood has decreased and the victim has awakened, irreversible damage may have occurred. For example, a patient who ingested approximately 100 ml of carbon tetrachloride (an otherwise lethal dose) awoke after 7 hr of hemoperfusion, but irreversible pulmonary insufficiency and hepatic damage appeared weeks later (52).

These procedures should never replace more specific antidotes. For example, they would not be necessary for a patient with an acute narcotic overdose, because of the availability and specificity of the narcotic antagonist, naloxone. They would also be of little value in treating acute ingestions of cytotoxic poisons, such as cyanide, which produce their toxic effects very rapidly, often within minutes. Furthermore, if the ingested drug has a high therapeutic index and, consequently, has little potential for causing intense, severe symptoms, these procedures would have questionable value.

Dialysis is governed by the laws of osmosis, whereby a diffusible chemical dissolved in water partitions across a semipermeable membrane, with the solution moving from an area of higher concentration (i.e., the blood) to one of lower concentration (i.e., a dialyzing solution). Its utility in treating drug and chemical intoxications has expanded over the past decade. The literature now documents numerous studies that compare the efficacy of one or another of the dialytic procedures for removing toxic substances. A partial list of dialyzable poisons is shown in Table 8.

Peritoneal Dialysis

Peritoneal dialysis is the easiest performed of methods and is associated with the lowest risk for causing complications. However, it is also the least effective method.

The procedure is undertaken by inserting a tube through a small incision made in the mid-abdomen area into the peritoneum (Fig. 8). The peritoneal membrane thus serves as the semipermeable (dialyzing) membrane. In this way, the dialyzable chemical will diffuse from the blood across the peritoneal membrane into the dialyzing fluid (from an area of higher to lower concentration). A warmed dialyzing solution (up to 2 L for adults and 1 L for children) is introduced into the peritoneal cavity over a period of 15 to 20 min. The fluid is left in place for 45 to 60 min for equilibration to occur, then removed. A fresh solution is reintroduced and the process is repeated again and again. Up to 30 L or more of dialysis fluid may be used.

The dialysis solution normally consists of a balanced electrolyte solution, although various solutions from different manufacturers will vary in composition. The osmotic pressure of the fluid is maintained above that of extracellular fluid with dextrose. By making the dialysis fluid hypertonic, there should be an increased recovery of water-soluble chemicals. For chemicals that are highly protein-bound, addition of al-bumin to the dialyzing solution may be helpful to increase recovery of drugs which have an affinity for proteins. The dialysis solution may also be modified by adjusting pH. For example, in acute phenobarbital ingestion, using an alkaline solution may considerably increase total drug recovery. Some dialysis procedures call for the addition of lipid (e.g., peanut oil) to attract chemicals (e.g., glutethimide) that are highly lipid-soluble.

In general, peritoneal dialysis is 5 to 10 times less efficient than hemodialysis (11,48). It is not the procedure of choice when rapid removal of a toxic substance is needed. On the other hand, peritoneal dialysis does not require elaborate equipment and needs little medical supervision. It seems to be more generally applicable for acute ingestions in children, because of their large peritoneal surface area in relation to body size. Also, their abdominal wall is much easier to penetrate than trying to isolate an appropriate vein in their small arm.

Some of the complications of peritoneal dialysis include abdominal pain, intraperitoneal bleeding; intestinal, bladder, liver, or spleen perforation; peritonitis; water and electrolyte imbalance; and protein loss.

Hemodialysis

The same basic principles as for peritoneal dialysis apply to hemodialysis. For peritoneal dialysis, an *in vivo* (peritoneal) membrane is utilized, whereas in hemodialysis, a cellophane bag (artificial kidney) forms the semipermeable membrane).

Two catheters are inserted into the patient's femoral vein, about 2 inches apart. Blood is pumped from one catheter through the dialysis unit, across the semipermeable membrane, and returned through the other catheter. The procedure is usually continued for 6 to 8 hr. Again, as for peritoneal dialysis, the solubilized drug or chemical will diffuse across the semipermeable membrane into the dialysis solution, its rate based upon the difference in osmotic and concentration gradients.

TABLE 8. *Commonly known dialyzable poisons*

Barbiturates	Analgesics	Miscellaneous substances
Barbital	Aspirin	Thiocyanate
Phenobarbital	Methyl salicylate	Aniline
Amobarbital	Phenacetin	Sodium chlorate
Pentobarbital	Dextropropoxyphene	Potassium chlorate
Butabarbital	Acetaminophen	Eucalyptus oil
Secobarbital	Antibiotics	Boric acid
Depressants, sedatives,	Streptomycin	Potassium dichromate
and tranquilizers	Kanamycin	Digoxin
Phenytoin	Neomycin	Sodium citrate
Primidone	Vancomycin	Amantia phalloides
Meprobamate	Penicillin	Carbon tetrachloride
Ethchlorvynol	Ampicillin	Ergotamine
Ethinamate	Sulfonamides	Cyclophosphamide
Methylprylon	Cephalosporins	5-Fluorouracil
Diphenhydramine	Chloramphenicol	Methotrexate
Methaqualone	Tetracycline	Camphor
Heroin	Nitrofurantoin	Trichlorethylene
Paraldehyde	Polymyxin	Carbon monoxide
Chloral hydrate	Isoniazid	Chlorpropamide
Chlordiazepoxide	Metals	Quinine
Glutethimide	Arsenic	
Antidepressants	Copper	
Amphetamine	Calcium	
Methamphetamine	Iron	
Tricyclic amines	Lead	
Monoamine oxidase	Lithium	
inhibitors	Magnesium	
Tranylcypromine	Mercury	
Pargyline	Potassium	
Phenelzine	Sodium	
Isocarboxazid	Halides	
Alcohols	Bromide	
Ethanol	Chloride	
Methanol	Iodide	
Isopropanol	Fluoride	
Ethylene glycol		

From ref. 46.

If a drug or chemical is to be effectively removed by dialysis, it must have a low molecular weight and small molecular size to passively diffuse across the dialyzing membrane. Usually, drugs with molecular weights greater than 350 do not cross the membrane. Since only free drug will diffuse from the blood into the dialysis solution (proteins are too large to pass through the membrane), hemodialysis is limited for those drugs that are highly protein-bound.

The effectiveness of hemodialysis is determined by the rate of clearance, the plasma concentration of the drug, and the duration of dialysis. This means that there are certain pharmacokinetic parameters which may be helpful in estimating whether or not a particular chemical can be dialyzed. For example, if the volume of distribution (V_d) is greater than 250 to 300 L, then less chemical per unit of blood is available for elimination by dialysis. On the other hand, chemicals that have a small volume of distribution (e.g., salicylates) are more readily removed by dialysis because the plasma concentrations are greater in relation to the total amount of drug in the body and, additionally, there is a high concentration gradient between the blood and dialysis solution. In other words, hemodialysis is virtually useless for chemicals that are extensively taken up by tissues because, at steady state, they circulate only at very small

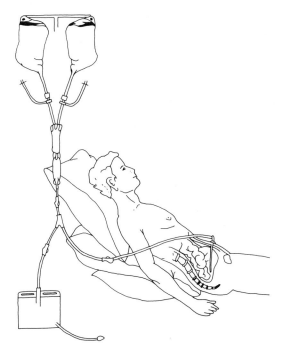

FIG. 8. Procedure for peritoneal dialysis.

concentrations. Also, unless the overall clearance of a chemical with dialysis is much greater than the total body clearance rate, the elimination half-life of the drug is not significantly shortened.

Complications include clotting and leaking of blood from around connections, hypotension, convulsions, arrhythmias, infection, and hematologic defects.

Hemoperfusion

Hemoperfusion is significantly more effective than peritoneal dialysis and hemodialysis (Table 9) for removing intoxicating compounds, particularly those which are lipid-soluble or protein-bound, or for those which for other reasons are poorly dialyzable. A list of common poisonous substances which are easily removed by hemoperfusion is shown in Table 10.

The ability of activated charcoal to adsorb toxic substances has been recognized for many years. Also, numerous analytical procedures have used anion exchange resins, as well as nonion resins, such as Amerlite XAD-2, to separate drugs. Consequently, either one of the resins may be used.

Regardless of the type of adsorbent used, blood is withdrawn from the patient via an arteriovenous or venovenous shunt (Fig. 9) and passed directly over the adsorbing material contained in sterile columns (Fig. 10) The procedure is a rather simple one and columns are

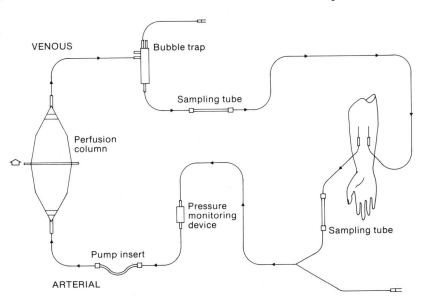

FIG. 9. Diagram illustrating hemoperfusion technique for removing poisonous compounds from the blood.

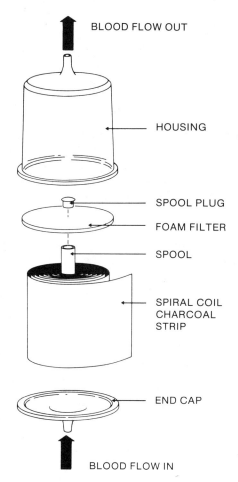

BLOOD FLOW OUT

HOUSING

SPOOL PLUG

FOAM FILTER

SPOOL

SPIRAL COIL
CHARCOAL
STRIP

END CAP

BLOOD FLOW IN

FIG. 10. Illustration showing the components of a hemoperfusion cartridge.

commercially available. The charcoal columns have been coated with acrylic hydrogel in order to decrease the risk of embolism and damage to blood cells.

The indications for using hemoperfusion in severe intoxications are evaluated by two important criteria. The first consideration is whether the adsorbent will eliminate the chemical from the blood. Second, the volume of distribution must be small and the half-life of the intoxicant must be relatively long, so the drug can continue to be drawn from the tissues to the blood and consequently be removed.

The primary complications include trapping of white blood cells (WBC) and platelets, and microembolization. However, these problems have largely been eliminated with the newer systems. When thrombocytopenia (decreased platelets) does occur, it seldom poses a significant clinical hazard.

SPECIFIC ANTIDOTES

Although a great number of specific antidotes exist based on their pharmacologic activities (6), there are relatively few that are actually employed for treatment of poisoning. Specific antidotes are discussed only briefly in this chapter but are discussed in more detail in later chapters on specific poisonings.

Classification of Specific Antidotes

Specific antidotes can be briefly classified into one of four categories: chemical, receptor, dispositional, and functional.

Chemical antidotes react with the poisonous chemical to produce a compound of lesser toxicity, or one that is absorbed to a lesser degree than the parent compound. In oxalic acid poisoning, the acid is absorbed and produces renal damage. Administering a calcium salt to react with the oxalic acid before absorption yields the poorly soluble compound, calcium oxalate. This largely passes through the intestines without being absorbed.

Antidotes such as dimercaprol (BAL) and deferoxamine form chemical chelates with certain heavy metals in the blood. Chelated complexes are soluble in urine and are readily excreted from the body, resulting in a lowering of the blood level of the heavy metal.

Receptor antidotes are substances that compete with a poison for the same receptor site, and thus reduce the undesired effect. Examples include naloxone reversal of morphine-induced respiratory depression, and atropine blockade of muscarinic activity.

For atropine or other compounds that cause symptoms of muscarinic receptor blockade, physostigmine is a specific antidote. Physostigmine is a reversible cholinesterase inhibitor. While it does not directly block atropine's effects by competing with it for muscarinic receptors, it inhibits the activity of the plasma

TABLE 9. *Comparison of hemodialysis with hemoperfusion*

Drug	Hemodialysis[a]	Charcoal hemoperfusion[a]	Resin hemoperfusion[a]
Phenobarbital	0.27	0.5	0.8–0.9
Amobarbital	0.26	0.3	0.9
Paraquat	0.5	0.6	0.9
Carbromal	0.25–0.4	0.5–0.6	1
Digoxin	0.15	0.3–0.6	0.4
Glutethimide	0.16	0.6–0.7	0.8
Methaqualone	0.13	0.4–1	0.5–1

[a]Expressed as plasma extraction ratio: PER = inlet concentration − outlet concentration/inlet concentration.
From ref. 52.

enzyme, pseudocholinesterase. This inhibition results in an increase in acetylcholine levels which then compete with atropine for its receptor sites.

Dispositional antagonism involves the alteration of a poison's absorption, metabolism, distribution, or excretion to reduce the amount available to tissues.

For example, when acetaminophen is taken in overdose, it is metabolized, in part, to a toxic metabolite which causes lethal hepatotoxicity. Conversion of this toxic intermediate to a nontoxic form proceeds by conjugation with glutathione, a sulfhydryl (− SH) group donor. When the liver's reserve of glutathione is depleted, as it is following massive overdoses of acetaminophen, the toxic manifestations appear. However, *N*-acetylcysteine is also a source of sulfhydryl groups and will serve the same function as endogenous glutathione. Acetaminophen and its toxic metabolite are, therefore, detoxified and the liver cells are not subjected to prolonged toxicity.

A *functional (physiologic) antagonist* is a chemical that acts on one biochemical system to produce effects that are opposite from those being produced on another system. For example, during an anaphylactic reaction following administration of a drug, the individual experiences severe breathing difficulties, due in part to intense bronchoconstriction. Epinephrine reverses this effect and breathing is normalized.

SUMMARY

Common sense is the dictum that governs most of the procedures discussed in this chapter. Successful antidoting of poisons is an art, but one that is not beyond our reach. Before proceeding to the next chapter, review the important antidotal procedures learned thus far. Take special effort to understand when a treatment should be used, and when treatment would be considered detrimental to the patient.

Case Studies

CASE STUDY: FATAL POISONING FROM A SALT EMETIC

History

A 3-year-old boy was given an unmeasured quantity of salt in water to induce emesis after his mother discovered he had ingested 36 baby aspirin tablets. The boy did not vomit, so he was taken to the hospital. Three hours after receiving the salt solution, he was lavaged with a saline solution. Shortly thereafter, he lost consciousness. Approximately 3 hr after the lavage procedure, he had a tonic-clonic convulsion. Although convulsions were managed with anticonvulsant therapy, he died 2 days later of cardiac arrest.

During his hospitalization, the victim's serum sodium level was approximately 180 mEq/L and re-

TABLE 10. *Common poisonous substances removed by hemoperfusion*

Barbiturates
  Amobarbital
  Butabarbital
  Carbromal
  Pentobarbital
  Phenobarbital
  Secobarbital

Nonbarbiturate sedatives
  Ethchlorvynol
  Glutethimide
  Methylprylon
  Methaqualone
  Diazepam
  Chloral hydrate
  Chlorpromazine
  Promazine
  Meprobamate

Analgesics
  Aspirin
  Methyl salicylate
  Acetaminophen

Antidepressants
  Amitriptyline
  Desipramine

Alcohols
  Ethanol
  Methanol (and its metabolites)

Cardiovascular
  Digoxin
  Procainamide

Miscellaneous
  Amanita phalloides (poisonous
    mushrooms)
  Carbon tetrachloride
  Chlorinated insecticides
  Ethylene oxide
  Methotrexate
  Paraquat
  Polychlorinated biphenyls
  Selected organophosphate
    insecticides

From ref. 52.

mained elevated throughout the period. His heart rate had increased to 220 beats/min. There were no murmurs or signs of cardiac enlargement; thus, no history of congestive heart failure. Toward the end he developed respiratory arrest and required mechanical ventilation. Two separate electroencephalograms, taken 24 hr apart, showed no evidence of electrical activity. Symptoms of aspirin intoxication were present, but not severe, and aspirin was not considered to be a major factor in his death. (See ref. 9.)

Autopsy permission was not given, but all sequelae were consistent with CNS abnormalities caused by hypernatremia.

Discussion

1. Explain how hypernatremia could lead to CNS abnormalities and be the cause of death of this child. Why do you suppose he died from cardiac failure?

2. Was lavage with saline (approximately 3 hr after the victim was first given the salt solution) wise or probably unwise?

3. It has been calculated that a level tablespoonful of salt contains at least 250 mEq solution. This is a sufficient quantity to raise the serum sodium in a 3-year-old child, if retained, by 25 mEq/L. (The child's mother did not recall how much salt she had given the boy; we can only guess it was excessive.) Knowing that this sodium level is inconsistent with life, what conclusions can you draw about recommending a salt solution for emesis?

CASE STUDY: EFFECTIVENESS OF CHARCOAL HEMOPERFUSION

History

A 48-year-old female was brought to the emergency department 2 hr after ingesting 50 200-mg aminophylline tablets (10 g aminophylline containing 8.5 g theophylline) prescribed for her asthmatic condition. On admission, she was lethargic and confused, but coherent. Her blood pressure had "bottomed-out" (50/0 mm Hg) and cardiac arrhythmias were present.

Initial treatment consisted of lavage, followed by activated charcoal and then a saline cathartic (magnesium citrate). Lidocaine was used to control the arrhythmias. She was in severe metabolic acidosis with an arterial pH of 6.59. She became nonresponsive, anuric, and had a grand mal seizure. Her serum theophylline level was 190 μg/ml (50 μg/ml is frequently associated with seizures, hypotension, and arrhythmias), and her prognosis grave.

At this point, approximately 9 hr after admission (see Fig. 11), she was placed on charcoal hemoperfusion. Within 1 hr her blood pressure and urine output improved, as well as all other signs of theophylline toxicity. Charcoal hemoperfusion was continued for 5 additional hr. She recovered with some residual neurological deficiency due to the cerebral anoxia. (See ref. 26.)

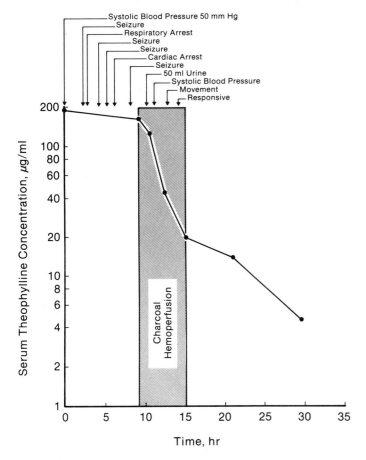

FIG. 11. Correlation between signs and symptoms of theophylline toxicity with serum theophylline levels, and the effect of charcoal hemoperfusion. (From ref. 26.)

Discussion

1. Explain the meaning of the patient's blood pressure, described as "bottomed-out." What caused this to occur?

2. Explain how the anuric state and metabolic acidosis are related to theophylline overdose.

3. Compare the rate of elimination of serum theophylline before, during, and after charcoal hemoperfusion. Are you convinced hemoperfusion was of benefit? If so, what specific event(s) led you to your decision?

CASE STUDIES: IPECAC MISUSE

History: Case 1

Ipecac syrup was administered to a 23-month-old female after she swallowed 10 to 12 5-mg pipamazine tablets (an antiemetic preparation no longer marketed). The baby-sitter was told by a physician to give the child one teaspoonful every 5 min until she

vomited, and a 120 ml bottle of syrup of ipecac was dispensed.

Two hours later, the baby-sitter was worried because the baby had become very drowsy and still had not vomited. It was estimated that 90 ml of syrup of ipecac had been given to the child by this time.

On admission to the emergency room, the child was very drowsy, but responsive to stimuli. Her pupils were constricted; blood pressure was 95/65; respirations 20/min, and pulse 120/min. Gastric lavage was performed, followed by a dose of magnesium sulfate.

The next morning she began to display some cardiac arrhythmias, but she was alert about 6 hr after admission and recovered uneventfully. (See ref. 1.)

History: Case 2

A 26-year-old female presented to the emergency room with palpitations, chest tightness, exertional dyspnea, and extreme fatigue which had been persistent for the past 10 days. Her medications included oral contraceptives (discontinued 1 month prior to admission) and amphetamines which she discontinued 10 days before admission. In order to lose weight she had been consuming 3 to 4 bottles of syrup of ipecac daily, after meals, for 3 months.

On admission, her blood pressure was 75/60 mm Hg, the pulse was 150/min, respirations 20/min, and temperature 36.7°C. Electrocardiogram (ECG) recordings showed a supraventricular tachycardia (150 beats/min). She became severely hypotensive and dyspneic, and steadily worsened. Despite intensive medical treatment, she died of ventricular arrhythmias. (See ref. 12.)

History: Case 3

An 18-year-old female had been suffering with anorexia nervosa for several years. Her adolescent desire to decrease food intake gradually turned into periods of starvation and bulimia (constant craving for food; abnormal eating binges). Her obsession with dieting was probably due to some deeply rooted emotional process. To increase her weight loss, she began indiscriminately to use about 60 Ex-Lax® tablets per day. Over a period of 2.5 years the patient lost approximatley 35% of her original body weight (71 kg).

For the next 5 months, she proceeded to use syrup of ipecac for its emetic effects. On a weekly basis, she probably ingested close to 300 ml of ipecac in doses up to 85 ml. This made her extremely weak and she was constantly fatigued.

She was finally admitted to the hospital by her family physician because of tiredness, slurred speech, dysphagia, and weight loss. On admission she weighed 54.5 kg. Her blood pressure was 80/44 mm Hg (supine) and pulse was 76 beats/min. She displayed severe skeletal muscular weakness. Laboratory results were unremarkable except for a mild neutropenia, lymphocytosis, transient increase in serum glutamate oxaloacetate transaminase (SGOT), and increase in creatine phosphokinase (CPK) and uric acid. Her ECG showed some minor T wave changes and sinus arrhythmias.

Treatment of this individual consisted of psychotherapy and discontinuing the use of the laxative and ipecac. She improved considerably by 5 months. (See ref. 34.)

History: Case 4

A 3-year-old male was admitted to an emergency facility with status epilepticus of unknown etiology. The previous evening the child had ingested 3 100-mg tablets of propoxyphene napsylate, and his mother promptly notified a poison control center. Instructions from the PCC were to obtain a bottle of syrup of ipecac, give the child one tablespoonful followed by water, and repeat only once if vomiting did not occur within 15 to 20 min.

Following these instructions, she sent her 12-year-old nephew to the local pharmacy. The pharmacist was unable to find any small bottles of syrup of ipecac, but he did find an old, half-filled bottle in the backroom labeled "Ipecac." He dispensed this preparation to the boy. The substance was eventually identified as fluid extract of ipecac.

The victim was given one tablespoonful of this preparation. Twenty minutes later, the mother tried unsuccessfully to give him another tablespoonful, since he had not vomited with the initial tablespoonful. He began to vomit and continued for the next 12 hr. Six hours prior to his hospital admission, he had an episode of profuse watery diarrhea. Also, opisthotonic generalized convulsions occurred about an hour before he was brought to the hospital.

On admission the child presented with tachypnea, pulse of 140 beats/min, respirations 35/min, blood pressure 110/80 mm Hg, and a temperature of 101.7°F. There was generalized abdominal tenderness, and bowel sounds were normal. Watery diarrhea persisted for several days. ECG monitoring revealed T wave inversion, and the child had extreme muscular weakness.

The following laboratory results were obtained:

Na^+	= 153 mEq/L	BUN	=	42 mg%
K^+	= 4.5 mEq/L	SGOT	=	47 IU
Cl^-	= 119 mEq/L	SGPT	=	12 IU
HCO_3^-	= 9 mEq/L	pH	=	7.32
Glucose	= 3 mg%	Pco_2	=	27 mm Hg
WBC	= 45,800/mm³	Po_2	=	75 mm Hg
Shift to the left				

The child was treated with phenobarbital to control seizures and was given glucose intravenously. He remained in the hospital for 2½ weeks and was given supportive and symptomatic care. Follow-up examination revealed normal growth, development, and hematological profiles. (See ref. 38.)

Discussion

1. In all cases, cardiac arrhythmias were present. Why did they occur?

2. In Case 2, how many milliliters of syrup of ipecac did the patient ingest per day? How does this compare to Case 3? Syrup of ipecac contains approximately 0.17 mg/ml emetine. What was her dose of emetine per day?

3. How many equivalent teaspoonfuls of syrup of ipecac did the victim in Case 4 receive with one tablespoonful of fluid extract of ipecac?

4. How does syrup of ipecac induce vomiting? What is the most logical explanation why it did not induce vomiting in Case 1?

5. In Case 4, which laboratory results were abnormal? How do they correlate with the toxic effects of ipecac? Give a specific reason for each of the abnormal values.

6. There are many lessons to be learned from these case studies. For example, in Case 1, what specific instructions on dosing syrup of ipecac should the physician have stated to the baby-sitter? In Case 4, what could the pharmacist who dispensed the fluid extract product have done to prevent this poisoning?

Review Questions

1. The text states that it is just as important to know when not to antidote a victim of poisoning, as it is to know when antidotal treatment should be given. What does this mean?

2. A patient presenting with deep tendon reflexes present, but without response to painful stimuli, is in which of the following stages of CNS depression?
   A. Stage 1
   B. Stage 2
   C. Stage 3
   D. Stage 4

3. Which of the following is true about milk given along with syrup of ipecac?
   A. It prevents ipecac's emetic action.
   B. It prolongs ipecac's activity.
   C. Milk reduces ipecac-induced diarrhea.
   D. Milk prolongs onset of emetic action.

4. Tannic acid has been shown to cause toxic problems to which of the following systems?
   A. Heart
   B. Brain
   C. Liver
   D. Blood

5. Compare the advantages and disadvantages of apomorphine to syrup of ipecac.

6. Why is apomorphine not controlled by the same regulatory standards as are other narcotics?

7. Fuller's earth has been shown to have a significant adsorbent action on a specific poison. What is it?

8. Which of the following is a true statement about activated charcoal?
   A. It should be administered in adult dosages of 10 to 20 g.
   B. The best antidotal grade is manufactured from powdered coal.
   C. It is a better antidote than the universal antidote.
   D. For best overall activity it should be taken in dry form.

9. A number of flavoring agents have been added to activated charcoal to improve palatability. Discuss the relative pros and cons of this practice.

10. Emesis can ordinarily be induced for all of the following poisonings *except*:
    A. Aspirin
    B. Barbiturates
    C. Hydrocarbons
    D. Insecticides

11. What advice should be given to a mother who asks about how much water should be given to her child to dilute an ingested poison? Comment on use of (a) milk and (b) carbonated beverages for use in diluting a poison.

12. State the pros and cons of giving syrup of ipecac to antidote an ingestion of substance that has antiemetic action.

13. Generally, emesis should not be attempted in children less than 6 months of age.
    A. True
    B. False

14. Discuss the mechanism of action of syrup of ipecac. Why might a second dose given within 20 to 30 min be considered of little additional value over the first dose?

15. Two to 3 tablespoonfuls of liquid detergent mixed with 6 to 8 ounces of water provides emesis by direct stimulation of the gastrointestinal mucosa.
    A. True
    B. False

16. Which of the following is a true statement about salt solution used as an emetic?

A. It is safe and effective.
B. It should not be used.

17. Comment on the use of zinc and copper sulfate used for emetic purposes. What are their advantages and drawbacks?

18. Burnt toast scrapings are an acceptable substitute for activated charcoal.
A. True
B. False

19. Administration of ammonium chloride will induce a urine pH that is:
A. Acidic
B. Alkaline

20. What urine flow rate is strived for by forced diuresis during antidoting of an ingested poison?

21. Phenobarbital excretion in the urine can be increased by making the urine:
A. Acidic
B. Alkaline

22. Explain why the following substances are sometimes added to peritoneal dialysis solutions:
A. Albumin
B. Lipid

23. How do chelating antidotes, such as dimercaprol, reduce blood levels of certain poisons? In general, for what specific class of toxic poisons are chelators most useful?

24. Discuss the role of demulcents in antidoting an ingested poison (e.g., their validity, limitations, etc.).

25. What specific physiological condition contraindicates use of activated charcoal?

26. Which of the following is not adsorbed onto activated charcoal: cyanide (I), iron salts (II), or salicylates (III)?
A. I only
B. I and II only
C. I and III only
D. II and III only

27. Name the specific antidote for treating phenol ingestions.

28. When undergoing gastric lavage, the patient should lie on his:

A. Right side
B. Left side
C. Back

29. Cite several risks associated with gastric lavage.

30. All of the following statements about syrup of ipecac are true *except*:
A. It is 14 times stronger than fluid extract of ipecac.
B. It causes emetic action by a direct stimulation of the gastrointestinal tract.
C. If given along with activated charcoal, it should precede the latter by at least 30 min.
D. Ipecac has demonstrated toxicity on the heart and neuromuscular junctions.

31. Following administration of syrup of ipecac, the patient should be kept:
A. Quiet and still
B. Active and alert

32. Drug-induced emesis is generally less traumatic than gastric lavage.
A. True
B. False

33. When a cathartic is indicated to antidote an ingested poison, the class of cathartic should be:
A. Stimulant
B. Lubricant
C. Softener
D. Saline

34. Hemoperfusion is more effective for removing most poisons from the blood than hemodialysis.
A. True
B. False

35. Discuss the role of activated charcoal in reducing blood levels of poisons that are excreted via the enterohepatic circulation. What is the enterohepatic circulation?

References

1. Adler, A. G., Walinksy, P., Krall, R. A., and Cho, S. Y. (1980): Death resulting from ipecac syrup poisoning. *JAMA*, 243:1927–1928.
2. Allan, B. C. (1961): The role of gastric lavage in the treatment of patients suffering from barbiturate overdose. *Med. J. Aust.*, 2:513–514.
3. American Association of Poison Control Centers and

American Academy of Clinical Toxicology Policy Statement: Universal antidote (1982): *J. Toxicol.-Clin. Toxicol.*, 19:527–529.

4. American Association of Poison Control Centers Policy Statement: Gastrointestinal dilution with water as a first aid procedure in poisoning (1982): *J. Toxicol.-Clin. Toxicol.*, 19:531–532.

5. Arena, J. M. (1970): Aspirin poisoning: Gastric lavage, ipecac or activated charcoal? *JAMA*, 212:327–328.

6. Arena, J. M. (1975): Poisoning—general treatment and prevention. Pt. 2. *JAMA*, 233:358–363.

7. Arieff, A. I., and Friedman, E. A. (1973): Coma following non-narcotic drug overdose: Management of 208 adult patients. *Am. J. Med. Sci.*, 266:405–426.

8. Atkinson, J. P., and Azarnoff, D. L. (1971): Comparison of charcoal and attapulgite as gastrointestinal sequestrants in acute drug ingestions. *Clin. Toxicol.*, 4:31–38.

9. Barer, J., Hill, L. L., Hill, R. M., and Martinez, W. M. (1973): Fatal poisoning from salt used as an emetic. *Am. J. Dis. Child.*, 125:889–890.

10. Berman, J. B. (1978): The art and science of clinical toxicology. *JAMA*, 240:265–267.

11. Boen, S. T. (1961): Kinetics of peritoneal dialysis. *Medicine*, 40:243–287.

12. Brotman, M. C., Forbath, N., Garfinkel, P. E., and Humphrey, J. G. (1981): Myopathy due to ipecac syrup poisoning in a patient with anorexia nervosa. *CMA Journal*, 125:453–454.

13. Cafruny, E. J. (1968): Renal pharmacology. *Ann. Rev. Pharmacol.*, 8:131–150.

14. Calvert, W. E., Corby, D. G., Herbertson, L. M., and Decker, W. J. (1971): Orally administered activated charcoal: Acceptance by children. *JAMA*, 215:641–645.

15. Cashman, T. M., and Shirkey, H. C. (1970): Emergency management of poisoning. *Pediatr. Clin. North Am.*, 17:525–534.

16. Chin, L. (1971): Gastrointestinal dilution of poisons with water—An irrational and potentially harmful procedure. *Am. J. Hosp. Pharm.*, 28:712–714.

17. Chin, L., Picchioni, A. L., and Gillespie, T. (1981): Saline cathartics and saline cathartics plus activated charcoal as antidotal treatments. *Clin. Toxicol.*, 18:865–871.

18. Comstock, E. G., Faulkner, T. P., Boisaubin, E. V., Olson, D. A., and Comstock, B. S. (1981): Studies on the efficacy of gastric lavage as practiced in a large metropolitan hospital. *Clin. Toxicol.*, 18:581–597.

19. Cooney, D. O. (1978): *In vitro* evidence for ipecac inactivation by activated charcoal. *J. Pharm. Sci.*, 67:426–427.

20. Crome, P., Dawling, S., Braithwaite, R. A., Masters, J., and Walkey, R. (1977): Effect of activated charcoal on absorption of nortriptyline. *Lancet*, 2:1204.

21. Dabbous, I. A., Bergman, A. B., and Robertson, W. O. (1965): The ineffectiveness of mechanically induced vomiting. *J. Pediatr.*, 66:952–954.

22. Daly, J. S., and Cooney, D. O. (1978): Interference by tannic acid with the effectiveness of activated charcoal in "universal antidote." *Clin. Toxicol.*, 12:515–522.

23. Decker, W. J., Shpall, R. A., Corby, D. G., Combs, H. F., and Payne, C. E. (1969): Inhibition of aspirin absorption by activated charcoal and apomorphine. *Clin. Pharmacol. Ther.*, 10:710–713.

24. DeGenaro, F., and Nyhan, W. L. (1971): Salt: A dangerous antidote. *J. Pediatr.*, 78:1048–1049.

25. DeNeve, R. (1976): Antidotal efficacy of activated charcoal in presence of jam, starch and milk. *Am. J. Hosp. Pharm.*, 33:965–966.

26. Ehlers, S. M., Zasko, D. E., and Sawchuk, R. J. (1978): Massive theophylline overdose. *JAMA*, 240:474–475.

27. Fane, L. R., Maetz, H. M., and Decker, W. J. (1971): Concurrent use of activated charcoal and ipecac in the treatment of poisoning. *Clin. Toxicol. Bull.*, 2:4–5.

28. Friedman, P. A. (1980): Chemical intoxication: General considerations and principles of management. In: *Principles of Internal Medicine*, 9th ed., pp. 949–953. McGraw-Hill, New York.

29. Gieseker, D. B., and Troutman, W. G. (1981): Emergency induction of emesis using liquid detergent products: A report of 15 cases. *Clin. Toxicol.*, 18:277–282.

30. Henderson, M. L., Picchioni, A. L., and Chin, L. (1966): Evaluation of oral dilution as a first aid measure in poisoning. *J. Pharm. Sci.*, 11:1311–1333.

31. Holt, L. E., and Holz, P. H. (1963): The black bottle. *J. Pediatr.*, 63:306–314.

32. Juhl, R. P. (1979): Comparison of kaolin-pectin and activated charcoal for inhibition of aspirin absorption. *Am. J. Hosp. Pharm.*, 36:1097–1098.

33. Levy, G., Soda, D. M., and Lampman, T. A. (1975): Inhibition by ice cream of the antidotal efficacy of activated charcoal. *Am. J. Hosp. Pharm.*, 32:289–291.

34. MacLeod, J. (1963): Ipecac intoxication—use of a cardiac pacemaker in management. *N. Engl. J. Med.*, 268:146–147.

35. Manno, B. R., and Manno, J. E. (1977): Toxicology of ipecac: A review. *Clin. Toxicol.*, 10:221–242.

36. Manoguerra, A. S., and Krenzelok, E. P. (1978): Rapid emesis from high dose ipecac syrup in adults and children intoxicated with antiemetics or other drugs. *Am. J. Hosp. Pharm.*, 35:1–6.

37. Mayersohn, M., Perrier, D., and Picchioni, A. L. (1977): Evaluation of a charcoal-sorbitol mixture as an antidote for oral aspirin overdose. *Clin. Toxicol.*, 11:561–567.

38. Miser, J. S., and Robertson, W. O. (1978): Ipecac poisoning. *West. J. Med.*, 128:440–443.

39. Morrelli, H. F. (1978): Rational therapy of poisoning. In: *Clinical Pharmacology—Basic Principles in Therapeutics*, 2nd ed., edited by K. L. Melmon and H. F. Morrelli, pp. 1028–1051. Macmillan, New York.

40. Neuvonen, P. J., and Elonen, E. (1980): Effect of activated charcoal on absorption and elimination of phenobarbitone, carbamazepine and phenylbutazone in man. *Eur. J. Clin. Pharmacol.*, 17:51–57.

41. Picchioni, A. L., Chin, L., Verhulst, H. L., and Dieterle, B. (1966): Activated charcoal versus "universal antidote" as an antidote for poisons. *Toxicol. Appl. Pharmacol.*, 8:447–454.

42. Robertson, W. O. (1971): A further warning on the use of salt as an emetic agent. *J. Pediatr.*, 79:877.

43. Rumack, B. H. (1977): Management of acute poisoning and overdose. In: *Management of the Poisoned*

Patient, edited by B. H. Rumack and A. R. Temple, pp. 250–280. Science Press, Princeton.

44. Rumack, B. F., and Peterson, R. G. (1979): Poisoning: Prevention of absorption. *Top. Emerg. Med.*, 1:13.

45. Saxena, K., and Kingston, R. (1982): Acute poisoning—management protocol. *Postgrad. Med.*, 71:67–77.

46. Schreiner, G. E. (1971): Dialysis of poisons and drugs. *Drug. Intell. Clin. Pharm.*, 5:322–339.

47. Schwartz, G. R. (1978): Emergency toxicology and general principles of medical management of the poisoned patient. In: *Principles and Practices of Emergency Medicine*, Vol. 2, edited by G. R. Schwartz, P. Safar, J. H. Stone, P. B. Storey, and D. K. Wagner, pp. 1317–1332. Saunders, Philadelphia.

48. Simon, N. M., and Krumlovsky, F. A. (1971): The role of dialysis in the treatment of poisonings. *Ration. Drug. Ther.*, 3:1–7.

49. Sketris, I. S., Moury, J. B., Czajka, P. A., Anderson, W. H., and Stafford, D. T. (1982): Saline catharsis: Effect on aspirin bioavailability in combination with activated charcoal. *J. Clin. Pharmacol.*, 22:59–64.

50. Varipapa, R. J., and Oderda, G. M. (1977): Effect of milk on ipecac-induced emesis. *J. Am. Pharm. Assoc.*, 17:510.

51. Weiner, I. M. (1967): Mechanisms of drug absorption and excretion: The renal excretion of drugs and related compounds. *Ann. Rev. Pharmacol.*, 7:39–56.

52. Winchester, J. F., Gelfand, M. C., and Tilstone, W. J. (1978): Hemoperfusion in drug intoxication: Clinical and laboratory aspects. *Drug. Metabol. Rev.*, 8:69–104.

53. Yancy, R. E., O'Barr, T. B., and Corby, D. G. (1977): *In vitro* and *in vivo* evaluation of the effect of cherry flavoring on the adsorptive capacity of activated charcoal for salicylic acid. *Vet. Hum. Toxicol.*, 19:163–165.

Alcohols, Glycols, and Aldehydes

4

Alcohols are hydroxy derivatives of straight or branched chain aliphatic hydrocarbons. The more common alcohols may include up to three hydroxyl groups with no more than one on each carbon. Lesser common alcohols may contain more than one hydroxyl group per carbon atom. Those alcohols that are most commonly encountered as causes of toxicity include ethanol (ethyl alcohol), methanol (methyl alcohol), and isopropanol (isopropyl alcohol). In general, the longer the carbon chain, the greater the toxicity. The one exception to this rule is methanol which is more toxic than ethanol.

The dihydroxy alcohols are called glycols (*glyc-* or *glyco-* from the Greek word meaning sweet), referring to their sweet taste. Dihydroxyethane is better known as ethylene glycol, the simplest glycol. It is even more commonly referred to as antifreeze, and is a frequently encountered toxic agent. Another glycol is trihydroxypropane (propylene glycol), a common constituent of numerous pharmaceutical products. For the most part, it is not toxic.

Alcohols and glycols are discussed together in this chapter, not solely because of their chemical similarities, but because of the close semblance of toxic symptoms of methanol and ethylene glycol. Ethanol and isopropyl alcohol also cause toxic symptoms which are similar to each other, when consumed in toxic amounts.

ETHANOL TOXICITY

Ethanol is the only alcohol that has widespread intentional internal human use. Ethanol is one of the oldest drugs recognized by man and is the primary alcohol present in beers, wines, and distilled spirits.

Ethanol is a clear, colorless liquid that imparts a burning sensation to the mouth and throat when swallowed. Pure ethanol has a very slight, pleasant odor. It is freely soluble in water. Contrary to popular belief, ethanol is a powerful CNS depressant that works primarily on the reticular activating system. In fact, its actions are qualitatively similar to those of the general anesthetics. It has a relatively low order of toxicity compared to methanol or isopropanol.

Ethanol is discussed first because it is the alcohol that is most frequently reported as a cause of toxicity, and because an understanding of certain aspects of its metabolic pathway and biological effects is necessary in order to understand the toxicity of methanol and ethylene glycol. As with all of the alcohols and glycols discussed in this chapter, only acute toxicological considerations will be discussed.

Mechanism of Action of Ethanol

The exact mechanism by which ethanol produces its actions is not entirely understood. The CNS is selectively affected. Ethanol is thought to act directly on neuronal membranes and not at the synapses. At the membrane, it may interfere with ion transport. *In vitro* studies indicate that Na^+, K^+-ATPase is inhibited by ethanol. Concentrations of 5 to 10% block the neuron's ability to produce electrical impulses. These concentrations are far greater than the concentration of ethanol in the CNS *in vivo*.

The effect of ethanol on the CNS is directly proportional to the blood concentration. The first region of the brain affected is the reticular activating system. This causes disruption of the motor and thought processes. In addition, suppressing the cerebral cortex with ethanol will cause behavioral changes. Which specific types of behavior will be suppressed and which will be released from inhibition depend on the individual. In general, complex, abstract, and poorly learned behaviors are disrupted at low alcohol concentrations.

Ethanol depresses the CNS irregularly in a descending order from the cortex to the medulla. Table 1 illustrates the correlation between blood alcohol concentration and the area of the brain which is affected. Also, subjective feelings are noted based on blood alcohol concentration and the area of the brain where ethanol produces its effect.

Kinetics of Acute Ethanol Ingestion

Absorption

Since ethanol is weakly polar and has a small molecular size and weak electronic charge, it is

TABLE 1. *Range of toxicity of ethanol*

Clinical description/ symptoms	Blood alcohol concentration	Brain
Mild	0.05–0.10%	Frontal lobe
Decreased inhibitions		
Slight visual impairment		
Slowing of reaction time		
Increased confidence		
Moderate	0.15–0.30%	
Ataxia		Parietal lobe
Slurred speech		
Decreased motor skills		
Decreased attention		Occipital lobe
Diplopia		
Altered perception		Cerebellum
Altered equilibrium		
Severe	0.03–0.5%	
Vision impairment		Occipital lobe
Equilibrium		Cerebellum
Stupor		Diencephalon
Coma	0.5%	
Respiratory failure		Medulla

miscible in water and soluble in lipids. Therefore, it can easily pass through cell membranes by simple diffusion. Alcohol is readily absorbed from the empty gastrointestinal tract. The principal site of absorption is the small intestine, and to a much lesser extent, the stomach and large intestine. Even though ethanol has a small molecular weight, it is quite lipid-soluble and generally is absorbed by passive diffusion. There are several factors which affect its absorption.

For example, the gastric emptying time is extremely important in regulating the absorption of alcohol. Gastric emptying time is influenced by the stomach contents and gastrointestinal motility. On an empty stomach, complete absorption will take place in about 1 to 2 hr, but on a full stomach, absorption can be delayed up to 6 hr. Beverage composition is also an important consideration with respect to ethanol absorption. Beer is more slowly absorbed than wine, and wine is more slowly absorbed than distilled spirits. In general, carbonated beverages are absorbed faster, because carbon dioxide promotes evacuation of the stomach.

Distribution

Following absorption, alcohol is uniformly distributed throughout all tissues and body fluids, and parallels the water content of each. Equilibrium is rapidly established between alcohol in the blood and the tissue compartment. It is especially important to remember that ethanol easily passes through both the blood-brain barrier and placenta. Recently, much attention has been focused on alcohol ingested during pregnancy and the occurrence of fetal alcohol syndrome. The distribution of alcohol between alveolar air and blood depends on the speed of diffusion, its vapor pressure, and the concentration of alcohol in the lung capillaries. The distribution ratio between alveolar air and the blood is 1:2,100. This consideration is utilized in the determination of blood alcohol concentration when using the breathalyzer.

The Swedish scientist Widmark developed a formula for estimating the amount of alcohol needed to produce a given blood alcohol concentration (BAC). Conversely, the formula can be used to estimate the BAC that will result from ingestion of a stated quantity of alcohol in an individual with a known body weight. The Widmark formula is expressed as:

$$A = \frac{Wr\,CT}{0.8}$$

where:

A = ethanol (ml) ingested
W = body weight (g)
r = distribution ratio of ethanol
    Men = 0.68
    Women = 0.55
CT = blood alcohol concentration (decimal equivalent)
0.8 = specific gravity of ethanol

The Widmark r factor is based on the distribution of alcohol in the blood, to that of the whole body, i.e.,

$$r = \frac{\% \text{ alcohol in body}}{\% \text{ alcohol in blood}}$$

For men, $r = 0.68$, and for women, $r = 0.55$ because women usually have less body water and a greater quantity of adipose tissue. To predict the BAC of an individual, consider the following example.

A man weighing 150 pounds who drinks one ounce (approximately 30 ml) of 100-proof (50% ethanol v/v) whiskey or other distilled spirit, or one 12-ounce can of beer (5% ethanol v/v) will obtain, after complete absorption, a blood alcohol concentration of 0.025% (2.5 mg%), i.e.,

$$A = \frac{Wr\,CT}{0.8}$$

$$A = \frac{68{,}100 \times 0.68 \times 0.025\%}{0.8}$$

$$A = \frac{11.58}{0.8}$$

$A =$ approximately 15 ml, or one-half ounce of pure ethanol, or one ounce of 50% ethanol

If we rearrange the equation, the BAC for a stated volume ingested can easily be estimated. For a man weighing more or less than 150 pounds, or if the alcoholic content of the beverage is different than 50%, the BAC would be proportionately altered. In any case, the BAC can be calculated by the following formula:

$$\frac{150}{\text{body weight}} \times \frac{\% \text{ EtOH}}{50} \times \frac{\text{Number ounces ingested}}{} \times 0.025\% = \frac{\text{Maximum}}{\text{BAC}}$$

In acute ethanol overdoses, it is sometimes helpful to be able to estimate the BAC when the intoxicated person was known to have ingested a certain quantity of alcoholic beverage. This value can then be used to verify the clinical signs and symptoms that follow an acute alcohol ingestion. For example, the physician attending a person who just arrived at the Emergency Department with decreased respiration and blood pressure, and was semicomatose, was told by friends of the victim that after two beers he began to pass out. Based on the history, we would not expect such a reduced state of consciousness (i.e., the BAC would not be high enough to induce unconsciousness). The problem is that either the history is incorrect, or the patient has also ingested some other CNS depressant. Whatever the case, the blood toxicology drug screen should clarify the situation. In this case the patient should be treated, not the "suspected" poison. For a comprehensive study of the pharmacokinetics of alcohols, consult the excellent reference by Walgreen (41).

Metabolism

Understanding the metabolism of ethanol is useful in predicting and managing the consequences of its ingestion. Between 90 and 98% of absorbed ethanol is removed from the body by enzymatic oxidation. Normally, about 2 to 10% is excreted unchanged, mainly through the lungs and kidneys. Small amounts can be detected in sweat, tears, bile, gastric juice, saliva, and other secretions. Remember, alcohol concentration parallels the water content of the organ system or biological fluid.

Enzymatic oxidation of ethanol occurs primarily in the liver, but to a smaller extent in the kidney. The metabolic process involves three enzymatic reactions, as shown in Fig. 1. During the first step, ethanol is oxidized to acetaldehyde by the enzyme, alcohol dehydrogenase, which requires NAD as a cofactor. This is the rate-limiting step in the dissipation of alcohol from the body. Hepatic alcohol dehydrogenase is a nonspecific enzyme that also catalyzes the conversion of other primary alcohols and aldehydes, as well as secondary alcohols and ketones.

Acetaldehyde, in the second step, is then converted by aldehyde dehydrogenase in the presence of NAD to acetic acid, which is then further converted to acetyl coenzyme A (CoA). Acetyl CoA enters the Kreb's cycle where it is eventually metabolized to CO_2 and water.

The metabolism of ethanol involves conversion of NAD to $NADH_2$, as shown in Figs. 1 and 2. This results in a significant decrease in

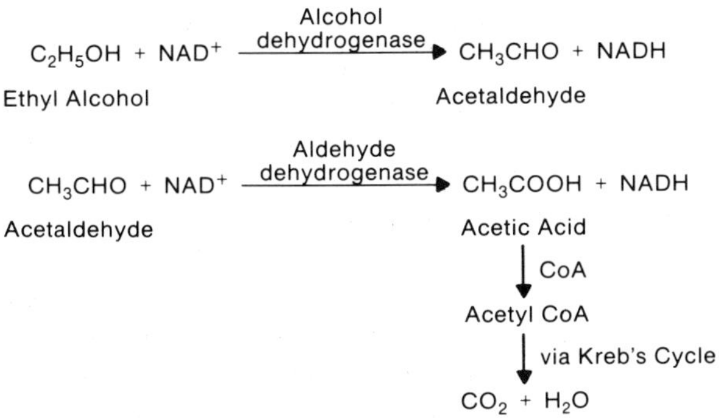

Alcohol dehydrogenase
C_2H_5OH + NAD^+
CH_3CHO + NADH
Ethyl Alcohol
Acetaldehyde
Aldehyde dehydrogenase
CH_3CHO + NAD^+
CH_3COOH + NADH
Acetaldehyde
Acetic Acid
CoA
Acetyl CoA
via Kreb's Cycle
CO_2 + H_2O

FIG. 1. Biochemical pathway for ethanol metabolism.

GLUCOSE
ETHANOL
FATS
GLYCOGEN
GLUCOSE-6-PHOSPHATE
NAD
$NADH_2$
ACETALDEHYDE
GLYCEROL
DIHYDROXY ACETONE-PHOSPHATE
GLYCERALDEHYDE-3-PHOSPHATE
ACETATE
LACTATE
PYRUVATE
ACETYL CoA
ACETOACETYL CoA
ACETOACETATE
AMINO ACIDS
β-HYDROXY-BUTYRATE
OXALOACETATE
CITRIC ACID CYCLE
CITRATE
AMINO ACIDS

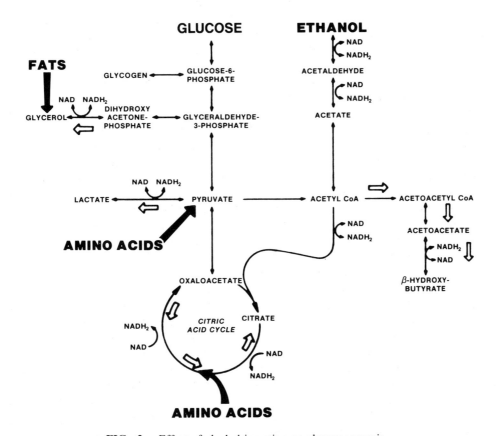

FIG. 2. Effect of alcohol ingestion on gluconeogenesis.

the $NAD/NADH_2$ ratio in the liver, and is responsible for some of the metabolic effects of ethanol intoxication. For example, significant hypoglycemia occurs following acute and chronic intoxication with ethanol. This can sometimes be extremely critical in children. Although the metabolic consequences of ethanol ingestion are complex, it is thought that they are partly due to the inhibition of gluconeogenesis by ethanol as a result of the depletion of NAD. This can be easily understood if we locate all the reactions in Fig. 2 that require NAD. Since NAD is depleted with ethanol, these reactions will proceed in the direction of the *open arrows*. Consequently, amino acids that usually enter the glycolysis pathway and tricarboxylic acid (TCA) cycle are shunted into other pathways. There is a decrease in oxaloacetate and pyruvate, and an accumulation of lactate and ketoacids. Also, there is a reduction in the metabolism of glycerol, resulting in the accumulation of fat in the liver.

Another important parameter to consider when dealing with acute ethanol ingestion is how long will it take the intoxicated person to sober up? Or, what is the rate of elimination? First-order elimination kinetics is the general rule for most drugs, i.e., most drugs are eliminated from the body at a rate which depends on the amount of drug present in the body, and the amount of drug remaining at any time in the body decreases exponentially to zero. For ethanol, this elimination rate occurs only for very low, clinically insignificant BAC levels of less than 20 mg% or 0.02%.

Studies have established the K_m, or Michaelis-Menton dissociation constant, for alcohol dehydrogenase to be 9.7 mg% (range of 8–14 mg%) and V_{max}, or the maximum velocity, to be 23.3 mg% (range of 22–24 mg%) (39,42). When the substrate (ethanol) concentration is less than the K_m, the rate of elimination is first-order. However, when the substrate concentration is much greater than the K_m, that is, the rate approaches the V_{max} or maximum velocity for the enzymatic reaction, the rate of elimination is constant, regardless of concentration, and is referred to as zero-order kinetics.

To apply these principles to acute ethanol ingestion, refer to Fig. 3. Plasma concentrations of ethanol which are commonly encountered are at least 100 mg% or 0.1%, which is about 10 times greater than the K_m. Therefore, the rate of elimination, or dissipation rate, for ethanol follows zero-order kinetics and is constant at 100 mg/kg/hr. For a man weighing 150 pounds, approximately 7 g of ethanol (approximately 10 ml of 100% EtOH) will be eliminated every hour. In terms of the BAC, the dissipation rate will average about 15 mg%/hr (0.015%/hr) which is referred to as the Widmark β factor in Fig.

4. From this information, we can then calculate the approximate length of time required to eliminate enough alcohol to be considered sober, or out of danger. To achieve a BAC of 100 mg% (0.1%), a 150-pound individual needs to ingest 55 ml of absolute ethanol. In a practical setting, this requires the ingestion of 120 ml or about 4 ounces of gin, whiskey, or vodka, but the maximum quantity that can be oxidized in the liver is 10 ml/hr. Consequently, it will take about 5 hr to eliminate the amount of alcohol ingested (55 ml absolute; 120 ml, 50–60 proof). Therefore, there is some validity to the suggestion that a safe "maintenance" dose of ethanol would be 10 ml/hr of absolute ethanol, which translates into one shot of liquor (20–25 ml).

Clinical Manifestations of Acute Ethanol Toxicity

Characteristics of ethanol intoxication include a wide variety of signs and symptoms that range from ataxia to coma.

The severely intoxicated patient appears to be stuporous or comatose. The skin is cold and clammy; the breath smells of alcohol; body temperature and respiration rate are decreased. There may be an increase in heart rate. Alcoholic coma usually occurs when the BAC exceeds 300 mg% or 0.3%. At concentrations less than 100 mg%, the frontal lobe shows a selective impairment.

The subjective effects include a decrease in inhibitions, increase in confidence, altered judgment, and decrease in attention span. As the blood alcohol concentration rises from 0.1 to 0.2%, the parietal lobe is affected. At these concentrations, there is a decrease in motor skill, slurred speech, tremor, and ataxia. Blood alcohol concentrations reaching 0.3% affect the cerebellum, as well as the occipital lobe of the cerebral hemisphere. These individuals exhibit altered equilibrium, perception, and possible diplopia. When the blood alcohol concentration reaches the LD_{50} value (about 0.45–0.5%), coma is evident with marked respiratory depression and peripheral vascular collapse. At this point the medulla has been affected, and the outcome may be critical.

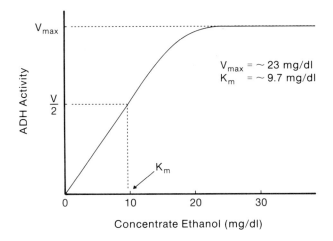

FIG. 3. The rate of enzymatic activity for alcohol dehydrogenase using ethanol as the substrate.

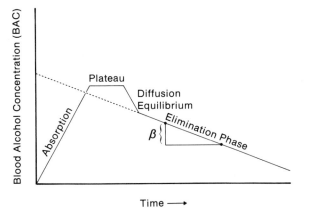

FIG. 4. Depiction of the pharmacokinetic profile of ethanol.

The degree of physical impairment observed in individuals that have been drinking alcoholic beverages is generally thought to parallel the level of ethanol in the blood.

Treatment of Acute Alcohol Ingestion

The severely intoxicated patient should be kept warm and the stomach contents should be evacuated. Top priority should include protection of the airway from aspiration, and intubation of the patient if necessary. Analeptics (stimulants) such as caffeine or pentylenetetrazole are not recommended and, in fact, should be avoided. The blood glucose level should be maintained by giving 10 to 50% dextrose solution intravenously. Sodium bicarbonate will correct the lactic acidosis. Hemodialysis may be indicated if symptoms are severe and the patient's BAC exceeds 0.4%.

Usually, specific therapy is not required for acute alcoholic intoxication. The patient is treated symptomatically and monitored carefully until the ingested alcohol is metabolized.

METHANOL

The alcohol with the simplest structure, but the one most likely to cause serious human toxicity, is methanol (wood alcohol, methyl alcohol, Columbian spirits, wood naphtha). Numerous studies over the years have investigated its toxicity potential, as well as the most beneficial means for treating acute toxicity.

Methanol is widely used in industry and around the home as a general solvent, paint thinner, antifreeze, fluid for desk "spirit" duplicating machines, and source of heat for fondue burners (e.g., Sterno®). Occasionally, at concentrations up to 5%, methanol is used as a denaturant for ethanol that is not intended for human consumption. It is called "wood" alcohol because formerly its primary source was from distillation of wood.

Most reports of methanol toxicity are due to ingesting methanol itself, or a methanol-containing product, although poisoning has been reported following absorption through the skin, and inhalation of as little as 0.2% in inspired air. Since yeast fermentation does not produce even trace quantities of methanol, pure "moonshine" liquor does not contain methanol (9). Cases that have been reported where consumers of this illicit beverage have developed severe intoxication to "shine" occasionally fail to mention that the cause of the poisoning was from methanol which was added to the substance in order to increase the quantity of salable product.

Methanol poisoning continues to be a worldwide (although regional) problem associated with high mortality and morbidity. Massive outbreaks of poisoning have been reported especially during wartime, ethanol shortages, and prohibition (6,37). Since new uses for methanol are currently being proposed (e.g., as an alternate fuel source), the problem will undoubtedly become more significant in future years.

Accidental ingestion is also related to the fact that methanol closely resembles ethanol in appearance and odor, is readily available, tax-free (thus cheaper) and, in general, is not understood by the public to be any more dangerous than ethanol. The lethal dose is near 30 ml although recovery following 500 ml has been recorded (29).

Mechanism of Methanol Toxicity

Methanol is absorbed and distributed through the body in a manner similar to ethanol. It is metabolized by the same enzymes, but at only one-seventh to one-fifth the rate of ethanol (35). This slow metabolic conversion rate accounts for the accumulation of methanol and its metabolites which cause delayed toxic effects.

Methanol metabolism proceeds as shown in Fig. 5, and like ethanol, this occurs independently of the blood concentration. Animal and human studies have shown that methanol is metabolized by alcohol dehydrogenase and aldehyde dehydrogenase to formaldehyde and formic acid, respectively (26). We should also note that the metabolic process may proceed along a variety of pathways depending on the animal species tested. Thus, in some lower animals, toxicity is due to the alcohol, per se, rather than to its various metabolites.

During its metabolism, methanol is oxidized to formaldehyde, which is 33 times more toxic than methanol. Some of this product reacts with body proteins and the rest is further oxidized.

Metabolic conversion is not the sole means for elimination of methanol. A significant amount may be excreted unchanged through the lungs and kidneys. However, metabolism is the major reaction.

Methanol, like ethanol, is distributed through the body in proportions equivalent to the amount of water in various tissues. This may help explain why the eye is at great vulnerability to damage from even small quantities of methanol.

Clinical Manifestations of Methanol Toxicity

Characteristics of methanol intoxication are qualitatively similar regardless of the quantity ingested. However, they do vary widely from person to person.

Symptoms initially resemble those of ethanol intoxication, although they are usually less severe. This is probably due to lower lipid solubility. These symptoms include euphoria, muscle weakness, and suppression of inhibitions. Inebriation, per se, is usually not a significant problem, except when larger quantities are consumed or ethanol has been concurrently ingested.

As should be expected, in cases of concomitant ethanol and methanol ingestion, initial symptoms of toxicity are predominantly those of ethanol. In persons suspected of concurrent consumption, methanol must be specifically looked for, even in the absence of immediate symptoms which are frequently delayed.

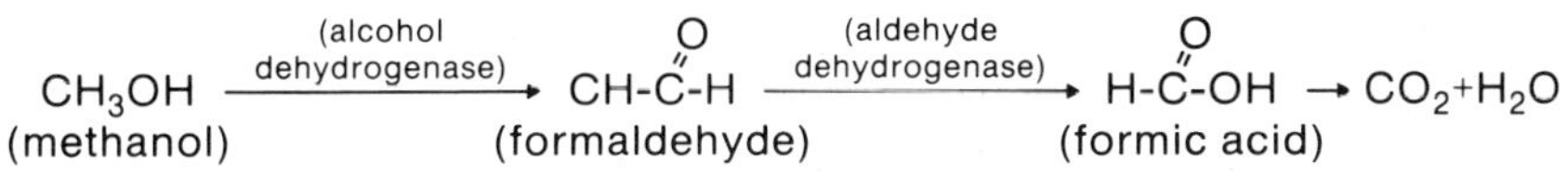

$$CH_3OH \xrightarrow[\text{dehydrogenase)}]{\text{(alcohol}} CH\text{-}\overset{\overset{O}{\|}}{C}\text{-}H \xrightarrow[\text{dehydrogenase)}]{\text{(aldehyde}} H\text{-}\overset{\overset{O}{\|}}{C}\text{-}OH \rightarrow CO_2 + H_2O$$

$$\text{(methanol)} \qquad\qquad \text{(formaldehyde)} \qquad\qquad \text{(formic acid)}$$

FIG. 5. Biochemical pathway for methanol metabolism.

Following a 3- to 36-hr latent interval, there is an abrupt onset of nausea with vomiting, dizziness, headache, delirium, intense gastrointestinal pain, and perhaps diarrhea, back pain and cold, clammy extremities. The optic disc appears hyperemic.

In severe methanol poisoning, respiration and heart rate are depressed and these signal a grave prognosis. Acidosis is noted, but the patient usually does not experience Kussmaul breathing (slow, deep respirations). He may enter into a coma, and death can be sudden or delayed for hours. Convulsions and opisthotonos may precede death. Toxicity to the central nervous system is due to methanol, per se; whereas the severe metabolic sequelae and other toxic effects are caused by complications of acidosis (5).

When methanol is oxidized to formaldehyde and formic acid, there is a relative increased conversion of NAD^+ to NADH. The excess NADH favors the reduction of pyruvate to lactate. Thus, acidosis associated with methanol poisoning is caused by the formation and accumulation of both formic acid and lactic acid. Consequently, there is an increased anion gap (difference between total cations and total anions). The normal anion gap is 18 mmoles/L (calculated as $[Na^+ + K^+] - [Cl^- + HCO_3^-]$), but may be two or more times above normal following methanol intoxication.

Ocular damage is of special concern. Ingestion of as little as 4 ml of methanol has caused blindness. In fact, 6% of all blindness in the United States Armed Forces during World War II is reported to have been due to methanol consumption (15). Eye damage, in the form of retinal destruction and optic nerve degeneration, is due primarily to formaldehyde accumulation (20–22) and is enhanced by acidosis (7,24). In the event of survival, the victim may be totally blind, or at the very least, have some degree of visual impairment lasting several months.

Treatment of Methanol Toxicity

Whereas a wide variety of treatments for methanol poisoning have been proposed over the years, the major focus of treatment should involve correcting the acidosis. This must be treated first, since it may be life-threatening (19). The severity of ocular damage is also somewhat dependent on the rapidity and completeness of acidosis reversal. Therefore, infusion of sodium bicarbonate should be started immediately and maintained until the urinary pH is normal.

Ethanol is theoretically a specific antidote for methanol toxicity, although its effectiveness still remains to be fully established. Since ethanol has an affinity for alcohol dehydrogenase that is at least 20 times greater than that of methanol, it preferentially serves as the substrate for this enzyme. Ethanol treatment should be initiated orally or by intravenous injection as soon as possible. It is usually dosed so that the blood ethanol level remains at 0.1%. As stated earlier, metabolism of alcohols proceeds independently of the blood concentration. Consequently, this amount of ethanol is sufficient to reduce the rate of methanol metabolism to its more toxic metabolites and, thus, reduce its overall toxicity. Ethanol treatment may need to be continued for a week or longer in order to completely eliminate all of the methanol.

Hemodialysis or peritoneal dialysis will effectively hasten methanol elimination. Dialysis should be initiated if the blood methanol concentration is greater than 50 mg%, and should be continued until it drops below 20 mg%. Since ethanol will be removed along with methanol, it is imperative that the ethanol infusion rate be adjusted continuously.

Alternative therapeutic measures have been suggested to overcome the deficiencies of ethanol therapy. Leucovorin calcium, a folate analog, is reasoned to provide such a beneficial action since it enhances metabolism of formaldehyde to carbon dioxide via folate-dependent enzyme systems (30). 4-Methylpyrazole (4 MP), a potent inhibitor of alcohol dehydrogenase in animal studies, has also been suggested for use (4,27). At this time, these suggestions are still untested and unproven, and both need further clarification and clinical study. These hypotheses, if eventually proven valid, exemplify the age-old principle that when we understand the reasoning behind a physiological or biochemical event, it then becomes a much easier task to alter that event should it be necessary to do so.

ISOPROPYL ALCOHOL

Isopropyl alcohol is commonly used as a disinfectant and for rubbing onto the skin. It is a constituent of many perfumes and colognes, and personal products. Occasionally it is used as a beverage, then becoming a cause of poisoning. The fatal dose is reported to be approximately 4 to 8 ounces (10).

Initial symptoms are similar to those of ethanol intoxication, but are reported to be at least twice as severe (35). Its duration of action is also longer than ethanol. Isopropyl alcohol is converted to acetone which may be responsible for many of the symptoms of isopropyl alcohol poisoning. Manifestations of acetone toxicity and its treatment are given in Chapter 11.

GLYCOLS: ETHYLENE GLYCOL

There are numerous glycols used in many industrial applications, as hydraulic fluids and heat exchangers; in chemical syntheses; as solvents and as components of cosmetics, inks, lacquers, and various pharmaceuticals. Only ethylene glycol, however, is of current significant toxicological interest. Its toxicity is stated to be quantitatively between the extremely toxic substance, diethylene glycol, and the relatively nontoxic chemical, propylene glycol.

Diethylene glycol (Fig. 6) was the culprit that caused more than 100 deaths in 1937 when it was inadvertently used as a solvent for sulfanil-

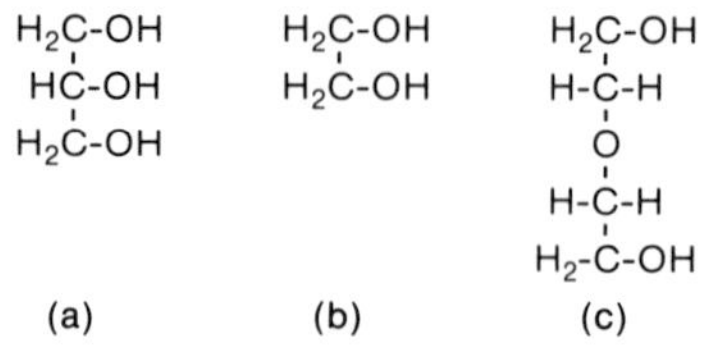

FIG. 6. Chemical structures for glycols shown in order of increasing toxicity. **(a)** Propylene glycol, **(b)** ethylene glycol, and **(c)** diethylene glycol.

amide in a pharmaceutical preparation (11,36). After 2 to 5 days of consuming this "elixir" which contained 72% diethylene glycol, patients complained of nausea with vomiting, intense gastrointestinal cramping and diarrhea, and back pain referred to the kidney area. These symptoms soon led to progressive liver necrosis, renal tubular degeneration, and death. Although diethylene glycol today is not a significant source of toxicity, it is still used in several industrial processes and must always be handled with special precaution.

Ethylene glycol is most generally encountered around the home as "permanent" automotive antifreeze. It is a colorless, nonvolatile liquid having a sweet taste. Antifreeze products are usually artificially colored. Ethylene glycol is a commonly ingested poison because of its sweet taste and the "lemonade" appearance of many antifreeze products, and because it is readily available to inquisitive children from carelessly stored containers of antifreeze in the garage. It is also consumed, on occasion, by adults, for purposes of inebriation which, in its early stages, closely resembles that of ethanol. Ingested ethylene glycol can produce extremely serious symptoms, even death, with toxic doses reported at approximately 100 ml, although survival has been reported with 240 ml (28). One of the case studies reported at the end of this chapter describes a massive ingestion of 2 L, with survival.

Mechanism of Ethylene Glycol Toxicity

Ethylene glycol, like methanol, is converted to metabolites that are more toxic than the parent compound. As with ethanol, methanol, and isopropanol, the same enzyme system, alcohol dehydrogenase, is involved. Not all of the metabolites have been identified, but Fig. 7 illustrates possible intermediates. These toxic intermediates are responsible for producing tissue destruction and severe metabolic acidosis. Tissue damage results from the deposition of calcium oxalate crystals. Acidosis results from the accumulation of lactic acid (due to the increased alcohol dehydrogenase activity), glycolic acid, glyoxylic acid, formic acid, and oxalic acid.

Clinical Manifestations of Ethylene Glycol Toxicity

Signs and symptoms of toxicity result from the direct toxic actions of ethylene glycol or its metabolites on these target systems: brain, cardiorespiratory, and renal.

Initially, central depression develops, perhaps as severe as with ethanol, and may persist for 12 or more hours. Depression is potentiated if the patient has also consumed alcohol (13). Other CNS effects include muscle paralysis, decreased tendon reflexes, convulsions, and tetany due to hypocalcemia. These effects are usually accom-

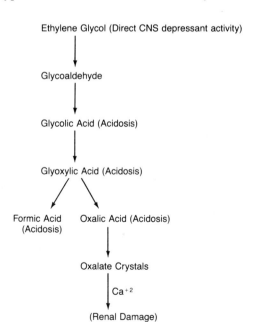

FIG. 7. Biochemical pathway for ethylene glycol metabolism.

panied by nausea and vomiting, ataxia, stupor, and, depending on the amount ingested, coma and death. If death occurs during the early phase of poisoning, it is due to respiratory and/or cardiac failure.

If the patient survives the initial effects, pulmonary edema (enhanced by CNS depression), congestive heart failure, tachycardia, and renal failure develop as a result of calcium deposition. The kidney is especially susceptible since the deposition of calcium in the renal tubules produces tubular epithelial necrosis with fat inclusion, particularly in the convoluted tubules (18). Glomeruli develop thickened basement membranes and granule deposits.

Treatment of Ethylene Glycol Toxicity

The principal goal in treating ethylene glycol poisoning is to correct the acidosis with sodium bicarbonate, enhance elimination of ethylene glycol by hemodialysis, and inhibit metabolism of ethylene glycol by providing ethanol as a competitive substrate for the enzyme alcohol dehydrogenase (33,40).

Animal studies have confirmed that ethanol inhibits ethylene glycol metabolism, thus reducing its toxicity potential following ingestion (14,34). Ethanol should be given within 8 hr of ethylene glycol ingestion, and be continued for at least 5 days.

Calcium salts (e.g., calcium lactate) are sometimes recommended to replace calcium which is lost from the blood through combining with oxalate. The rationale for this recommendation is not clear. Calcium is probably not needed for routine cases because the body can usually maintain a normal calcium homeostasis.

PROPYLENE GLYCOL

Propylene glycol is generally reported as having a low order of systemic toxicity and, in fact, is widely used as a solvent for numerous pharmaceutical products. However, reports in the literature suggest that propylene glycol may be toxic if it is used inappropriately (1,25). In a few susceptible children, ingesting a propylene-glycol-based product for long periods has caused seizures, tachypnea, diaphoresis, and unconsciousness. Such reports of toxicity are rare.

ALDEHYDES: FORMALDEHYDE

A large number of aldehydes are employed in numerous industrial processes. However, only two, formaldehyde and acetaldehyde, currently pose a significant toxicologic health hazard. Metaldehyde (snail bait) and paraldehyde are both polymers of acetaldehyde and presumably are slowly converted to acetaldehyde in the body. Toxic acetaldehyde levels do not accumulate following paraldehyde ingestion since acetaldehyde oxidation to nontoxic products (acetic acid, etc.) proceeds faster than decomposition of paraldehyde to acetaldehyde. For metaldehyde, decomposition to acetaldehyde progresses more quickly than the resulting intermediate can be oxidized.

Symptoms of acute toxicity from paraldehyde are largely extensions of its pharmacological use as a CNS sedative. Following a toxic dose of metaldehyde, symptoms are largely similar to acetaldehyde poisoning.

There has recently been renewed interest in accidental poisoning caused by formaldehyde. Most of this interest has centered on the release into the air of formaldehyde from insulation composed of urea formaldehyde (2,17). Additionally, formaldehyde may cause contact urticaria in susceptible individuals, and it is suspected of being a carcinogen and mutagen (23,32). Systemic intoxication also occurs. In this chapter, we will discuss important implications of formaldehyde poisoning by inhalation and ingestion.

Formaldehyde is a colorless, flammable gas with a strongly characteristic, objectionable odor. It is most commonly found as a 40% solution in water (formalin) for use as a disinfectant, antiseptic, and embalming fluid. Because it is highly reactive chemically, it is widely used in a variety of products such as paints and adhesives, dyes, fuels, paper, and other chemicals. It is a component of air, originating from numerous sources including incinerators and engine exhaust. Atmospheric levels of 0.06 ppm

have been reported near industrial sites or in areas of thick fog (32). Cigarette smoke contains high levels. Air concentration in some mobile homes and other dwellings where urea formaldehyde insulation has been used may approach 1.9 ppm. The current NIOSH standard for formaldehyde in the occupational environment is 1 ppm for any 30-min sampling period (31). Thus, we can see that an individual who breathes contaminated air over many hours each day in enclosed quarters, such as in a mobile home, may be exposed to nearly twice the amount set for safety.

Mechanism of Formaldehyde Toxicity

When formaldehyde is ingested in toxic amounts (60–90 ml is reported to be fatal), it produces a variety of effects. It is highly reactive with most cellular components and quickly suppresses all cellular activity leading to cell death. Tissue destruction is similar to that produced by mineral acids. Formaldehyde is oxidized to formic acid and this accumulates quickly; within minutes following ingestion, the victim may be in metabolic acidosis. All necrotic damage to gastrointestinal cells and other sites is secondary in importance to the acidosis which must be treated immediately.

Clinical Manifestations of Formaldehyde Toxicity

Inhaled formaldehyde induces a direct irritant effect on the eyes and respiratory tract. The patient typically complains of tearing, rhinitis, itchy eyes, coughing, and dyspnea. CNS effects include malaise, headache, insomnia, and anorexia. It has been suggested, but not proven, that inhalation of formaldehyde from urea-formaldehyde foam insulation may be responsible for a significant number of cases of upper respiratory and gastrointestinal tract irritation in Americans.

Ingestion brings on immediate and intense gastrointestinal tract irritation and severe abdominal cramping. This is quickly followed by metabolic acidosis, cardiovascular collapse, unconsciousness (due to CNS depression), and anuria (due to renal failure). Death usually occurs from circulatory collapse.

Treatment of Formaldehyde Toxicity

Treatment is aimed at maintaining the blood pressure and correcting the acid-base imbalance. Pressor amines may be given to achieve the former; sodium bicarbonate for the acidosis.

Dialysis is effective in removing formic acid from the blood, and this removal will significantly aid treatment of acidosis.

ACETALDEHYDE

Acetaldehyde (ethanol, acetic aldehyde) is a colorless liquid or gas with a strongly penetrating fruity odor. Acetaldehyde is used in manufacturing dyes, plastics, flavors and perfumes, vinegar, and numerous other products.

Like formaldehyde, acetaldehyde is a highly reactive chemical. It is extremely irritating to all cells and can quickly depress all cellular activity. Common routes of accidental exposure include inhalation of vapors and ingestion of the solution, although poisoning by the latter is rare. As stated previously, both paraldehyde and metaldehyde undergo .conversion in the body to acetaldehyde.

One other source of acetaldehyde that may produce clinical symptoms is encountered by an individual who is taking disulfiram (Antabuse®) and ingests ethanol. Typically, this person is an alcoholic attempting to reform, and is using disulfiram as a deterrent to drinking. Recall from pharmacology that disulfiram inhibits the enzyme aldehyde dehydrogenase. When ethanol is consumed, its metabolism is slowed at this step, and blood levels of acetaldehyde may increase 10-fold (35). This, then, causes the signs and symptoms that are reported to be "unpleasant" to the individual—those which the person attempts to avoid by not consuming alcohol. Collectively they are termed the "acetaldehyde syndrome" and include a hot and flushed feeling, throbbing pain in the head and neck, nausea and vomiting, dizziness, confusion, and hypotension.

Acetaldehyde intoxication by ingestion produces symptoms of narcosis. These are followed shortly by CNS depression, pulmonary edema, and albuminuria. Inhaled, it causes severe irritation of the eyes and respiratory system.

Treatment is purely symptomatic.

SUMMARY

Numerous products found around the home and workplace contain an alcohol or substance that reacts like an alcohol. Aldehydes and glycols are not as common as causes of poisoning, but this nevertheless does occur. Immediate antidoting with supportive therapy is required for all alcohol/glycol/aldehyde intoxications.

Case Studies

CASE STUDY: ETHANOL INTOXICATION

History

A 23-year-old female, weighing 45.8 kg, was involved in a hit-and-run automobile accident. She was arrested for suspicion of drunken driving. While in jail she became faint and passed out. Following recovery, she gave the following account of her activities.

On an empty stomach, the woman had consumed an entire fifth (26 ounces) of 100-proof bourbon over a 2-hr span. Just a few moments after she left the bar, the accident occurred. She also later admitted that she had a history of alcohol usage since she was 13 years old, and had been discharged from an alcoholic rehabilitation center a week prior to this incident.

On arrival at an emergency facility, the patient was in Stage I coma, responding to deep pain. Laboratory values were normal for pH, electrolytes, and glucose. Her blood alcohol concentration (BAC) was 780 mg%; the toxicological screen did not detect any other drugs. Gastric lavage was performed, followed by administration of activated charcoal. Within 2 hr, her BAC had come down to 730 mg%, and she began to respond to verbal commands. Three hours after admission, her BAC was 420 mg%, and at 11 hr, she was discharged with a BAC of 190 mg%. (See ref. 16.)

Discussion

1. Calculate the maximum BAC this individual should obtain after complete absorption of all she ingested. Does your value correspond to the BAC determined on admission to the ER? If it does not, suggest why the discrepancy exists.

2. How effective is forced diuresis in enhancing the elimination of ethanol?

3. With such high ethanol blood levels, why was the patient not dialyzed? Did there seem to be an apparent need for dialysis?

4. Plot the blood ethanol levels versus time. Comment on the dissipation. Does it follow zero-order kinetics or first-order kinetics? Calculate the theoretical amount that should have dissipated over 11 hr, and relate this to the patient's blood level at 11 hr after admission.

CASE STUDY: METHANOL INTOXICATION

History

A well-nourished, otherwise healthy female pathology resident complained of a "whiteness" to her vision, similar to "stepping out into a snow field." The previous evening she had drunk 2 to 3 ounces of 86-proof vodka, and two glassfuls of wine. There had been nothing unusual about her activities the previous evening. She was admitted to the emergency room with irregular, rapid respiration (30/min), blood pressure 170/105 mm Hg (previous history of labile hypertension), and a pulse rate of 110 beats/min.

Laboratory values were as indicated below:

Na^+	= 135 mEq/L
K^+	= 4.7 mEq/L
Cl^-	= 107 mEq/L
HCO_3^-	= 6 mEq/L
Serum osmolality	= 325 mOsm/kg water
Blood methanol	= 140 mg%
pH	= 7.21
P_{CO_2}	= 11 mm Hg
P_{O_2}	= 123 mm Hg
BUN	= 12 mg/dl
Creatinine	= 1.0 mg/dl

Treatment consisted of ethanol, sodium bicarbonate, and hemodialysis for 6 hr. The patient did not complain of further disturbances during dialysis. Blood methanol levels were negative at the end of the dialysis procedure. Ophthalmologic examination revealed only slight pallor of the optic disc; otherwise, recovery was complete. (See ref. 3.)

Discussion

1. What was the most likely source of methanol exposure?

2. Did the patient present in acidosis with a normal or elevated anion gap?

3. What is the significance in measuring the osmolality of the serum?

4. Why was gastric lavage not performed and activated charcoal not administered to this patient?

5. Give an explanation for the delayed onset of symptoms of methanol intoxication; i.e., visual disturbances.

6. When using a combination of ethanol and hemodialysis to antidote an intoxicated patient, why is it necessary to adjust the ethanol administration periodically?

CASE STUDIES: ETHYLENE GLYCOL POISONING

History: Case 1

A 51-year-old male was admitted to the emergency room 2.5 hr after ingesting 600 ml of an antifreeze solution containing 95% ethylene glycol. He was ataxic, dysarthric, and lethargic. Laboratory values are listed in Table 2.

Treatment. Initial treatment began with gastric lavage and activated charcoal followed by sodium bicarbonate and ethanol i.v. infusion (5% ethanol; 0.98 g/hr). After 2 hr treatment, blood concentration of ethylene glycol decreased to 325 mg%. Hemodialysis

TABLE 2. *Laboratory findings*

Measurement	Case 1	Case 2	Case 3
Quantity of ethylene glycol ingested	600 ml	Unknown	2 L
Arterial pH	7.18	7.03	7.31
P_{CO_2} (mm Hg)	14	13	39
P_{O_2} (mm Hg)	91	92	90
Anion gap (mEq/L)[a]	46	28.7	Normal
Osmolality (mOsm/kg)	422	331	383
Calculated osmolality (mOsm/kg)[b]	312	291	
Serum ethylene glycol (mg%)[c]	650	98	560

[a] Anion gap = $(Na^+ + K^+) - (HCO_3^- + Cl^-)$

[b] $Osm = 2(Na^+) + \dfrac{BUN}{2.8} + \dfrac{Glucose}{18}$

[c] Toxic concentration = 150 mg%

See Appendix I for a table of normal laboratory values.

was performed (Fig. 8) and ethylene glycol levels decreased to 60 mg% after 6 hr of dialysis, and were reduced to an undetectable quantity 80 hr after ingestion. Throughout the dialysis, ethanol levels were maintained between 100 and 140 mg% by hourly nasogastric doses of 20% ethanol. (See ref. 12.)

History: Case 2

This case involved an 18-year-old male who presented to the emergency department with symptoms of hysteria and hyperventilation. The patient gave a history which was essentially uneventful, and there was no indication of drug abuse. Laboratory tests for salicylates, methanol, and ethanol were negative, and urinalysis showed a large number of unidentifiable crystals.

Treatment. Based upon the laboratory findings listed in Table 2, the patient was treated for acidosis. When bicarbonate therapy was unsuccessful, dialysis was initiated. Despite dialysis, the patient died less than 16 hr after he was admitted. (See ref. 33.)

History: Case 3

A 33-year-old female with suicidal tendencies ingested 2 L of ethylene glycol. Upon admittance to the emergency room, she showed signs of mild intoxication. Her laboratory values are presented in Table 2.

Treatment. Gastric lavage recovered approximately 1 L of ethylene glycol. She was then given activated charcoal, castor oil, and was infused with ethanol (absolute) at an initial volume of 60 ml,

followed by 10 ml/hr for 25 hr. Serum ethylene glycol concentration dropped from 560 mg% to less than 100 mg% during the dialysis period. The patient completely recovered. (See ref. 38.)

Discussion

1. Compare Case 3 to Cases 1 and 2; the amount ingested was greater than the other two, but why was there not a significant metabolic acidosis or elevated anion gap?

2. What are some probable reasons why the patient in Case 2 died, even though the blood ethylene glycol levels, when admitted to the emergency room, was less than the other two cases?

3. If Patient 3 actually ingested 2 L of substance as reported, but half was still recovered, give the most probable explanation for why she still did not die.

4. Comment on the effectiveness of hemodialysis in each of the cases presented.

CASE STUDY: FORMALDEHYDE POISONING

History

A 41-year-old female ingested 120 ml of a formaldehyde solution containing 37% (w/v) formaldehyde, and 12.5% (v/v) methanol. No formic acid was present in the solution. On admission to the emergency room one-half hour after ingesting the solution, the patient was cyanotic, apneic, and hypotensive.

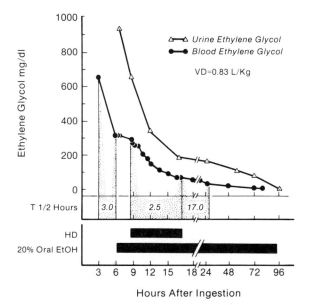

FIG. 8. The effect of hemodialysis and oral ethanol on the rate of elimination of blood ethylene glycol. Note that when hemodialysis is stopped, the half-life of ethylene glycol was prolonged. (From ref. 33.)

Treatment. When the patient was lavaged, there was a noticeable odor of formaldehyde. Fluid replacement included: lactated Ringer's solution and 5% dextrose in water. Control of acidosis was attempted with sodium bicarbonate, 132 mEg/L. Her blood pressure was maintained with dopamine hydrochloride.

Laboratory values are listed below:

Blood:

Formaldehyde	= 0.48 mg/dl
Methanol	= 42.5 mg/dl
Formic acid	= 42 mg/dl
pH	= 6.87
HCO_3^-	= 10 mEq/L
Cl^-	= 60 mEq/L
Na^+	= 92 mEq/L
K^+	= 5.1 mEq/L
Serum creatinine	= 2.9 mg/dl
BUN	= 12.0 mg/dl
Pco_2	= 35 mm Hg
Po_2	= 54 mm Hg

Liver enzymes:

LDH	= 1,830 units/dl
SGOT	= 1,520 units/dl

Despite efforts to maintain her acid-base balance and blood pressure, the patient died 28 hr after admission to the hospital. (See ref. 8.)

Discussion

1. If the patient ingested 120 ml of a formaldehyde solution containing methanol, why is the initial blood level for formaldehyde so low? What was the source of the high formic acid level?

2. Which laboratory values demonstrate that the patient presented with metabolic acidosis? Is the anion gap normal, or elevated?

3. What was the probable cause of death?

4. Would hemodialysis have been of any benefit?

Review Questions

1. Discuss the factors involved in causing eye damage, following a toxic dose of methanol.

2. Cite the reasons why ethanol is an antidote for methanol and ethylene glycol poisoning. What blood level of ethanol is recommended? How is it administered?

3. A significant toxicologic event occurred in 1937 that caused the drug laws to be changed which then reduced the chances for drug toxicity to occur. What was this event?

4. To which of the following is isopropyl alcohol metabolized?
   A. Acetic acid
   B. Formaldehyde
   C. Ethanol
   D. Acetone

5. Describe the toxicologic relevance of ethanol metabolism proceeding by zero-order kinetics.

6. Analeptic therapy is an important component of the antidoting procedures for ethanol intoxication.
   A. True
   B. False

7. A victim of poisoning by Columbian spirits should receive treatment for which of the following substances?
   A. Ethanol
   B. Methanol
   C. Ethylene glycol
   D. Isopropyl alcohol

8. Which of the following symptoms is seen when the blood level of ethanol is 0.05%?
   A. Visual impairment
   B. Altered equilibrium
   C. Stupor
   D. Coma

9. Discuss the relevance of using the anion gap value in assessing the probable cause of poisoning.

10. List, in decreasing order of toxicity, the following glycols: ethylene glycol, diethylene glycol, propylene glycol.

11. The term "glycol" was coined from a Greek word that describes the taste of these substances. What is that taste?

12. In general, increasing the number of carbon atoms for a series of alcohols decreases the toxicity of the substance.
    A. True
    B. False

13. A victim of "snail bait" intoxication has been poisoned by which of the following substances?
    A. Paraldehyde
    B. Formaldehyde
    C. Metaldehyde
    D. Acetaldehyde

14. In recent years urea formaldehyde has been the cause of toxicologic concern. What is this substance, where is it found, and what is the medical problem?

15. Which of the following is the most commonly reported cause of poisoning in a general population?
    A. Ethanol
    B. Methanol
    C. Isopropanol
    D. Butanol

16. Describe how the CNS toxic symptoms of ethanol are presented.

17. The rate of absorption of alcoholic beverages can be an important factor in determining the overall toxic profile. List, in decreasing order of rate of absorption, the following beverages: wine, distilled spirits, beer.

18. Discuss what information the Widmark equation provides. Why is the formula different for men and women?

19. Ethanol and methanol are metabolized by oxidative enzymes to less toxic substances.
    A. True
    B. False

20. Pure "moonshine" liquor is a rich source of methanol.
    A. True
    B. False

21. Methanol is metabolized by the same enzymes that metabolize ethanol.
    A. True
    B. False

22. Describe the treatment protocol for methanol intoxication. What is the significance of keeping a methanol-poisoned patient in a darkened room?

23. The most potentially dangerous symptom of methanol intoxication is not the CNS sedation. What is it, and how is it specifically treated?

24. Oxalic acid is a toxic substance produced when which of the following poisons is metabolized?
    A. Methanol
    B. Ethylene glycol
    C. Acetaldehyde
    D. Isopropyl alcohol

References

1. Arulamantham, K. (1978): Central nervous system toxicity associated with ingestion of propylene glycol. *J. Pediatr.*, 93:515–516.
2. Anderson, R. C., Stock, M. F., and Sawin, R. (1979): Toxicity of thermal decomposition products of urea formaldehyde and phenol formaldehyde foams. *Toxicol. Appl. Pharmacol.*, 51:9–17.
3. Becker, C. E. (1981): Acute methanol poisoning— The blind drunk. *West. J. Med.*, 135:122–128.
4. Chow, J. Y., and Richardson, K. E. (1978): The effect of pyrazole in ethylene glycol toxicity and metabolism in the rat. *Toxicol. Appl. Pharmacol.*, 43:33–44.
5. Clay, K. L., Murphy, R. C., and Watkins, W. D. (1975): Experimental methanol toxicity in the primate: Analysis of metabolic acidosis. *Toxicol. Appl. Pharmacol.*, 34:49–61.
6. Cooper, M. N., Mitchell, G. W., Bennett, I. L., and Cary, F. N. (1952): Methyl alcohol poisoning: An account of the 1951 Atlanta epidemic. *JAMA*, 141:48–51.
7. Cooper, J. R., and Kini, M. M. (1962): Biochemical aspects of methanol poisoning. *Biochem. Pharmacol.*, 11:405–406.
8. Eells, J. T., McMartin, K. E., Black, K., Virayotha, V., Tisdell, R. H., and Tephley, T. R. (1981): Formaldehyde poisoning—Rapid metabolism to formic acid. *JAMA*, 246:1237–1238.
9. Forney, R. B., and Harger, R. N. (1971): The alcohols. In: *Pharmacology in Medicine*, 4th ed., edited by J. R. DiPalma, p. 275. McGraw-Hill, New York.
10. Freireich, A. W., Cinque, T. J., Xanthary, G., and Landaw, D. (1967): Hemodialysis for isoproterenol poisoning. *N. Engl. J. Med.*, 277:699.
11. Geiling, E. M. K., and Cannon, P. R. (1938): Pathologic effects of elixir of sulfanilamide (diethylene glycol) poisoning. *JAMA*, 111:919–926.
12. Godolphin, W., Meagher, E. P., Sanders, H. D., and Frohlich, J. (1980): Unusual calcium oxalate crystals in ethylene glycol poisoning. *Clin. Toxicol.*, 16:479–486.
13. Goldsher, M., and Better, O. S. (1979): Antifreeze poisoning during the October 1973 war in the middleeast. *Military Medicine*, May.
14. Gosselin, R. E., Hodge, H. C., Smith, R. P., and Gleason, M. N. (1976): *Clinical Toxicology of Commercial Products*, 4th ed. Williams & Wilkins, Baltimore.
15. Greear, J. N. (1950): The causes of blindness. In: *Blindness: Modern Approaches to the Unseen Environment*, edited by P. A. Zahl, p. 130. Princeton University Press, Princeton, NJ.
16. Hammond, K. B., Rumack, B. H., and Rodgerson, D. O. (1973): Blood ethanol—A report of unusually high levels in a living patient. *JAMA*, 226:63–64.
17. Harris, J. C., Rumack, B. H., and Aldrich, F. D. (1981): Toxicology of urea formaldehyde and polyurethane foam insulation. *JAMA*, 245:243–246.
18. Holck, H. G. O. (1937): Glycerin, ethylene glycol, propylene glycol and diethylene glycol. *JAMA*, 109:19.
19. Kenny, A. H., and Mellinkoff, S. M. (1958): Methyl alcohol poisoning. *Ann. Intern. Med.*, 34:331–338.

20. Kini, M. M., and Cooper, J. R. (1962): Biochemistry of methanol poisoning. 4. The effect of methanol and its metabolites on retinal metabolism. *Biochem. J.*, 82:164–172.

21. Kini, M. M., King, D. W., and Cooper, J. R. (1962): Biochemistry of methanol poisoning. 5. Histological and biochemical correlates of effects of methanol and its metabolites on the rabbit retina. *J. Neurochem.*, 9:119–124.

22. Koivusalo, M. (1970): Methanol. In: *Alcohols and Derivatives*, Vol. 2, edited by J. Tremolieres, pp. 465–505. Pergamon Press, London.

23. Lewis, B. B., and Chestner, S.B. (1981): Formaldehyde in dentistry: A review of mutagenic and carcinogenic potential. *J. Am. Dent. Assoc.*, 103:429–434.

24. Mardones, J. (1963): The alcohols. In: *Physiological Pharmacology*, Vol. 1, edited by W. S. Root and F. G. Hofmann, pp. 105–107. Academic Press, New York.

25. Martin, G., and Finberg, L. (1970): Propylene glycol: A potentially toxic vehicle in liquid dosage forms. *J. Pediatr.*, 77:877.

26. McMartin, K. E., Ambre, J. J., and Tephley, T. R. (1980): Methanol poisoning in human subjects. *Am. J. Med.*, 68:414.

27. McMartin, K. E., Hedstrom, K. G., Tolf, B. R., Ostling-Wintzel, H., and Blomstrand, R. (1980): Studies on the metabolic interactions between 4-methyl-pyrazole and methanol using the monkey as an animal model. *Arch. Biochem. Biophys.*, 199:606–614.

28. Milles, G. (1946): Ethylene glycol poisoning with suggestions for its treatment as oxalate poisoning. *Arch. Pathol.*, 41:631–632.

29. Naragi, S., Dethlefs, R. F., and Slobodniuk, R. A. (1979): An outbreak of acute methyl alcohol intoxication in New Guinea. *Aust. NZ J. Med.*, 9:65–68.

30. NIH Report (1979): Use of folate analogue in treatment of methyl alcohol toxic reactions is studied. *JAMA*, 242:1961.

31. NIOSH Report (1976): Criteria for a recommended standard . . . Occupational exposure to formaldehyde. *DHEW Publication* No. 77–126.

32. NIOSH Report (1981): Formaldehyde: Evidence of carcinogenicity. *Curr. Intell. Bull.*, 34.

33. Peterson, C. D., Collins, A. J., Himes, J. M., Bullock, M. L., and Keane, W. F. (1981): Ethylene glycol poisoning. *N. Engl. J. Med.*, 304:21–23.

34. Peterson, D. I., Peterson, J. E., Hardinge, M. D., and Wacker, E. C. (1963): Experimental treatment of ethylene glycol poisoning. *JAMA*, 186:955–957.

35. Ritchie, J. M. (1980): The aliphatic alcohols. In: *The Pharmacological Basis of Therapeutics*, 6th ed., edited by A. G. Gilman, L. S. Goodman, and A. Gilman, pp. 376–390. Macmillan, New York.

36. Ruprecht, H. A., and Nelson, I. A. (1937): Preliminary toxicity reports on diethylene glycol and sulfanilamide. 5. Clinical and pathologic observations. *JAMA*, 109:1537–1540.

37. Scrimgeour, E. M. (1980): Outbreak of methanol and isopropanol poisoning in New Britain, Papua New Guinea. *Med. J. Aust.*, 2:36–38.

38. Stokes, J. B., and Aueron, F. (1980): Prevention of organ damage in massive ethylene glycol ingestion. *JAMA*, 243:2065–2066.

39. Wagner, J. G., Wilkinson, P. K., and Sedman, A. J. (1976): Elimination of alcohol from human blood. *J. Pharm. Sci.*, 60:152–154.

40. Wacker, W. E. C., Haynes, H., Druyan, R., Fisher, W., and Coleman, J. E. (1965): Treatment of ethylene glycol poisoning with ethyl alcohol. *JAMA*, 194:1231.

41. Walgreen, H. (1970): Absorption, diffusion, distribution, and elimination of ethanol. Effect on biological membranes. In: *Alcohols and Derivatives*, Vol. 1, edited by J. Tremolieres, pp. 161–188. Pergamon Press, Oxford.

42. Wilkinson, P. K., Sedman, A. J., and Sakmar, E. (1977): Pharmacokinetics of ethanol after oral administration in the fasting state. *J. Pharmacokinetics Biopharm.*, 5:207–224.

Nitrates and Nitrites

5

Nitrates represent one of the inorganic ions that have caused considerable recent concern among environmentalists and toxicologists (13,17,18). Nitrates, along with phosphates and several other ions, can persist in the environment for long periods. Nitrates are being used with increasing frequency, as synthetic nitrogen-gased fertilizers are becoming more popular. Nitrates are used in food production and processing to prevent botulism, and are essential starting products, components, or intermediates produced in formation of thousands of different chemicals and drugs. Animal waste products are also rich in nitrates.

The result is that high levels of nitrates have now contaminated the soil and water supplies of many regions, especially in rural areas. Because of their high water solubility, they eventually leach into the soil and water supplies of adjacent areas. The day may be near when nitrate poisoning from drinking water will be a normally encountered occurrence, rather than an unusual one. In a sampling of the nation's water supplies in 1977, water from about 3% of the country contained concentrations of nitrate that exceeded the level generally accepted as safe (14).

The use of amyl, butyl, and isobutyl nitrite as recreational drugs has also become a major problem. Each year a reported 250,000,000 doses of these nitrites are sold in the United States (11). These volatile nitrites are inhaled directly from their containers, or are first allowed to volatilize in an enclosed area from which they are then inhaled, to enhance the perception of certain social activities. While no fatalities have been reported to date, we can consider the illicit use of these drug items to be potentially dangerous and should be curtailed (8).

A special concern involves possible nitrosation of nitrites with amines (3). The resulting nitrosamines constitute one of the most potent classes of carcinogenic chemicals known to mankind. They cause tumor growth in most animal models studied so far, including humans (20). The special problem is that nitrates readily undergo biologic conversion to nitrites, and nitrites may be subjected to nitrosamine formation *in vivo*. This has been demonstrated to occur in animals. At this point, whether such a reaction actually occurs *in vivo* in humans has not been definitely proven (5). The possibility that it does certainly must be taken seriously and cannot be brushed aside. So the concern is real. This is why vitamin C, vitamin E, sulfamate, and antioxidants such as butylated hydroxytoluene (BHT) and butylated hydroxyanisole (BHA) are frequently added to nitrite-treated foods and to some drug products that have the potential for nitrosamine formation. These substances reduce the nitrosation process.

In the meantime, our consideration of nitrate/nitrite poisoning will not focus on suspected carcinogen formation. Rather, we will concentrate on acute poisoning from the nitrogenous substances that may be found around the home or work place. We will also consider, in infants, nitrate poisoning from drinking contaminated water or ingesting foods that are rich in nitrate.

MECHANISMS OF NITRATE TOXICITY AND CLINICAL MANIFESTATIONS

The major toxic effects of nitrate poisoning are cardiovascular collapse and methemoglobinemia. Either can be fatal. Their mechanisms and clinical manifestations are described below.

When we consider the cardiovascular effects of nitrate toxicity, recall that nitrates produce nonspecific relaxation of all smooth muscle,

including that which comprises the vasculature. Although this action is generalized throughout the body, the effect on postcapillary vessels is somewhat more prominent and results in venous pooling. At therapeutic doses of nitrates, neither inotropy nor chronotropy is affected to any significant degree, but at high doses the heart is depressed.

As opposed to the therapeutic actions of nitrates, when they are used in toxic quantities they produce intense vasodilation. This then can precipitate several effects ranging from a throbbing headache and flushed face to a rapid fall in blood pressure and cardiogenic shock. Normally, the heart would compensate for the venous pooling and decreased blood pressure as a result of reflex sympathetic stimulation which stimulates it. But when toxic levels of nitrates are present, the myocardium is unable to respond. The appropriate cardiac-related signs and symptoms of nitrate poisoning are listed in Table 1.

In addition to cardiovascular collapse, the other major toxic action of nitrate toxicity is the formation of methemoglobinemia. Methemoglobinemia is a condition characterized by oxidation of ferrous (Fe^{2+}) iron in hemoglobin to the ferric (Fe^{3+}) state. This form of hemoglobin is no longer able to bind oxygen and, consequently, oxygen transport is interrupted resulting in cyanosis which is unresponsive to oxygen therapy. As a result of this oxidation reaction, arterial blood will have a "chocolate-brown" appearance which is pathognomonic (distinctively characteristic) for methemoglobinemia. The formation of methemoglobin also causes the ox-

TABLE 1. *Signs and symptoms of nitrate poisoning*

Headache, pulsation feeling in head
Palpitations
Tachycardia
Hypotension, shock
Cardiovascular collapse
Dizziness, fainting
Weakness
Cyanosis
Shallow respirations
Methemoglobinemia

ygen dissociation curve to shift to the left, as will be discussed with cyanide and carbon monoxide in Chapter 6. While the mechanisms are different, the end result, anoxia, is the same. The clinical characteristics of methemoglobinemia are listed in Table 2 and all can be related to the inability of oxygen to bind to hemoglobin.

Any chemical that oxidizes ferrous iron to its ferric state can cause methemoglobinemia. This includes nitrates and nitrites, as well as the substances listed in Table 3. Heme group oxidation also occurs spontaneously, probably due to environmental influences or from certain foods. At any time, approximately 1 to 2% of total hemoglobin exists in the oxidized methemoglobin form.

Erythrocytes contain several enzymes that are responsible for reduction of methemoglobin (Fig. 1) (9,12). The most important of these is methemoglobin reductase (diaphorase I). A second methemoglobin reductase enzyme (diaphorase II) is dependent on levels of nicotinamide adenine dinucleotide phosphate (NADP, NADPH) for its action (2). This second system is ordinarily of little importance, since the former nor-

mally maintains levels below 1 to 2%, and when methemoglobin concentration increases, diaphorase II can increase in activity by 60-fold (2). Normal erythrocytic methemoglobin reductase is capable of reducing methemoglobin to hemoglobin at a rate 250 times its rate of formation (16). As long as an individual can maintain an adequate level of these enzymes, or does not ingest large quantities of oxidizing chemicals, blood levels of methemoglobin remain around 1 to 2%. It is only when the enzyme becomes saturated, as occurs when large amounts of oxidizing substances are ingested, that methemoglobin accumulates in sufficient quantities to induce clinical symptoms.

There are several other ways in which the concentration of methemoglobin can be raised above the normal, in addition to the oxidizing agents mentioned. For example, toxic methemoglobin levels can result from a congenital disorder, hereditary methemoglobinemia. This condition is characterized by an absence of NADH-dependent methemoglobin reductase (15). The disorder is usually detected by the presence of cyanosis at birth.

The results of a study which was designed to illustrate the effects of a challenge dose of sodium nitrite in an individual with hereditary methemoglobinemia versus a normal person is depicted in Fig.. 2. Both individuals were given a single 500-mg intravenous dose of sodium nitrite. From the figure, we see that 6 hr after injection the methemoglobin level had returned to near the base line in the normal person, but it still remained abnormally elevated in the individual who lacked the enzyme. The total amount of methemoglobin formed in both subjects was essentially the same.

Nitrate-induced methemoglobinemia is of special concern in infants less than 6 months of age for several reasons. First, the gastric pH of young children is characteristically less acidic than it is in older children and adults. Normally, when the pH is low, this helps retard the growth of certain microorganisms (e.g., *Escherichia coli*) which convert nitrate to its more toxic form, nitrite. However, when there is less acid, this permits these bacteria to proliferate (1,7).

TABLE 2. *Characteristics of methemoglobinemia*

Gray cyanosis, persistent even with oxygen therapy
Easy fatigability
Dyspnea; respiratory distress
Tachycardia
Dizziness with exertion
Venous blood is chocolate-brown in color
Oxygen-carrying capacity of arterial blood is decreased. Shift to the left of oxygen and dissociation curve

TABLE 3. *Drugs reported to cause methemoglobinemia*

Acetanilid
Acetophenetidin
Aniline
Arylamino and arylnitro compounds
Chlorates
Methylene blue (high doses)
Nitrites and nitrates
Nitrobenzenes
Nitrotoluenes
Quinones
Sulfonamides

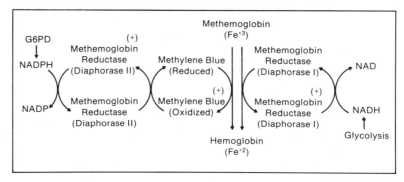

FIG. 1. Mechanisms of methemoglobin reduction.

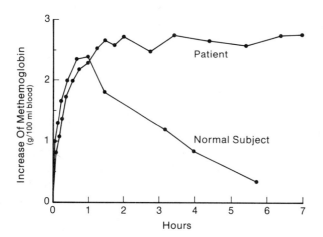

FIG. 2. The response of a patient with hereditary methemoglobinemia compared to the response by a normal person. (From ref. 6.)

Therefore, when foods rich in nitrate (e.g., spinach or carrots) are given to these infants in excess, or when baby formula is prepared from water containing high levels of nitrates, there is a possibility of nitrate poisoning occurring, resulting in methemoglobinemia (7,19). To illustrate the extent of the problem from these infants, it has been reported that water concentrations of 10 ppm are considered unsafe for infants. The same concentration typically causes no problems in older children or adults (2,17).

Second, fetal hemoglobin is more susceptible to oxidation to methemoglobin than adult hemoglobin. This is because methemoglobin reductase is less active in infants less than 3 months old (17). Therefore, any excessive amount of nitrates will cause methemoglobinemia.

The third reason infants are more prone to methemoglobinemia is because they have an incompletely developed hepatic microsomal en-

zyme system. Therefore, when the ingested nitrates are converted to nitrites by the intestinal bacteria, the absorbed nitrite is not metabolized by the liver to its inactive form as rapidly as it is in older children and adults. Consequently, nitrite blood levels are elevated and the chance of oxidizing hemoglobin to methemoglobin is enhanced.

TREATMENT OF METHEMOGLOBINEMIA

Whenever cyanosis is present and unresponsive to treatment with oxygen, methemoglobinemia should be suspected. Diagnosis is strengthened when arterial blood appears chocolate-brown. This color is present when methemoglobin levels are greater than 15%. Definite confirmation can then be made by analyzing the blood for methemoglobin.

Cyanosis may be noticed at a methemoglobin concentration of 10%, although levels less than 20 to 30% are usually asymptomatic and do not require immediate treatment (9). Levels as high as 55% may be manifested by little more than shortness of breath in certain individuals (19). The offending agent should be identified and removed, of course, if possible.

Blood levels of 30% or more usually dictate that specific treatment should be initiated. A 60 to 70% blood concentration is considered to be lethal. Oxygen, alone or with methylene blue, is the treatment of choice.

Methylene blue is a dye that serves as an intermediate in electron transfer between methemoglobin reductase (diaphorase II) and methemoglobin. The mechanism of action is outlined in Fig. 1 (9). A reversal of the toxic effects of methemoglobinemia should then be noted within an hour of initiation of methylene blue therapy. Special care is needed when using methylene blue, since large doses may actually produce methemoglobinemia by a reverse action. That is, large doses oxidize ferrous ion to the ferric form (10).

The suggestion is sometimes made that another reducing agent, ascorbic acid, will substitute for methylene blue in treatment of methemoglobinemia. Whereas this substance is occasionally used with some success, it normally is not suitable for serious cases since it does not reduce methemoglobin to hemoglobin quickly enough (9).

SUMMARY

Symptoms of nitrate/nitrite poisoning are, for the most part, similar, regardless of the nature of the poison. Likewise, these poisons are antidoted in the same manner. It is important to understand what these symptoms are and how they are treated.

Case Studies

CASE STUDIES: NITRITES AND METHEMOGLOBINEMIA

History: Case 1

Following a suggestion from a relative, a parent of twin boys, 4 months of age, administered "sweet spirits of nitre" (4% ethyl nitrite in ethanol) to the boys because they had an upper respiratory infection, and the spirits of nitre would supposedly control their fussiness. A "small amount" was added to each of the children's milk bottles.

After ingesting the entire contents of the bottle, one of the twins developed signs of severe respiratory distress. He was cyanotic and unresponsive. On admission to an emergency facility, the baby was resuscitated. Arterial blood was a chocolate-brown color when dried. Blood gases were: P_{O_2} 280 mm Hg, P_{CO_2} 176 mm Hg, and the blood pH was 6.71. Methemoglobin level was 80%.

Ten milligrams of methylene blue were administered; however, the baby died 12 hr later.

The other baby, who did not finish his bottle, had a methemoglobin level of 38%. He was also given 10 mg of methylene blue i.v., and he completely recovered. (See ref. 4.)

History: Cases 2 and 3

Two men were showered with molten chemicals in an industrial accident when a chamber, containing 50% sodium nitrate and 50% potassium nitrate heated to 246°C, exploded. Their clothing was immediately removed at the site and they were rushed to the hospital.

On admission, Patient 1, aged 23 years, had third degree burns over 70% of his body. These areas were coated with a white, salt-like crust. The patient was alert and able to speak coherently. His vital signs included: blood pressure 90/60 mm Hg, and pulse rate 110 beats/min. His respiration was normal, although he admitted some subjective breathing difficulty. The patient complained of pain, but no narcotics were given because of his hypotension. The crust was washed away, but the damaged tissue was not debrided.

Within 10 to 15 min of arrival, the patient suddenly became cyanotic. He lapsed into unconsciousness and experienced a grand mal seizure. He was given 100% oxygen, but suffered a cardiac arrest several minutes later and died. A postmortem blood sample showed a methemoglobin level of 65%.

The second patient, aged 49 years, was also alert and oriented when admitted. His burns were determined to be first and second degree, with 40% of his body affected. Burned areas were also coated with a white crust. His vital signs were all within normal limits except for a pulse rate of 100 beats/min.

Attendants began to wash the white crust away, but approximately 20 min after arrival the patient experienced a generalized seizure. He then became intensely cyanotic.

Oxygen was administered, but the cyanosis did not respond. A blood sample appeared chocolate-brown in color, so methylene blue was administered, intravenously. Despite this treatment, his cyanosis continued.

Therefore, the patient was transferred to an intensive care unit where he received an exchange transfusion with 30 units of whole blood. Prior to exchange, his methemoglobin level was measured at 56%.

The patient tolerated the procedure well and by 16 hr post-admission, he was awake, alert, and oriented. He received further treatment for his thermal burns and was eventually released without further complications.

Both of these victims illustrate that severe poisoning can occur by absorbing a toxic agent(s) through the skin. Absorption in these victims was no doubt enhanced by the hot temperature of the chemicals. (See ref. 9.)

Discussion

1. What is the mechanism for inducing methemoglobinemia by "spirits of nitre" and sodium or potassium nitrate?

2. What is considered to be a toxic concentration of methemoglobin?

3. Why was the arterial blood of these patients chocolate-brown?

4. Is it likely that the 10-mg dose of methylene blue given in Case 1 was too high, and actually caused the infant's death? Why or why not was it to blame?

5. The first victim in Cases 2 and 3 most likely died before the attending physicians realized what was needed to be done to save his life. Since his blood methemoglobin level was approximately equal to the level of the other victim, do you suppose the first patient would have survived his ordeal had he received methylene blue? Why or why not?

Review Questions

1. Cite the most probable cause of death in an individual poisoned with a massive overdose of a nitrate.

2. What is the toxicologic concern of nitrosamines and how are they formed?

3. Which of the following is a true statement?
   A. Methemoglobinemia exists when heme containing iron is in its oxidized state.
   B. Methemoglobinemia is best antidoted with ascorbic acid.
   C. The enzyme diaphorase I converts hemoglobin to methemoglobin.
   D. A methemoglobin blood level of 30% is usually fatal.

4. Infants have been reported to be more seriously affected by excessive nitrate ingestion than adults. Discuss the factors that promote this action.

5. Discuss the consequences of administering nitrites to an individual with hereditary methemoglobinemia.

6. The dosage of methylene blue must be closely regulated for what reason?

7. Most people have a normal blood methemoglobin level of 1 to 2%.
   A. True
   B. False

8. Dried methemoglobin appears green in color.
   A. True
   B. False

9. At what blood level of methemoglobin should treatment be initiated?

10. What is "sweet spirits of nitre," and what is the special toxic problem it causes?

References

1. Abramowicz, M. (1974): Nitrates and nitrites in food. *Med. Lett. Drugs Ther.*, 16:75–76.
2. Angelakos, E. T. (1975): Coronary vasodilators. In: *Drill's Pharmacology in Medicine*, 4th ed., edited by J. R. DiPalma, pp. 809–823. McGraw-Hill, New York.
3. Brunnemann, K. D., Hecht, S. S., and Hoffman, D. (1982–83): *N*-Nitrosamines: Environmental occurrence, *in vivo* formation and metabolism. *J. Toxicol.-Clin. Toxicol.*, 19:661–688.
4. Chilcote, R. C., Williams, B., Wolff, L. J., and Baehner, R. R. (1977): Sudden death in an infant from methemoglobinemia after administration of "sweet spirits of nitre." *Pediatrics*, 59:280–282.

5. Doll, R., and Peto, R. (1981): Avoidable risks of cancer in the U.S. *J. Natl. Cancer Inst.*, 66:1196.

6. Eder, H. A., Finch, C., and McKee, R. W. (1949): Congenital methemoglobinemia. A clinical and biochemical study of a case. *J. Clin. Invest.*, 28:265.

7. Geffner, M. E., Powars, D. R., and Choctaw, W. T. (1981): Acquired methemoglobinemia. *West. J. Med.*, 134:7–10.

8. Haley, T. J. (1980): Review of the physiological effects of amyl, butyl, and isobutyl nitrites. *Clin. Toxicol.*, 16:317–329.

9. Harris, J. C., Rumack, B. H., Peterson, R. G., and McGuire, B. M. (1979): Methemoglobinemia resulting from absorption of nitrates. *JAMA*, 242:2869–2871.

10. Harvey, S. C. (1980): Antiseptics and disinfectants; fungicides; ectoparasiticides. In: *The Pharmacological Basis of Therapeutics*, 6th ed., edited by A. G. Gilman, L. S. Goodman, and A. Gilman, pp. 964–987. Macmillan, New York.

11. Lowry, T. P. (1979): Amylnitrite: an old high comes back to visit. *Behavioral Med.*, 6:19–21.

12. McGilvery, R. W., and Goldstein, G. W. (1983): *Biochemistry—A Functional Approach*, 3rd ed. Saunders, Philadelphia.

13. Menzer, R. E., and Nelson, J. D. (1980): Water and soil pollutants. In: *Toxicology—The Basic Science of Poisons*, 2nd ed., edited by J. Doull, C. D. Klaassen, and M. O. Amdur, pp. 632–658. Macmillan, New York.

14. National Research Council (1977): *Drinking Water and Health*. National Academy of Sciences, Washington, D.C.

15. Scott, E. M. (1960): The relation of diaphorase on human erythrocytes to inheritance of methemoglobinemia. *J. Clin. Invest.*, 39:1176–1186.

16. Scott, E. M. (1968): Congenital methemoglobinemia due to DPNH diaphorase deficiency. In: *Hereditary Disorders to Erythrocyte Metabolism*, edited by E. Bentler, pp. 102–113. Grune & Stratton, New York.

17. Shearer, L. A., Goldsmith, J. R., Young, C., Kearns, O. A., and Tamplin, B. R. (1972): Methemoglobin levels in infants in an area with high nitrate water supply. *Am. J. Public Health*, 9:1174–1180.

18. Smith, R. J. (1980): Nitrites: FDA beats a surprising retreat. *Science*, 209:1100–1101.

19. Ten Brink, W. A. G., Luijpen, A. F. M. G., Van Heijst, A. N. P., Pikaar, S. A., and Seldenrijk, R. (1982): Nitrate poisoning caused by food contaminated with cooling fluid. *J. Toxicol. Clin. Toxicol*, 19:139–147.

20. Weisburger, J. H., and Williams, G. M. (1980): Chemical carcinogens. In: *Toxicology—The Basic Science of Poisons*, 2nd ed., edited by J. Doull, C. D. Klaassen, and M. O. Amdur, pp. 84–138. Macmillan, New York.

Carbon Monoxide, Cyanides, and Sulfides

6

Air may contain a variety of substances which, if inhaled, can cause symptoms of toxicity to the lungs and respiratory passages, as well as systemic effects and certainly death. These substances include particulate matter such as dusts, fumes, and smokes; and gaseous products including carbon monoxide, cyanide, sulfides, and other vapors and solvents.

Many environments are such that we continually breathe low levels of numerous solid and gaseous poisons without experiencing clinically discernible symptoms. Most airborne particles are either trapped by nasal hair or are deposited on the moist walls of respiratory structures, to be removed by coughing and sneezing, and by the action of respiratory secretions aided by ciliary movement.

Even many of the gases that are inhaled are expired with the next breath. If absorbed into the blood, their concentraton there must approach a critical level before symptoms of poisoning are seen. In fact, most Americans probably have detectable levels of potentially toxic gases in their blood that, at these low levels, have not yet been proven to pose a serious health hazard. This may change someday as we learn more about potential toxicity from chronic exposure.

This chapter concentrates on three gases that exhibit special toxicity problems. In each illustration, you, as a health professional, may be called on to assist in antidoting them. These poisons include carbon monoxide, cyanide, and sulfides. Other gaseous or volatile substances that are associated with toxicity by inhalation will be discussed in subsequent chapters (e.g., formaldehyde, gasoline, etc.).

CARBON MONOXIDE

Acute carbon monoxide (CO) poisoning is reported to account for over 3,500 accidental or intentional deaths each year in the United States (58). Chronic exposure is also reported to be the cause of a wide variety of common complaints of many Americans, including tiredness and lethargy, shortness of breath, irritability, and vision impairment. Chronic CO exposure has been suggested as a cause of heart disease and atherosclerosis, as well as numerous other pathological events (2). It should be pointed out, however, that most of these suggestions are based on animal studies or inferential data and have not yet been proven in humans.

Toxic effects of CO are primarily due to its preferential affinity (compared to oxygen) for hemoglobin and subsequent interference with the oxygen-carrying capacity of hemoglobin (27). In order to appreciate the significance of this "silent killer," it is necessary to recall that a constant oxygen supply is essential for all basic body functions. Some tissues have a greater oxygen requirement than others. For example, the cells of the CNS and myocardium become significantly impaired when their oxygen requirement is compromised, even for short periods of time.

Atmospheric air contains approximately 21% oxygen. Oxygen is made accessible to body tissues by respiration. As oxygen diffuses across the alveolar membranes, it combines with hemoglobin and then is transported to the various tissues.

CO is a ubiquitous product of incomplete combustion. Since the gas is odorless, colorless, tasteless, nonirritating, and readily mixes with air in all proportions, it is referred to as the "silent killer." These features often prevent the victim from recognizing its potential danger. A very dangerous misconception occurs when a person believes that "as long as you can't smell smoke, there is no carbon monoxide."

Worldwide CO production is estimated to be in excess of 250 million tons a year (3). CO is normally present in the atmosphere at less than 0.001% because most CO formed by incomplete combustion rises high into the atmosphere where it is quickly oxidized to carbon dioxide. However, it is still the most abundant pollutant found in the air we breathe. Natural gas (methane) does not contain CO, but its incomplete combustion, of course, will produce it. It should be pointed out that natural gas is not the same as CO. Whereas CO produces its toxic effects by combining with hemoglobin, as will be described shortly, methane causes asphyxiation by simple competition with oxygen for alveolar spaces. Charcoal fires also produce CO, and this creates a potential hazard when hibachis and other forms of charcoal grills are used in closed, poorly ventilated areas such as camping trailers or apartments. It is generally agreed that more people die in fire-related accidents from CO poisoning than by heat or burns. Internal combustion automobile engine exhaust is the major source of CO (2).

Another source of CO is methylene chloride (CH_2Cl_2, dichloromethane). This is a common industrial solvent and is the major component of many paint thinners and paint removers (44,45). Additionally, its use is increasing as a solvent in personal-care aerosol products. Unfortunately, methylene chloride is readily absorbed and promotes formation of carboxyhemoglobin.

A frequent source of inhaled CO is tobacco smoke. Cigarette smoke contains 3 to 6% CO, producing air concentrations that are up to eight times the level allowable by industry, while smoking from pipes and cigars, which normally burn at lower temperatures, may contain up to 15%. Smoking one or two packs of cigarettes per day produces CO blood concentrations of 1.9% and 3%, respectively (4). Also, individuals of certain occupations (e.g., firemen and tunnel workers) who do not smoke have blood levels in excess of the mean of other persons residing in the same area (8,38).

The blood normally contains low levels of CO that are less than 1%. This is believed to occur through endogenous CO formation from metabolism of hemoglobin and other tetrapyrroles (15,20,39). These low levels are probably insignificant to an otherwise normal, healthy individual.

Mechanism of Carbon Monoxide Toxicity

The toxic effects of CO have been known for thousands of years. Indeed, important political prisoners of Hippocrates' time were put to death with CO. However, it has only been since the last decade of the 19th century that its physiological and biochemical effects have been systematically studied.

The mechanism by which CO causes its toxic effect is by producing tissue hypoxia. This is achieved by two means: (a) by decreasing the amount of oxygen bound to erythrocytes, thus causing a reduction in tissue oxygenation, and (b) by shifting the oxyhemoglobin dissociation curve to the left, thus lowering the partial pressure at which oxygen is available to tissues.

CO reversibly combines with hemoglobin to produce carboxyhemoglobin (COHb) (27). This binding is approximately 240 times greater than that of oxygen. Consequently, inhalation of relatively low concentrations of this gas can produce a clinically significant decrease in the oxygen-carrying capacity of red blood cells. In other words, this means that a 50% COHb concentration will be achieved when the concentration of CO in ambient air is only 1/240 that of oxygen, or about 0.08% (800 ppm).[1]

The binding of oxygen to hemoglobin displays a sigmoidal relationship with oxygen partial pressure. That is, the binding of one oxygen molecule produces an allosteric modification of the heme protein to enhance binding of the succeeding three oxygen molecules.

CO not only interferes with this association, or binding of oxygen to hemoglobin, but it also interferes with the dissociation, or release of oxygen from hemoglobin. As stated above, CO shifts the oxyhemoglobin dissociation curve to the left. Graphically this means that the normal oxygen association-dissociation curve now changes from a sigmoidal to a hyperbolic relationship. The sigmoidal curve shows that oxygen can be readily released from hemoglobin when it is needed by the tissue. Figure 1 shows that the slope of the S-curve is steep when the P_{O_2} is low, and levels off when the P_{O_2} is high. When CO binds to the hemoglobin molecule, shifting the dissociation curve to the left producing a hyperbolic curve, less oxygen is available to the tissues or is only available at a low P_{O_2}. Thus, it produces a hypoxic state.

It should also be pointed out that, to a lesser degree, CO also binds to muscle myoglobin (a

---

[1]ppm = Parts per million: 1 ppm = 1×10^{-4} = 0.001% = 1.29 mg/m^3.

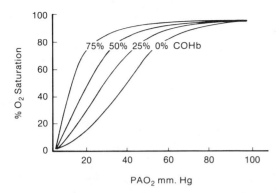

FIG. 1. Oxyhemoglobin dissociation curve in the presence of CO.

TABLE 1. *Carboxyhemoglobin equilibrium at one atmosphere*

CO inhaled (ppm)	COHb (% saturation)
1	0.49
10	1.94
100	14.45
1,000	62.41
10,000	94.31
100,000	99.40
900,000	99.93

heme-containing protein that transports oxygen in skeletal and cardiac muscle) and to intracellular cytochrome oxidases (intracellular enzymes for respiration) which can contribute to tissue and cellular hypoxia (49).

Absorption, Metabolism, and Excretion of Carbon Monoxide

The concentration of COHb in the blood is a function of CO concentration of the inspired air, the duration of exposure, and the volume of pulmonary ventilation (tidal volume). Aqueous solubility of CO is low, but is significantly high in the blood because of its binding affinity to hemoglobin. Table 1 correlates concentrations of CO in inspired air with the corresponding percent COHb saturation reached at equilibrium. From this table we can estimate the COHb concentration after a known amount of CO has been inhaled for a given time period and respiratory activity by the following equation:

$$\text{Resting state: } \%\text{COHb} = 6 \text{ L/min} \times \%\text{CO} \times \text{min exposure}$$

Of course, this relationship applies to an otherwise healthy individual, and there are several factors which can influence the percent COHb saturation and, thus, the degree of tissue hypoxia. For example, infants and other persons with increased metabolic rates, patients with anemia (lower oxygen reserve), chronic obstructive pulmonary disease (COPD), and those with arteriosclerotic cardiovascular heart disease will be much more susceptible to the toxic effects of CO. The increased metabolic rates make for a greater chance of toxicity. This is the reason for placing canaries in mines: They are much more susceptible to reduced oxygen concentrations. If the birds die, oxygen concentration is too low to sustain human life, or perhaps a toxic gas (i.e., methane) is present and the miners must leave.

CO is eliminated from the lungs unchanged in an exponential manner. The rate of elimination can be increased by exercise or administration of pure oxygen. Less than 1% is oxidized endogenously to carbon dioxide. The biological half-life of CO in a healthy, sedentary adult at sea level is 4 to 5 hr. This half-life decreases to approximately 80 min with administration of 100% oxygen, and to 23 min if hyperbaric oxygen is used (27).

Acute Carbon Monoxide Poisoning

Signs and Symptoms

Each year there are numerous acute CO poisonings, both intentional and accidental, cited in the literature. It has been previously pointed out that the concentration of CO in ambient air does not need to be great for an acute toxic exposure to occur. Table 2 lists the COHb levels at which certain signs and symptoms have been correlated. These signs and symptoms correlate with tissues that have the greatest oxygen consumption, the brain and heart. Keep in mind that not all signs will necessarily be observed in everyone exposed to CO. Also, remember that persons have survived breathing large quantities of CO, while others have succumbed from breathing low levels.

TABLE 2. *Signs and symptoms at various concentrations of carboxyhemoglobin*

% COHb	Signs and symptoms
0–10	No symptoms; asymptomatic
10–20	Tightness across the forehead, possibly slight headache, dilation of the cutaneous blood vessels, exertional dyspnea
20–30	Headache and throbbing in the temples, easily fatigued, possible dizziness
30–40	Severe headache, weakness, dizziness, confusion, dimness of vision, nausea, vomiting, and collapse
40–50	Same as above, a greater possibility of collapse, syncope, and increased pulse and respiratory rate
50–60	Syncope, increased respiratory and pulse rate, coma, intermittent convulsions, and Cheyne-Stokes respiration
60–70	Coma, intermittent convulsions, depressed heart action and respiratory rate, and possibly death
70–80	Weak pulse, slow respirations, respiratory failure, and death within a few hours
80–90	Death in less than an hour
90–	Death within a few minutes

Typically, individuals with COHb levels less than 1% are asymptomatic, and even COHb levels between 10 to 20% produce effects that are sometimes vague and nondescriptive.

Effects of CO become increasingly severe as COHb levels rise to the 30 to 50% range, with the victim showing irritability, headache, dizziness, confusion, disturbance of judgment, collapse, and fainting on exertion. The intense headache that often follows CO poisoning probably results from cerebral edema. It is also potentiated by increased intracranial pressure. Unconsciousness rarely occurs in individuals with COHb levels less than 50%. If the duration of exposure to CO is prolonged or if an acute exposure to high concentrations of CO (0.5–1.0%) occurs and the resultant COHb increases to 60 to 70%, then pulse rate, cardiac output, and respirations will be critically compromised, and death can follow.

Whereas it is common knowledge that CO causes deleterious effects on the CNS, its actions on the myocardium are less well under-stood. In actuality, death often occurs as a result of myocardial ischemia.

To illustrate that the heart is readily affected by CO levels, a study, using monkeys placed in a chamber containing CO, showed that 25% of the animals quickly developed ventricular arrhythmias and other ECG abnormalities (19). In another investigation, 40% of a group of individuals who had preexisting heart disease, and who were exposed to CO emissions on a freeway in a major metropolitan area, experienced significant ECG abnormalities and increased anginal pain. Blood CO concentrations in all affected individuals were below 5% (6), and yet, in still another study, 7 of 21 persons, aged 41 to 60 years, who were exposed to CO resulting in blood levels of 5 to 9% COHb, experienced ECG irregularities, with arrhythmias developing in 2 patients (28).

It is believed that persons with coronary heart disease are at special risk because their hearts cannot compensate for CO-induced increased myocardial oxygen demand (5,7). Normal patients, breathing CO for short periods, showed increased coronary blood flow and increased myocardial oxygen extraction. Patients with coronary heart disease had increased oxygen extraction by myocardial tissue, but no increased coronary blood flow.

Various animal studies have demonstrated that focal areas of necrosis can be seen on the myocardium following prolonged CO exposure, but these necroses are usually reversible. Evidence from a few animal studies suggests that permanent cardiac damage may occur, but the studies are not yet correlated to humans. It has been shown that when COHb concentration is 5% or higher, people are 21 times more likely to develop atherosclerosis than when COHb is decreased to 3% (52).

Nonfatal cases of CO exposure usually result in complete recovery within 2 to 4 days. It is usually reported that survivors will show little or no residual effects. It is only when the victim remains comatose for more than 24 hr that serious neurological symptoms can occur. As a result of the prolonged hypoxia, twitching, choreiform movements, and convulsive seizures may occur.

A feared late complication of CO poisoning is a delayed neuropathy characterized by demyelination of nerves within the CNS. Patients may appear to be well off immediately after recovery from the acute effects, only to show neurologic deficits later. One study has demonstrated that, of patients poisoned by CO who were evaluated 3 years after recovery, 13% displayed gross neuropsychiatric damage, 33% showed "deterioration of personality," and 43% had some degree of memory impairment (41).

Other complications include visual and hearing impairment, neurologic and muscular deficiencies, blood and kidney damage, and skin lesions including erythema, blisters, and bullae.

The fetus is especially vulnerable to CO poisoning. The gas readily crosses the placental barrier. Longo (29) demonstrated that infants born of women who had survived CO poisoning had a higher tendency toward neurological deficiencies than infants born of mothers not exposed.

CO classically produces a bright cherry-red discoloration of the skin. It begins around the mouth, when COHb levels exceed 25%, and spreads over the face and extremities as the percent saturation increases. In fatal CO poisonings, the cherry-red discoloration persists and can be readily demonstrated on autopsy.

This red color can also be a detriment to early detection of CO poisoning. Whereas a victim's COHb level increases with exposure to cause increasingly severe hypoxia and cyanosis, the cyanotic ashen skin color may be overshadowed by the red color of COHb. During these early stages, before other more readily discernible signs appear, the patient's poisoning may thus go unnoticed.

Treatment of Carbon Monoxide Poisoning

The specific goals in treating CO poisoning are, first, to relieve cerebral and cardiac ischemia and, second, to promote the dissociation of COHb, thus increasing the CO elimination rate and replacing CO on the hemoglobin molecule with oxygen. Each goal is readily achieved by administering oxygen. The initial step, therefore, is to remove the victim from the CO source and then administer pure oxygen. The victim should be kept quiet, and not allowed to move about so as to avoid increasing muscular demand for oxygen. If this occurs, oxygen extraction from the blood by muscles would increase, leaving even less oxygen available for the CNS. Antidoting CO poisoning is one of those rare situations where a direct antagonist, oxygen, is available for treatment, and, in general, the more oxygen that is given, the better the outcome. COHb levels can be easily determined in the laboratory, but the presence of signs and symptoms and positive conditions of exposure indicate that treatment is required, and should not be delayed until the laboratory results are ready.

When COHb levels are less than 15%, fresh air and rest are all that is usually indicated. If COHb levels are above 15%, 100% oxygen should be given since the dissociation of 50% of the COHb will be achieved in 40 min as compared to 4.1 hr in ambient air (36).

The use of hyperbaric oxygen (oxygen at increased pressure) is recommended when the COHb level reaches 40% or greater. Oxygen at two atmospheres will cause an almost instantaneous reversal of tissue hypoxia. This occurs because oxygen dissolved in the plasma will oxygenate the tissues directly. Also, it accelerates the rate of dissociation of COHb and shifts the oxyhemoglobin dissociation curve back to the right.

Recall that oxygen is transported through the body bound to hemoglobin, and also in lesser concentration in a dissolved form. Normally, the concentration of dissolved form is low, but this can be increased if the oxygen tension is increased. Breathing 100% oxygen can result in a dissolved oxygen concentration of 2.09 vol%. The body's normal arterial-to-venous oxygen difference is approximately 6%; so, forcing oxygen at 100% concentration can supply up to one-third the body's oxygen requirements (58). Giving oxygen at 2.5 atmospheres pressure can result in a dissolved oxygen concentration of 5.62 vol% (17).

At high COHb levels, oxygen therapy at 100% concentration may be administered over a prolonged period ranging to 4 hr at normal atmospheric pressure, and 1 hr at 2.5 atmospheric pressure. While prolonged therapy with high concentrations of oxygen can be toxic in its own right, treatment of CO poisoning with high concentrations at prolonged periods is not usually associated with seizures and other symptoms of oxygen poisoning (57).

From all indications, addition of 5 to 7% carbon dioxide to oxygen offers little advantage in treatment of CO poisoning. It is the opinion of some that carbon dioxide would stimulate breathing and compensate for the decreased carbon dioxide concentration in the blood. But others have shown that any possible advantage that carbon dioxide might have is overcome by the benefit that pure oxygen has on the dissociation of COHb.

Cerebral edema may result from central hypoxia. Thus, diuretics and glucocorticoids may be appropriate to prevent its appearance or reduce its severity.

CYANIDE

Cyanide (hydrocyanic acid, prussic acid) is not a frequently encountered poison, although today the public is more aware of its occurrence than in the past. Most cyanide ingestions occur from accidental exposure or intentional ingestion of a cyanide-containing compound. There has also been an increasing frequency in the number of case reports dealing with accidental cyanide poisonings since the use of laetrile became popularized (10,32,37). Occasionally, fruit seeds are ingested as part of a health food diet plan, and toxic levels of cyanide are consumed. In addition, the public was grimly reminded of its rapidly induced toxicity when more than 900 suicide-murders occurred in Jonestown, Guyana in 1978, as a result of drinking a cyanide-containing beverage.

The more conventional means of cyanide exposure occur in industry. Hydrogen cyanide and its derivatives are used in electroplating, metallurgy, and extraction of gold and silver metals from ores; production of synthetic fibers and plastics; and as a fumigant and fertilizer. Table 3 lists many of the cyanide-containing compounds with their appropriate chemical formulas and names, as well as other relevant information.

A common error regarding cyanide poisoning is that it occurs only from ingestion; that is, from swallowing some substances containing cyanide. Actually, intoxication can occur from inhalation and also absorption through the skin. In the presence of cyanide gases, a gas mask will offer little protection from intoxication.

At the top of the list is the most rapidly acting cyanide compound, hydrocyanic acid, which is readily volatilized to hydrogen cyanide producing the characteristic odor of bitter almonds. The cyanide salts are the most frequently encountered of all the cyanide-containing compounds. The LD_{50} for these compounds is approximately 2 mg/kg, with ingestion of 50 to 75 mg of any one of these salts usually resulting in syncope and respiratory difficulty within a few minutes (25). The halogenated cyanides are irritating gases and produce pulmonary edema, tearing, and excessive salivation.

It is not uncommon on autopsy to find cyanide concentrations in the blood, as well as CO, in individuals who have succumbed to smoke inhalation (30,47). Many plastics and polyacrylic fibers produce cyanide-containing gases when they are burned. These may be inhaled and absorbed through the skin, and cyanide toxicity possibly contributes to the cause of death in many fire victims.

Another source of exposure to cyanide is from ingestion of cyanogenic glycosides found in the seeds of several fruits. Amygdalin (Fig. 2), one such cyanogenic glycoside, is present in apple, peach, plum, apricot, cherry, and almond seeds. As shown in Fig. 3, amygdalin is hydrolyzed to hydrogen cyanide.

Mechanism of Cyanide Toxicity

Cyanide produces its toxic effects by binding to the trivalent (ferric) form of iron (Fe^{3+}). The

TABLE 3. *Examples of cyanide-containing compounds*

Name	Formula	Commercial use	Fatal dose (TLV)[a]
Acetone cyanohydrin	$(CH_3)_2C(OH)CN$	—	15 mg/kg
Acetonitrile	CH_3CN	Solvent	120 mg/kg
Acrylonitrile	$CH_2{:}CHCN$	Synthetic fibers and plastics	35–90 mg/kg (20 ppm)
Calcium cyanamide	$CaCN_2$	Fertilizer	40–50 g
Calcium cyanide	$Ca(CN)_2$	Fumigant, pesticide	5 mg/cu
Cyanogen	$N{:}CC{:}N$	Fumigant, blast furnace	13 ppm
Cyanogen bromide	$CNBr$	Fumigant	13 ppm
Cyanogen chloride	$CNCl$	Organic synthesis	13 ppm
Dimethyl cyanamide	$(CH_3)_2NCN$	Organic synthesis	75 mg/kg
Hydrocyanic acid	HCN	Fumigant	0.5 mg/kg (10 ppm)[a]
Nitroprusside	$Na_2[Fe(NO)(CN)_5] \cdot H_2O$	Antihypertensive, analytical reagent	10 mg/kg
Potassium cyanate	$COCN$	Herbicide, chemical reagent	1 g/kg
Potassium cyanide	KCN	Electroplating, organic synthesis	2 mg/kg
Potassium ferrocyanide	$K_4Fe(CN)_6 \cdot 3H_2O$	Metallurgy, graphic arts	1.6 g/kg
Sodium cyanide	$NaCN$	Electroplating, organic synthesis	2 mg/kg

[a]TLV = Threshold limit value.
From ref. 25.

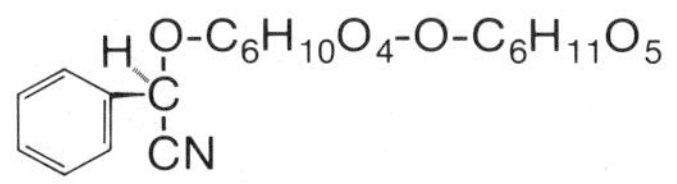

FIG. 2. Structural formula for amygdalin.

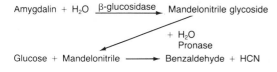

Amygdalin + H_2O → (β-glucosidase) → Mandelonitrile glycoside
+ H_2O
Pronase
Glucose + Mandelonitrile → Benzaldehyde + HCN

FIG. 3. Biochemical pathway for amygdalin metabolism.

body has over 40 enzyme systems which are reported to be inactivated by cyanide. The most significant of these, however, is the cytochrome oxidase system which consists of the cytochrome a-a_3 complex of the electron transport system (40). When cyanide binds to this enzyme complex, electron transport is inhibited; that is, electron transfer from cytochrome a_3 to molecular oxygen is blocked. This results in a reduction of cellular utilization of oxygen and an increase in venous Po_2.

Cyanide has the same physiologic effect as a complete lack of oxygen, and all cofactors in the cytochromes of the respiratory chain are in a reduced state. Consequently, no ATP can be generated since this is dependent on cyto-

chrome oxidase at the last step in oxidative phosphorylation (55).

Since there are several metabolic pathways converging on the electron transport system, the impairment of the cell to utilize oxygen reduces aerobic respiration in the cell. This causes a histotoxic (cellular) hypoxia. When this occurs, the quantity of oxygen that reaches the tissues is normal, but the cell is unable to utilize it. Recall that this event differs from CO poisoning where tissue hypoxia is due to an insufficient amount of oxygen available for tissue utilization. In essence, a victim of cyanide poison suffocates from an inability to use oxygen.

In cyanide toxicity, since it is only cellular utilization of oxygen that is impaired, venous blood becomes almost as oxygenated as arterial blood. Consequently, cyanosis is not usually observed.

Clinical Manifestations of Cyanide Poisoning

Cyanide is an extremely rapidly acting poison which is capable of causing death within minutes. The classical odor of bitter almonds is not detected by everyone and the ability to do so seems to be genetically determined (9). Onset of symptoms of cyanide poisoning depends on the type of exposure. For example, hydrogen cyanide vapors are the most rapidly acting, and symptoms can occur within seconds and death within minutes. When the cyanide salts are ingested, they are less rapidly acting because they are slowly absorbed. The severity of acute poisoning is determined, of course, by the dose and time-lapse since exposure. Symptoms of a mild cyanide poisoning are generally limited to weakness, dizziness, headache, nausea, and vomiting. These occur rapidly and are obviously rather nonspecific. A summary of signs and symptoms of cyanide poisoning is shown in Table 4.

Cyanide, by its inhibitory action on cytochrome oxidase, interferes with tissue use of oxygen producing an effect on the carotid and aortic bodies in the same manner as would a decrease in Po_2. That is, it stimulates the chemoreceptors to send a message to the respiratory center in the brain resulting in an increase in respiration (hyperpnea). This results in an increase in tidal volume and frequency, and minute volume of breathing.

In general, the cellular hypoxia produced by cyanide causes cells to die; but the lack of oxygen in the specialized cells of the carotid and aortic bodies stimulates them. This causes hyperpnea followed by dyspnea. Nausea and vomiting associated with cyanide poisoning are probably due to local irritation to the gastric mucosa from the cyanide salts. Tachycardia is produced with moderate cyanide poisoning by reflex actions resulting from stimulation of the chemoreceptors of the carotid and aortic bodies in response to cellular anoxia. It should again be noted that the patient usually does not appear cyanotic because of the oxygenated venous blood.

As cyanide blood concentration increases, the respiration rate becomes slower and gasping occurs, but cyanosis is still usually absent. Some believe the presence of bradycardia and absence of cyanosis are strong evidence to support a suspected cyanide poisoning. As blood levels of cyanide increase, sufficient oxygen deprivation occurs in the brain, and hypoxic convulsions occur followed by death due to respiratory arrest. Also, the lactic acidosis with a wide anion gap (see Chapter 4) should not be overlooked in these patients because the inhibition of aerobic respiration is going to shift the glucose metabolism scheme to anaerobic glycolysis. This causes pyruvate to be reduced to lactate and the consequent increase in lactic acid to cause lactic acidosis.

Treatment of Cyanide Poisoning

The treatment of acute cyanide poisoning continues to be a significant clinical problem because current methods are, for the most part, ineffective. Also, it should be remembered that present methods have their own inherent morbidity and mortality problems. Development of newer methods for antidoting cyanide has been slow.

Treatment is aimed at decreasing the amount of cyanide available for cellular binding. It must be initiated immediately to be effective. The primary objective is to maintain cellular utilization of oxygen by sequestering or interfering with cyanide in order to prevent its interaction with cytochrome oxidase.

Unlike most other toxic exposures, however, cyanide poisoning is a good example of a situation where specific antidotal treatment is avail-

TABLE 4. *Correlation between blood cyanide levels and clinical manifestations of poisoning*

CN level (mg/L)	Degree of poisoning	Signs and symptoms
0.5–1.0	Mild	Conscious, flushed, rapid pulse, headache
1.0–2.5	Moderate	Stuporous but responsive to stimuli, tachycardia, tachypnea
2.5 and greater	Severe	Comatose, unresponsive, hypotension, respirations slow and gasping, dilated pupils, cyanosis at high levels, death unless treated immediately

From ref. 51.

able, but the key to successful treatment is limited by how rapidly this treatment can be initiated. Many situations do not lend themselves to a rapid, straightforward diagnosis of cyanide poisoning, and therefore specific treatment is further delayed. In fact, it is a rare event for an intentional ingestion of cyanide to be discovered prior to death because this toxic agent acts so rapidly.

With sublethal concentrations, cyanide is released from its ferric iron binding sites and converted to thiocyanate by the enzyme sulfur transferase and an endogenous source of thiosulfate as shown in Fig. 4. The thiocyanate that is formed is, for all practical purposes, nontoxic and is rapidly excreted by the kidney. When greater concentrations of cyanide are present, this built-in detoxification system becomes saturated, and death will result unless some specific measures are taken.

Over the years there have been several antidotes suggested for cyanide poisoning. Pedigo (34) reported, in 1888, that amyl nitrite was effective in antidoting cyanide-poisoned dogs. Methylene blue was later reported effective (18). Methylene blue is an aniline dye which produces methemoglobin when taken in large doses. Methemoglobin contains iron in its oxidized form (Fe^{3+}), and thus competes with cytochrome oxidase for the binding of cyanide. In a series of experiments it was subsequently shown that nitrites were successful antidotes (12–14). It was later confirmed by animal data that amyl nitrite and sodium nitrite were much more effective in producing methemoglobinemia, and if a sufficient source of sulfur was in supply in the form of thiosulfate, the combination of nitrite and thiosulfate provided an effective antidotal regimen.

This then formed the basis for the Cyanide Antidote Package (Fig. 5) which contains amyl nitrite inhalant, 3% sodium nitrite solution, and 25% sodium thiosulfate solution. First, amyl nitrite is administered by inhalation, followed by sodium nitrite by intravenous administration. The purpose of these two agents is to oxidize the ferrous iron of hemoglobin to its ferric form, thus producing methemoglobin as shown in Fig. 6, Equation A. Methemoglobin (Fe^{3+}) can now compete with cytochrome oxidase for circulating cyanide.

Since amyl nitrite alone produces only about 5% methemoglobin, it must be combined with sodium nitrite to produce an adequate concentration of methemoglobin to bind with the cyanide. In practice, a methemoglobin level close to 40% is desirable. Caution should be exercised not to exceed this level, because methemoglobinemia toxicity will result and compromise the situation.

Methemoglobin has a greater affinity for cyanide than does cytochrome oxidase. Therefore, methemoglobin can bind to free cyanide (Fig. 6, Equation B), as well as cause dissociation of the cyanide-cytochrome oxidase complex. This results in the release of the enzyme, allowing it to resume its activity in the electron transport system. In addition, the released intracellular cyanide will now bind to methemoglobin forming cyanomethemoglobin as shown in Fig. 6, Equation C.

We should be aware of the fact that all the discussed reactions which involve cyanide and its complexes are reversible and may shift in either direction, depending on the circumstances. In the same light, cyanomethemoglobin also has the potential to dissociate. This is partly the reason for applying the second phase of the Cyanide Antidote Package. This step involves the binding of cyanomethemoglobin with thiosulfate in the presence of sulfur transferase (rhodanese) to form a relatively nontoxic compound, thiocyanate, which is readily excreted by the kidney (Fig. 6, Equation D).

Here we should recall a fundamental concept of antidotal therapy. We are using a drug (sodium nitrite), which usually has undesirable properties of its own, to antidote another sub-

$$\text{CYANIDE} + \text{THIOSULFATE} \xrightarrow{\text{(sulfur transferase)}} \text{THIOCYANATE} + \text{SULFITE}$$

FIG. 4. Reaction of cyanide with thiosulfate in the presence of sulfur transferase.

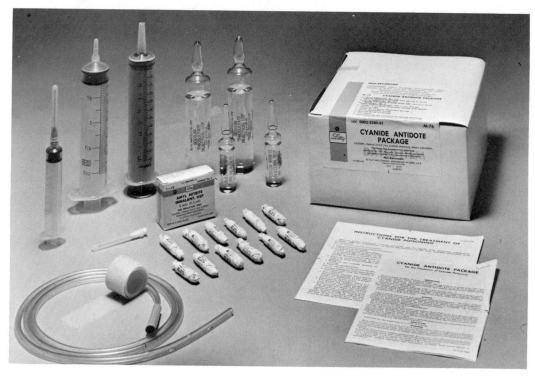

FIG. 5.   Cyanide Antidote Package. (Photograph courtesy of Eli Lilly Company.)

HEMOGLOBIN   AMYL NITRITE   METHEMOGLOBIN
(Fe^{+2})   +   or   →   (Fe^{+3})
SODIUM NITRITE

(Equation A)

CYANIDE + METHEMOGLOBIN ⇌ CYANOMETHEMOGLOBIN

(Equation B)

CYANIDE - CYTOCHROME   METHEMOGLOBIN ⇌ CYANOMETHEMOGLOBIN
OXIDASE COMPLEX   +   +
CYTOCHROME OXIDASE

(Equation C)

CYANOMETHEMOGLOBIN + THIOSULFATE ⇌ THIOCYANATE
                                                            +
SULFITE
+
METHEMOGLOBIN

(Equation D)

FIG. 6.   Steps involved in antidoting cyanide intoxication.

stance; therefore, extreme caution must be exercised.

Although the treatment regimen previously described for cyanide poisoning merits recognition, it does have considerable drawbacks. For example, when hemoglobin is converted to methemoglobin, it loses its ability to bind oxygen. This causes the oxygen dissociation curve to shift to the left. As a result, the body may be placed in a double jeopardy. That is, cellular oxygen utilization has first of all been diminished by cyanide, and with the production of methemoglobin, the amount of oxygen available for tissues to utilize is potentially diminished. As can be expected, there is a fine line between reversing the toxicity of one agent and inadvertently initiating toxicity by another agent. In practice, it appears that the production of methemoglobin does not severely compromise the cyanide-poisoned patient unless methemoglobin levels reach 40 to 50% or greater, but this potential danger should not go unrecognized.

Another caution to note is the possibility of drastically lowering blood pressure with the use of the nitrites. Both agents induce severe vasodilation and the procedure may run the risk of causing cardiovascular collapse which would, of course, be detrimental and render the treatment completely ineffective.

Oxygen is not a specific antidote for cyanide, but it has been advocated as a necessary adjunct in the treatment of cyanide toxicity (53,54). Oxygen therapy may be useful for two reasons: (a) It may displace cyanide from cytochrome oxidase, and (b) the increased intracellular oxygen tension may be sufficient to nonenzymatically convert reduced cytochrome to oxidized cytochrome enabling the electron transport system to function again. It has been recommended that oxygen be given after treatment with nitrites because of the formation of methemoglobin which causes decreased binding of oxygen to hemoglobin.

Unlike treating CO poisoning, oxygen administration, even at increased pressures, does not produce significant benefits. To illustrate, a study was conducted using mice that were given potassium cyanide followed by nitrite and/or thiosulfate, and air and/or oxygen (54). Oxygen was given under atmospheric conditions and at hyperbaric pressures. Table 5 shows that oxygen at 4 atmospheric pressures reduces cyanide mortality in mice more so than air (not given along with nitrite and thiosulfate). But when oxygen at 1 atmospheric pressure was compared to oxygen at 4 atmospheric pressures (Fig. 7), there was no significant difference between the two treatments.

SULFIDES

Sulfide poisonings usually occur following exposure to hydrogen sulfide (H_2S), carbon disulfide (CS_2), or one of the mercaptans. These compounds can produce systemic effects by inhalation or absorption through the skin.

H_2S is a colorless gas which is heavier than air (S.G. = 1.192). For this reason, H_2S accumulates in underground locations such as sewers and wells. This gas has a characteristic odor of rotten eggs and is found any place where putrefaction occurs. It is also generated in several industrial settings including petroleum refineries, tanneries, and rubber and rayon factories (Table 6). H_2S has been the cause of intoxication from liquid manure tanks in agricultural settings, and in rural latrines connected directly to septic tanks (16,31,33). H_2S is classified as a primary irritant and, when inhaled in high concentrations, produces its toxic effects almost as rapidly as hydrocyanic acid (23,24). The TLV (threshold limit value, i.e., the amount of substance a worker can be exposed to for 8 hr a day, 5 days a week) for H_2S has been set at 10 ppm. Inhalation of 1,000 ppm can cause coma after a single breath and become fatal (46). A victim typically loses consciousness without warning, and without crying out. The presence of apnea is a serious prognostic sign. Once respiration ceases, it generally does not begin again spontaneously. Apnea is quickly followed by hypoxic convulsions, cardiovascular collapse, and death (42).

CS_2 is a colorless liquid which boils at 46°C but volatilizes at room temperature. In its pure state it has a sweetish aromatic odor, but most

TABLE 5. *Effect of hyperbaric oxygen, sodium nitrite, and sodium thiosulfate on the LD_{50} of potassium cyanide in mice*

Experiment no.			Treatment before KCN (s.e.)		LD_{50} values[b] (mg/kg)
	Air	HBO[a]	$NaNO_2$(s.c.) (g/kg)	Na_2S_2O(i.p.) (g/kg)	
1	+	0	0	0	11.8
2	0	+	0	0	11.2
3	+	0	0.1	0	21.2
4	0	+	0.1	0	21.3
5	+	0	0	1.0	34.8
6	0	+	0	1.0	39.0
7	+	0	0.1	1.0	51.7
8	0	+	0.1	1.0	73.0

[a]HBO = 100% oxygen at 4 atmospheres.
[b]Each LD_{50} value was obtained from 5 graded doses of KCN administered to 5 or more groups of 10 mice each; $p < 0.05$.
s.c. = subcutaneous, i.p. = intraperitoneal.
From ref. 54.

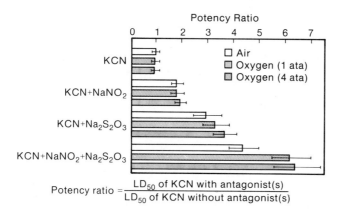

FIG. 7. Effect of hyperbaric oxygen (4 ata), oxygen, and air on the LD_{50} of KCN. (From ref. 54.)

$$\text{Potency ratio} = \frac{LD_{50} \text{ of KCN with antagonist(s)}}{LD_{50} \text{ of KCN without antagonist(s)}}$$

commercial grades smell somewhat like decaying cabbage or radishes. It is widely used as an insecticide, soil fumigant, and as a solvent for lipids, sulfur, rubber, phosphorus, waxes, and resins. Most exposures occur in industry, where it is used in production of viscose rayon fibers. The TLV for CS_2 has been set at 20 ppm to prevent serious systemic effects, especially damage to the central and peripheral nervous systems. This value may be lowered soon, perhaps to a low of 1 ppm. The World Health Organization has stated that over 20,000 workers are regularly exposed to CS_2 (50).

Inhalation of CS_2 is the major route of toxic exposure. Reports of skin contamination or ingestion are rare.

Both ethyl and methyl mercaptans are quite toxic flammable gases with a TLV set at 0.5 ppm. These compounds are used in the production of jet fuels, plastics, and pesticides. They are extremely foul-smelling, and have been used in minimal concentrations as "warning agents" for propane, butane, and natural gases. Mercaptan odors can be detected well below the concentrations necessary to produce toxicity.

Sulfides are not generally viewed by the public as being extremely toxic, and this is probably the major reason they are so dangerous. Also, the olfactory responses are quickly paralyzed when the gases are inhaled in lethal concentrations, so the victim often fails to recognize the danger.

TABLE 6. *Sites of exposure of victims of hydrogen sulfide poisoning*[a]

Site	% (Of all cases)
Gas plant	52
Pumping station	24
Oil rig	12
Sulfuric acid production plant	2
Oil refinery	1
Sewer	1
Other	8

[a]Total number of victims = 221.
From ref. 11.

Mechanism of Sulfide Toxicity

H_2S manifests its toxicity in a manner similar to hydrogen cyanide, by inhibiting the enzyme cytochrome oxidase (40). It thus produces cellular anoxia. *In vitro* experiments have shown that sulfide is an even more potent enzyme inhibitor than cyanide (42). Also, the hydrosulfide anion (HS^-) forms a dissociable complex with ferric heme groups to produce sulfmethemoglobin. Sulfmethemoglobin is nontoxic and is reduced to hemoglobin by polysulfides, thiosulfate, or sulfate. In addition to the cellular anoxia produced by H_2S, the gas also exerts a direct depressant effect on the CNS, producing complete paralysis of all parts including the respiratory center. The heart continues to beat for several minutes, so artificial respiration with a mixture of oxygen and carbon dioxide may be beneficial, if given quickly.

CS_2 has a greater affinity for the CNS and cardiovascular system than does H_2S. Damage to the cranial nerves, and peripheral neuropathies are prevalent in occupational exposures to CS_2. It has also been shown that CS_2 poisoning may accelerate the atherosclerotic process and, thus, contribute to the onset of coronary heart disease. Recent epidemiological studies of viscose rayon workers have shown a two- to five-fold increase in the risk of coronary heart disease, as compared to workers not exposed to carbon disulfide (48).

Clinical Manifestations of Sulfide Poisoning

In low concentrations, H_2S is relatively harmless except for its unpleasant odor and irritation to the eyes, respiratory tract, and gastrointestinal system. It produces significant hyperpnea by direct chemostimulation of the carotid body (26).

Exposure to levels of 50 ppm for 1 hr or more can produce the effects listed in Table 7. These may include acute conjunctivitis with pain, lacrimation, and photophobia. Prolonged exposure can also cause irritation of the mucosal membranes of the respiratory tract causing inflammatory reactions along the full length of the respiratory tract, culminating with pulmonary edema.

Inhalation of higher concentrations (greater than 700 ppm) results in instantaneous paralysis of the entire nervous system and can be rapidly fatal.

In deaths associated with H_2S, the viscera and the brain will have a greenish-blue discoloration. Unlike CO, H_2S does not combine with hemoglobin during life. The formation of sulfhemoglobin occurs after death, as a result of decomposition of tissues. It is this sulfur-containing hemoglobin complex that is thought to be responsible for the discoloration of the tissues at autopsy (1).

CS_2 intoxication can involve all areas of the central and peripheral nervous systems. Centrally, it produces damage to the cranial nerves, caudate nucleus, and the putamen. In the periphery, CS_2 causes axonal degeneration which may be delayed in producing symptoms. The peripheral neuropathies can produce paresthesias, muscle weakness in the extremities, unsteady gait, and dysphagia. In extreme cases of CS_2 intoxication, a Parkinsonism-like syndrome including tremors, loss of memory, mental depression, speech disturbances, and muscle twitches can occur. Table 8 lists some of the other reported effects of exposure to CS_2. Splashes of the liquid in the eyes cause immediate and severe irritation. Exposure of the skin can produce dermatitis and vesiculation. CS_2 is reported to be one of the strongest skin irritants known, causing third degree irritant burns within minutes (43).

TABLE 7. *Effects of hydrogen sulfide exposure*

Exposure to 50 ppm H$_2$S for 1 hr or more		Exposure to >700 ppm H$_2$S (high concentration)
Mucous membranes	Respiratory tract	
Conjunctivitis	Rhinitis	Respiratory collapse
Keratitis	Tracheitis	Sudden collapse
Photophobia	Bronchitis	Convulsions
	Pneumonia	Death
	Pulmonary edema	
	Greenish cyanosis	

Treatment of Sulfide Poisoning

Since H$_2$S produces its toxic effects in a manner similar to hydrogen cyanide, the same treatment procedure has been proposed for H$_2$S poisonings. This involves production of methemoglobin with nitrites (46). Sulfide ions combine with methemoglobin to form sulfmethemoglobin, and (it is hoped) spare intracellular cytochrome oxidase. The sulfmethemoglobin produced is excreted through the kidneys, or is gradually metabolized to nontoxic products. The sodium thiosulfate step may or may not be omitted. Other treatment is symptomatic.

There is still significant doubt that nitrite therapy is beneficial. Animal studies have shown that LD$_{50}$ doses of sulfide salts are increased when animals receive sodium nitrite immediately after exposure (22). Once cytochrome oxidase has been affected, even for a short period, death is likely. To be effective, nitrite would have to be given before or immediately after exposure. Also, because of methemoglobin production with resultant decrease in oxygen-carrying capacity of blood, the chance for producing cellular hypoxia is increased even more.

Oxygen is usually considered to be an antidote of choice, but, again, studies have failed to demonstrate a protective effect greater than breathing air alone.

H$_2$S is an intense irritant of tissues, such as the conjunctiva and respiratory epithelium, and causes severe injury; oxygen seems to retard this damage.

Recall that the antidoting of cyanide requires thiosulfate to convert cyanide to the less toxic thiocyanate. For sulfide, no comparable detox-ification pathway exists. Still, thiosulfate is recommended by some authorities because of a slight protective effect shown in animal studies. Until this phenomenon is better understood, thiosulfate is not considered to be a regular part of sulfide treatment.

For any sulfide, if exposure is not immediately fatal and if adequate treatment is given, recovery is probable (11).

SUMMARY

One of the important points presented in this chapter is that poisoning by gases may occur indiscreetly, with symptoms appearing without prior warning. Chances should not be taken when working in any environment where these poisonous gases may be formed. Also, be prepared to offer quick assistance to others who may be victimized by a gas poisoning.

Case Studies

CASE STUDIES: CYANIDE POISONING

History: Case 1

A 21-year-old male was admitted to an emergency facility unconscious, cyanotic, and with evidence of previous vomiting. His blood pressure was 168/112 mm Hg. The pulse rate was 68 beats/min, and respirations (gasping) were 24/min. A routine toxicological laboratory analysis for toxic substances in the blood and stomach was negative. The laboratory results are listed in Table 9. Pulmonary edema and lactic acidosis were characteristic throughout the clinical course.

TABLE 8. *Effects of carbon disulfide exposure*

Nervous system
  Paresthesias
  Unsteady gait
  Dysphagia
  Parkinson-like syndrome

Ocular changes
  Corneal anesthesia
  Decreased pupillary reflex
  Nystagmus

Gastrointestinal disturbances
  Chronic gastritis
  Achlorhydria

Renal impairment
  Albuminuria
  Elevated BUN

TABLE 9. *Laboratory findings in 2 cases of cyanide poisoning*

Measurements	Case 1[a]	Case 2[b]
Amount of cyanide ingested	600 mg	Unknown
Respiration/min	24	20 (gasping)
Anion gap (mEq/L)	35	38
BUN (mg%)	21	9
Glucose (mg%)	245	313
Po_2 (mm Hg)	115	139
Pco_2 (mm Hg)	12	11
HCO_3^- (mEq/L)	5.6	—
pH	7.27	7.32
CN (μg/ml)	12 hr = 2.0	2.3
	22 hr = 1.6	
	84 hr = 1.2	

[a]From ref. 21.
[b]From ref. 51.

Treatment. The patient was ventilated and diuresis was initiated with furosemide. Nine hours post-admission, it was discovered that he had ingested three capsules, each containing 200 mg of potassium cyanide. Blood levels for cyanide are listed in Table 9. In addition, the following ketoacids were elevated: β-hydroxybutyrate 1.2 mEq/L (normal 0.6), acetoacetic acid 1.6 mEq/L (normal 0.8), and lactic acid 3.3 mEq/L (normal 0.8). Also, make note of the high anion gap. (See ref. 21.)

History: Case 2

A 31-year-old male biochemist, with a previous history of alcohol abuse, was found comatose. He had been undergoing treatment for hypertension and an ulcer. It was not revealed until 6 hr after admission that he had ingested an unknown quantity of potassium cyanide from his laboratory.

Laboratory values for this patient are reported in Table 9. A routine toxicological drug screen was negative, although his blood alcohol concentration was 290 mg%.

Treatment. Since at the time of admission it was not known what the toxic agent may have been, he was given naloxone (Narcan®, a narcotic antagonist), but no improvement was shown. Supportive treatment was continued. Three hours later, he was fully responsive. It was not until 3 hr after that time that he admitted to ingesting some cyanide. Specific antidoting for cyanide was not performed. (See ref. 51.)

Discussion

1. In Case 1, gasping for air was noted. What is the reason for this?

2. The patient in Case 1 ingested more than the lethal dose of cyanide, but survived. What is the most likely reason for his survival?

3. Neither patient was antidoted with nitrite and thiosulfate, even after the nature of their intoxication was determined. Why not?

4. What is the mechanism of cyanide-induced toxicity?

5. Explain the elevated anion gap in these patients.

CASE STUDIES: CARBON MONOXIDE INHALATION

History: Case 1

On a cold night, a hibachi grill was used by a husband-and-wife camping team to cook their evening meal. After eating, the hibachi was taken inside the camping trailer to add heat. The trailer was well insulated and closed, since it was rather cool that evening.

During the night, the wife was awakened with nausea and went to the bathroom to vomit. There, she collapsed. Later she awakened only to find her husband in bed was dead. She reported they had never before used the hibachi inside the trailer.

On autopsy, the husband's COHb concentration was 71%. Also, mitral valve damage from a previous episode of rheumatic heart disease was observed. (See ref. 56.)

History: Case 2

A 13-year-old boy was found unconscious on the garage floor, wedged between the car and the garage door. When he was found, the car's engine was not running and there were no noticeable exhaust fumes. There did not appear to be open containers of gasoline, kerosene, or other volatile hydrocarbons sitting around. Previous to this incident, the boy had been in excellent health and there were no reasons to suspect drug abuse. He often worked on his motorbike in the garage without experiencing difficulties.

He was admitted to the hospital in a comatose state. His breathing was rapid and labored, which progressively worsened, requiring intubation. His pupils were equal and reactive, but a few retinal hemorrhages were present. There was no response to painful stimuli. Brief episodes of tonic contractions were periodically noted.

The following laboratory data were obtained on admission and at a time period corresponding to 13 hr after his discovery:

	On admission	13 hr after discovery
Na^+ (mEq/L)	141	138
K^+ (mEq/L)	5.7	5.9
Cl^- (mEq/L)	90	100
HCO_3^- (mEq/L)	8	24
BUN (mg%)	28	42
Glucose (mg%)	155	183
Arterial pH	7.21	7.50
Po_2 (mm Hg)	97	88
Pco_2 (mm Hg)	16	25

The initial toxicology drug screen was negative for barbiturates and salicylates. The ECG showed sinus tachycardia, but computerized tomography (CT) scans and X-rays were normal. CO was suspected. The patient's hospital stay was marked by anuria, pulmonary edema, ventricular tachycardia, hyperkalemia, and hypocalcemia.

Treatment. Treatment included sodium polystyrene sulfonate, glucose, insulin, and calcium gluconate. Due to the elevated BUN (78 mg%) and serum creatinine (6.0 mg%) values on Day 6, peritoneal dialysis was started and maintained for 21 days. The boy remained intubated and dependent on the respirator for 11 days and was neurologically comatose for 12 days.

The patient was then able to respond to vocal commands. He could feed himself by the 18th day, but it was not until the 21st day that he could speak and remembered going into the garage to work on his bike. His memory improved over the next 5 weeks and he was able to move his lower extremities.

He was then transferred to a rehabilitation facility where he remained for the next 14 weeks. He made substantial progress during this time. At the time of discharge, he was speaking normally although he had a poor ability to concentrate. He was able to walk with the aid of a walker and braces. (See ref. 59.)

Discussion

1. In both case studies, the fact that carbon monoxide is a "silent killer" became evident. What precautions should have been taken to prevent the exposure to CO?

2. In Case 1, give a probable reason why the woman was not as acutely affected by the CO. Why did she not die? Why was she not treated at an emergency room?

3. Comment on the role of the husband's heart disease (from Case 1) as a factor in his susceptibility to CO.

4. What was the purpose of the peritoneal dialysis used in Case 2?

5. Comment on the possible use of hyperbaric oxygen in Case 2.

6. The victim in Case 2 showeed periods of tonic contractions, even though he was comatose. Based on the information presented, what is the most likely cause of this event?

7. In the description of Case 2, something was mentioned that suggested CO as the probable cause of poisoning. What was this?

CASE STUDY: INTOXICATION FROM HYDROGEN SULFIDE

History

A 45-year-old male was overcome by fumes from a drain trap to which he was adding sulfuric acid (90%). The sink was located in a small basement cubicle of a hospital, which was used to prepare plaster of Paris casts. The drain had not been previously cleaned by chemical means because of the high sludge content. Three other workers and a physician were less seriously affected when attempting to remove him from the area.

The man inhaled fumes for 2 or 3 min before being removed to fresh air. At that time he was apneic, cyanotic, comatose, and displayed generalized tremors.

The following laboratory results were obtained:

HCO_3^-	=	15 mEq/L
K^+	=	3.4 mEq/L
Na^+	=	152 mEq/L
Cl^-	=	108 mEq/L
Anion gap	=	29
Sulfhemoglobin	=	7.9% (normal $<0.5\%$)

Blood gases (mm Hg)	P_{O_2}	P_{CO_2}	pH
Initial	127	26	7.27
After treatment with 100% O_2	270	32	7.30

Treatment. Poisoning by H_2S was strongly suspected because of the strong odor of gas in the room. Initial treatment consisted of sodium bicarbonate (44 mEq) and 100% oxygen. Five amyl nitrite ampules were broken over his airway during a 10 to 15 min span. He was given 300 mg sodium nitrite, and 12.5 g of sodium thiosulfate. He was also given dexamethasone (20 mg) and diazepam (15 mg), in divided doses. After 3 to 4 hr, the patient was able to breathe on his own, and after several more hours most symptoms disappeared except for headache and chest pains. (See ref. 35.)

Discussion

1. It was later discovered that sulfuric acid had been added to a drain blocked by calcium sulfide sludge which had been produced by bacterial action on the plaster of Paris. The acid caused release of H_2S gas. Discuss why the worker may not have smelled this gas, even though other persons who entered the room afterwards were able to detect it. What is the characteristic odor?

2. How was the acidosis produced from this toxic exposure?

3. What was the purpose of using amyl nitrite/sodium nitrite and sodium thiosulfate in treating this case?

4. Why did symptoms of headache and chest pains persist in this patient?

Review Questions

1. To what substance does the term "silent killer" refer, and why is it used?

2. Discuss the physiological barriers that normally prevent airborne particles from entering the lungs.

3. Which of the following produces carboxyhemoglobin?
   A. Hydrogen sulfide
   B. Cyanide
   C. Methane
   D. Methylene chloride

4. Infants are more susceptible than adults to the toxic effects of CO. Cite the reason why this is so.

5. Which of the following is an antidote for CO poisoning: oxygen (I), sodium nitrite (II), sodium thiosulfate (III)?
   A. I only
   B. II only
   C. III only
   D. II and III only

6. CO causes a characteristic discoloration of the skin. State the color and discuss why it appears.

7. State the probable cause(s) of headache in persons with CO intoxication.

8. What is meant by the term hyperbaric oxygen? At what blood concentration of CO is it recommended that hyperbaric oxygen be used?

9. The binding affinity of hemoglobin with CO compared to its affinity with oxygen is:
   A. One-fourth as great
   B. Approximately the same
   C. About 100 times greater
   D. More than 200 times greater

10. Describe the shape of the curve which depicts the binding of oxygen to hemoglobin, and discuss why the curve assumes this shape.

11. On a graph depicting the oxyhemoglobin dissociation curve, when CO binds to hemoglobin and the amount of oxygen available to the tissues is reduced, the curve shifts:
    A. Left
    B. Right

12. Smoking two packs of cigarettes per day will produce CO blood concentrations that are closest to:
    A. 1 to 2%
    B. 3 to 4%
    C. 7 to 8%
    D. 10 to 12%

13. The blood normally has a low level of CO always present. What is this level, and what is its source?

14. Poisoning can occur through absorption of cyanide through the skin.
    A. True
    B. False

15. Sodium cyanide is the most rapidly acting (toxic) form of cyanide.
    A. True
    B. False

16. Describe the odor that is strongly suggestive of cyanide intoxication.

17. Although cyanide possesses affinity for binding to a number of different enzyme systems, it has strongest affinity toward one specific system. Which of the following systems is it?
    A. Sulfur transferase
    B. Carboxyhemoglobin reductase
    C. Cytochrome oxidase
    D. Acetylcholine esterase

18. Name the most common source of human exposure to amygdalin.

19. Cyanosis is a usual outcome of cyanide poisoning.
    A. True
    B. False

20. Cyanide is more tightly bound to iron in which of its valence states?
    A. Fe^{2+}
    B. Fe^{3+}

21. Treatment of cyanide poisoning involves two primary antidotal steps. Name them, and specify the precise purpose of each step.

22. Oxygen is not a specific antidote for cyanide intoxication, although it may be administered. Cite the specific reasons why oxygen may be of benefit.

23. CS_2 is a strong skin irritant.
    A. True
    B. False

24. Which of the following is a true statement?
    A. H_2S produces cellular anoxia by reacting with sulfur transferase (rhodanese) enzyme.
    B. Hydrosulfide ions readily combine with hemoglobin during life.
    C. CS_2 has a greater affinity for the CNS than does H_2S.
    D. After death by H_2S poisoning, the brain will appear dark red in color.

25. Commercial grades of CS_2 have a characteristic odor. Describe it.

26. H_2S has a characteristic odor. Describe it.

27. Describe the steps taken to antidote sulfide poisoning. Cite the goals of each step.

References

1. Adelson, L., and Sunshine, I. (1966): Fatal hydrogen sulfide intoxication. *Arch. Pathol.*, 81:375–380.
2. Amdur, M. O. (1980): Air pollutants. In: *The Basic Science of Poisons*, edited by J. Doull, C. D. Klaassen, and M. O. Amdur, pp. 608–631. Macmillan, New York.
3. Astrup, P., and Kjeldsen, K. (1973): Carbon monoxide, smoking and atherosclerosis. *Med. Clin. North Am.*, 58:323–350.
4. Ayres, S. M., Mueller, H. S., Gregory, J. J., Giannelli, S., and Penny, J. V. (1969): Systemic and myocardial hemodynamic responses to relatively small concentrations of carboxyhemoglobin (COHb). *Arch. Environ. Health*, 18:699–709.
5. Ayres, S. M., Giannelli, S., and Mueller, H. (1970): Myocardial and systemic responses to carboxyhemoglobin. *Ann. NY Acad. Sci.*, 174:268–293.
6. Ayres, S. M., Evans, R., and Light, D. (1973): Health effects of exposure to high concentrations of automobile emissions. *Arch. Environ. Health*, 27:168–177.
7. Ayres, S. M., Giannelli, S., Mueller, H., and Criscitiello, A. (1973): Myocardial and systemic vascular responses to low concentrations of carboxyhemoglobin. *Ann. Clin. Lab. Sci.*, 3:440–447.
8. Barnard, R. J., and Weber, J. S. (1979): Carbon monoxide: A hazard to fire fighters. *Arch. Environ. Health*, 34:255–257.
9. Bonnichsen, R., and Maehly, A. C. (1966): Poisoning by volatile compounds. *J. Forensic Sci.*, 11:516–527.

10. Braico, K. T., Humbert, J. R., Terplan, K. L., and Lehotay, J. M. (1979): Laetrile intoxication: Report of a fatal case. *N. Engl. J. Med.*, 300:238–240.
11. Burnett, W. W., King, E. G., Grace, M., and Hall, W. F. (1977): Hydrogen sulfide poisoning: Review of 5 years' experience. *CMA Journal*, 117:1277–1280.
12. Chen, K. K., Rose, C. L., and Clowes, G. H. (1933): Amyl nitrite and cyanide poisoning. *JAMA*, 11:1920–1922.
13. Chen, K. K., and Rose, C. L. (1952): Nitrite and thiosulfate therapy in cyanide poisoning. *JAMA*, 149:113–119.
14. Chen, I. K., and Rose, C. L. (1956): Treatment of acute cyanide poisoning. *JAMA*, 162:1154–1155.
15. Coburn, R. F. (1970): Endogenous carbon monoxide production. *N. Engl. J. Med.*, 282:207–209.
16. Donham, K. J., Knapp, L. W., Monson, R., and Gustafson, K. (1982): Acute toxic exposure to gases from liquid manure. *J. Occup. Med.*, 24:142–145.
17. End, E., and Long, C. W. (1942): Oxygen under pressure in carbon monoxide poisoning. *J. Indust. Hyg. Toxicol.*, 24:302.
18. Geiger, J. C. (1932): Cyanide poisoning in San Francisco. *JAMA*, 99:1944–1945.
19. Ginsberg, M. D., and Myers, R. E. (1974): Experimental carbon monoxide encephalopathy in the primate. I. Physiologic and metabolic aspects. *Arch. Neurol.*, 30:202–208.
20. Goldsmith, J. R., and Landaw, S. A. (1968): Carbon monoxide and human health. *Science*, 162:1352–1359.
21. Graham, D. L., Laman, D., Theodore, J., and Robin, E. D. (1977): Acute cyanide poisoning complicated by lactic acidosis and pulmonary edema. *Arch. Intern. Med.*, 137:1051–1055.
22. Gunter, A. P. (1956): The therapy of acute hydrogen sulfide poisoning. *Chem. Abst.*, 50:5916f.
23. Haggard, H. W. (1925): Toxicology of hydrogen sulfide. *J. Indust. Hyg.*, 7:113–121.
24. Hamilton, A., and Hardy, H. L. (1949): *Industrial Toxicology*, 2nd ed. Paul B. Hoeber, New York.
25. Hanenson, I. B. (1980): *Quick Reference to Clinical Toxicology*. J.B. Lippincott Company, Philadelphia.
26. Heymans, C., and Neil, E. (1958): *Reflexogenic Areas of the Cardiovascular System*. Little, Brown, Boston.
27. Klaassen, C. D. (1980): Nonmetallic environmental toxicants: Air pollutants, solvents and vapors, and pesticides. In: *The Pharmacological Basis of Therapeutics*, 6th ed, edited by A. G. Gilman, L. S. Goodman, and A. Gilman, pp. 1638–1659. Macmillan, New York.
28. Knelsen, J. H. (1972): United States air quality criteria and ambient standards for carbon monoxide. *UDI. Berichte. Nr.*, 180:99–101.
29. Longo, L. D. (1977): The biological effects of carbon monoxide on the pregnant woman, fetus, and unborn infant. *Am. J. Obstet. Gynecol.*, 129:69–103.
30. Mohler, S. R. (1975): Air crash survival: Injuries and evacuation toxic hazards. *Aviat. Space Environ. Med.*, 46:86–88.
31. Morse, D. L., Woodbury, M. A., Rentmeester, K., and Farmer, D. (1981): Death caused by fermenting manure. *JAMA*, 245:63–64.
32. Ortega, J. A., and Creek, J. (1978): Acute cyanide poisoning following administration of laetrile enemas. *J. Pediatr.*, 93:1059.
33. Osbern, L. N., and Crapo, R. O. (1981): Dung lung: A report of toxic exposure to liquid manure. *Ann. Int. Med.*, 95:312–314.
34. Pedigo, L. (1888): Antagonism between amyl nitrite and prussic acid. *Med. Soc. Virginia*, 19:124–130.
35. Peters, J. W. (1981): Hydrogen sulfide poisoning in a hospital setting. *JAMA*, 246:1538–1539.
36. Roughton, F. J. W., and Root, W. S. (1945): The fate of carbon monoxide in the body from mild carbon monoxide poisoning in man. *Am. J. Physiol.*, 145:239–244.
37. Sadoff, L., Fuchs, K., and Hollander, J. (1978): Rapid death associated with laetrile ingestion. *JAMA*, 239:1532.
38. Sammons, J. H., and Coleman, R. L. (1974): Firefighters' occupational exposure to carbon monoxide. *J. Occup. Med.*, 16:543–546.
39. Sjostrand, T. (1949): Endogenous formation of carbon monoxide in man under normal and pathological conditions. *Scand. J. Clin. Lab. Invest.*, 1:201–204.
40. Smith, R. P. (1980): Toxic responses of the blood. In: *The Basic Science of Poisons*, edited by J. Doull, C. D. Klaassen, and M. O. Amdur, pp. 311–331. Macmillan, New York.
41. Smith, J., and Brandon, S. (1973): Morbidity from acute carbon monoxide poisoning at a three-year follow-up. *Br. Med. J.*, 1:318–321.
42. Smith, R. P., and Gosselin, R. E. (1979): Hydrogen sulfide poisoning. *J. Occup. Med.*, 21:93–97.
43. Spyker, D. A., Gallanosa, A. G., and Suratt, P. M. (1982): Health effects of acute carbon disulfide exposure. *J. Toxicol. Clin. Toxicol.*, 19:87–93.
44. Stewart, R. D. (1976): Paint-remover hazard. *JAMA*, 235:398.
45. Stevenson, M. F., Chenoweth, M. B., and Cooper, G. L. (1978): Effect on carboxyhemoglobin of exposure to aerosol spray paints with methylene chloride. *Clin. Toxicol.*, 12:551–561.
46. Stine, R. J., Slosberg, B., and Beacham, B. E. (1976): Hydrogen sulfide intoxication: A case report and discussion of treatment. *Ann. Intern. Med.*, 85:756–758.
47. Symington, I. S., Anderson, R. A., Oliver, J. S., Thomson, I., Harland, W. A., and Kerr, J. W. (1978): Cyanide exposure in fires. *Lancet*, 2:91–92.
48. Tolonem, M. (1975): Vascular effects of carbon disulfide: A review. *Scand. J. Work. Environ. Health*, 1:63–75.
49. Turino, G. M. (1981): Carbon monoxide toxicity: Physiology and biochemistry. *Circulation*, 63:253A–259A.
50. United Nations Environment Programme, World Health Organization (1977): *Environmental Health Criteria 10 for Carbon Disulfide*. World Health Organization, Geneva.
51. Vogel, S. N., Sultan, T. R., and TenEyck, R. P. (1981): Cyanide poisoning. *Clin. Toxicol.*, 18:367–383.
52. Wald, M., Howard, S., Smith, P. G., and Kjedlsen, K. (1973): Association between atherosclerotic diseases and carboxyhemoglobin levels in tobacco smokers. *Br. Med. J.*, 1:761–765.
53. Way, J. L., Gibbson, S. L., and Sheehy, M. (1966): Effect of oxygen on cyanide intoxication. I. Prophy-

lactic protection. *J. Pharmacol. Exp. Ther.*, 153:381–385.

54. Way, J. L., End, E., Sheehy, M. H., DeMiranda, P., Fertknecht, O. F., Bachand, R., Gibson, S. L., and Burrows, G. E. (1972): Effects of oxygen on cyanide intoxication. IV. Hyperbaric oxygen. *Toxicol. Appl. Pharmacol.*, 22:415–421.

55. White, A., Handler, P., and Smith, E. L. (1968): *Principles of Biochemistry*, 4th ed. McGraw-Hill, New York.

56. Wilson, E. F., Rich, T. H., and Messman, H. C. (1972): Carbon monoxide poisoning following use of charcoal. *JAMA*, 221:405–406.

57. Winter, P. M., and Smith, G. (1972): The toxicity of oxygen. *Anesthesiology*, 37:210–241.

58. Winter, P. M., and Miller, J. N. (1976): Carbon monoxide poisoning. *JAMA*, 236:1502–1504.

59. Zimmerman, S. S., and Truxal, B. (1981): Carbon monoxide poisoning. *Pediatrics*, 68:215–224.

Hydrocarbons

7

The hydrocarbon poisons are mixtures of aliphatic and aromatic hydrocarbons that vary in their molecular weight, and chemical and physical properties. Hydrocarbon products represent a diverse group of substances ranging from distillates of petroleum (e.g., gasoline, kerosene, mineral spirits, petroleum naphtha, petroleum ether, mineral seal oil), coal tar (benzene, toluene, xylene), to pine wood (turpentine). Table 1 lists many hydrocarbon substances and their common names. Although hydrocarbon ingestion involves a relatively small number of poisonings (variously reported to be approximately 5% of all cases), it does constitute a major cause of hospitalization of its victims. In 1976 it was the leading cause of mortality (29%) following accidental ingestion of household products by children under age 5 (21). While any hydrocarbon substance may be the source of toxicity, it is the liquid products that are more frequently reported. Some of these include lubricants, mineral seal oil (in furniture polishes), fuels, cigarette and charcoal lighter fluids, solvents, paint and varnish thinners, and paint removers. Gasoline sniffing as a means of intentional abuse has been shown to be a major cause of toxicity (4,13,19).

Hydrocarbon products represent a group of substances that are often stored in unmarked bottles or other containers in the home or workplace. It is largely because of this practice that these substances are within easy reach of an unsuspecting child who mistakes them for something more palatable (12). Also, the ubiq-

TABLE 1. *Examples of hydrocarbon substances*

Hydrocarbon substance	Synonym(s)	Composition
Benzin (benzine)	Petroleum ether	Low boiling point fractions (e.g., pentanes, hexanes)
Asphalt	Tar	
Diesel oil		$C_{20}H_{42}$ and heavier
Gasoline	Petroleum spirit	Heptanes, octanes, and other diverse hydrocarbons
Kerosene	Coal oil, kerosine, jet fuel, No. 1 heating oil	Decane to hexadecane
Lubricating oil	Auto engine oil, household lubricating oils	
Mineral seal oil	Signal oil, seal oil, red furniture polish	
Naphtha	Lighter fluid, racing fuel	
Paraffin	Wax	
Petrolatum	Petroleum jelly	
Petroleum	Mineral spirits	
Turpentine	Pine oil	Cyclic turpentines, wood distillate (aromatic compounds)

From ref. 8.

uitous nature of many household substances (e.g., lemon- or pine-scented furniture polish or room deodorants, or attractively colored and packaged cleaning aids) may invite more than a passing glance by a curious or inquisitive child. Table 2 lists some of the ways in which children have been exposed to kerosene, and illustrates the imaginative nature of children.

One of the major causes of hydrocarbon poisoning in adults is gasoline ingestion resulting from siphoning it from one container to another.

TABLE 2. *Means by which children ingest kerosene*

Sniffed from a 30-gallon drum from which the top was missing.
Drank from a coffee can used to catch drippings from a leaky fuel line connected to an oil stove.
Drank from a can in the woodshed used for soaking paint brushes.
Drank from a cup left on the kitchen table by mother who was treating the child for nits (lice eggs).
Sucked from an open vent pipe of an oil stove.
Drank from soda bottle left on kitchen floor.
Dipped fingers into the fuel container of an oil stove and sucked them about 30 min.
Drank from a can of fluid used to start fires.

From ref. 6.

During the world oil embargo of 1973 and, more recently, because of spurious gasoline shortages when supplies have been curtailed, the reported incidence of poisoning has increased significantly. It might even be predicted that this incidence will continue to rise and remain high for as long as fuel prices persist at inflated values.

Not all hydrocarbon-based products are sources of toxicity and not all ingested products cause toxicological problems. For example, highly viscous substances (paint, glues, asphalt, rubber cement, etc.) pose little significant hazard of aspiration. Obstruction would be the greatest concern following the ingestion of one of these highly viscous products.

On the other hand, compounds such as gasoline, kerosene, and lighter fluid contain a high percentage of aromatic hydrocarbons. These solutions have a low viscosity and low surface tension, and can spread over mucosal surfaces easily and rapidly. Consequently, their risk for aspiration is greatest. Table 3 illustrates some of the common petroleum distillates listed by decreasing order of volatility (and hence toxicity) or increasing order of viscosity.

TABLE 3. *Common petroleum distillates*[a]

Petroleum ether (benzine)
Gasoline
Turpentine
Mineral spirits
Kerosene
Fuel oil
Mineral seal oil
Petrolatum
Lubricating oils
Paraffin wax
Asphalt (tar)

[a]Listed in decreasing order of volatility, or increasing order of viscosity.

MECHANISM OF HYDROCARBON TOXICITY

The two most common routes of exposure for hydrocarbons are inhalation and ingestion. The clinical manifestations of hydrocarbon poisoning are, for the most part, similar, regardless of the hydrocarbon ingested.

Ingestion is the more common route of exposure encountered in acute accidental hydrocarbon poisonings. When ingested, hydrocarbons produce their toxic effects on several organ systems including the lung, CNS, gastrointestinal tract, liver, and heart. Among these, the greatest involvement occurs with the pulmonary system, and aspiration pneumonitis is the greatest cause of morbidity and mortality (5).

In the past, some authorities believed that CNS depression was a serious complication of hydrocarbon ingestion. Therefore, whenever a hydrocarbon ingestion occurred, it was thought that the poison should be quickly removed (the implications of this procedure will be discussed later). However, based on the clinical studies reported more recently, CNS depression occurs in fewer than 30% of the patients who have ingested a petroleum distillate (16). In fact, it is not clear if CNS involvement following hydrocarbon ingestion is due to a direct effect on the CNS or occurs secondary to hypoxic cerebral damage resulting from the chemical-induced pneumonitis (12,26). Animal studies have shown that ingested hydrocarbons are only absorbed in small amounts (15,23,25). This supports the theory that hypoxia is probably responsible for the major CNS effects associated with hydrocarbon aspiration.

From a chemical standpoint the highly volatile aromatic hydrocarbons (e.g., gasoline, petroleum ether, toluene, turpentine, xylene, etc.) are associated with a greater risk for CNS toxicity due to their high lipid solubility.

The most serious and potentially lethal complication of hydrocarbon ingestion is the development of a chemical pneumonitis (5,12). Pulmonary toxicity is primarily related to aspiration of the poison that occurs either during ingestion or vomiting (26).

Another controversy over the years regards whether or not hydrocarbons will reach the lungs in sufficient concentration to incite pulmonary toxicity following gastrointestinal absorption. There are four lines of evidence that suggest pulmonary damage results from aspiration of the hydrocarbon through the trachea, and not by circulating via the blood.

First of all, animal studies have shown that if a sublethal dose of a hydrocarbon is placed directly into the stomach, with the esophagus ligated to physically prevent the poison from coming into contact with the trachea, little or no pulmonary damage occurs (10,15,23,25). The second line of evidence is based on another series of animal studies by Gerarde (7). He showed that the LD_{50} ratio of oral-to-intratracheal instillation of kerosene is 140:1, and concluded that large quantities (amounts in excess of 100 ml) must be swallowed to note significant gastric absorption that would induce pulmonary damage. As we learned earlier, most victims, especially children whose volume of a swallow is estimated to be 4 to 5 ml (11), do not swallow these large quantities. The fact remains, aspiration-induced chemical pneumonitis is the most frequent complication in hydrocarbon ingestions (1,2,12,14).

The third factor is the time course of onset of pathological changes in the lung. It is rapid, which is more suggestive of aspiration rather than absorption (7).

The final line of evidence comes from chest roentgenographic findings showing that the lesions observed are more consistent with aspiration than systemic absorption and distribution to the lungs (7).

The results of animal studies provide further support for the theory that aspiration is the primary hazard associated with hydrocarbon ingestion (15,25). Using all the experimental data cited, the following can be concluded. Hydrocarbons are absorbed from the gastrointestinal tract in very small quantities. Aromatic hydrocarbons are absorbed to a greater degree than aliphatic hydrocarbons. Except for ingestion of large quantities (>15 ml/kg) of highly volatile aromatic hydrocarbons, the amount absorbed is not sufficient to be directly responsible for the CNS toxicity.

The physiochemical properties of hydrocarbons are also important factors which are responsible for the increased incidence of aspiration among certain hydrocarbons. From Gerarde's animal studies (7), the risk of aspiration and lung damage is directly proportional to volatility, and indirectly related to surface tension and viscosity. That is, hydrocarbons that are most likely to be aspirated are highly volatile and have a low surface tension and viscosity. These properties permit the hydrocarbon to "creep" up the wall of the esophagus and enter the trachea. Hydrocarbons are also gastric irritants, and spontaneous vomiting sometimes occurs during which there is a greater chance for entry into the trachea (see Fig. 3 in Chapter 3).

CLINICAL MANIFESTATIONS OF HYDROCARBON POISONING

Clinical symptoms are, for the most part, similar regardless of the hydrocarbon ingested. Not all substances cause clinically significant problems, however, and certain substances have greater affinity for one tissue site over another (Table 4).

A variety of organ systems are affected by hydrocarbons. The toxic effects associated with each of these systems are listed in Table 5. Following an acute ingestion, the most outstand-

TABLE 4. *Hydrocarbon tissue sensitivities*

Hydrocarbon substance	CNS depression	Pulmonary pathology
Turpentine	3+	1+
Petroleum ether	4+	0
Gasoline	3+	2+
Mineral spirit	3+	3+
Kerosene	1+	2+
Diesel oil	1+	1+
Mineral seal oil	1+	4+
Mineral oil (liquid petrolatum)	0	1+[a]
Lubricating oils		1+[a]

[a]Aspiration may cause low-grade pneumonia.
From ref. 26.

TABLE 5. *Characteristics of hydrocarbon inhalation and ingestion*

System	Effect
Blood	Aplastic anemia (especially if sickle cell disease present), leukopenia, thrombocytopenia, hemolysis, leukemia
Gastrointestinal	Burning and stinging in mouth, throat, esophagus, and stomach; gagging, nausea and vomiting, diarrhea, bloody vomiting and stool. Frequently have odor of substance (e.g., gasoline) on breath
Heart	Atrial flutter, nodal rhythms, ST–T wave changes, ventricular tachycardia, and fibrillation
Hepatic	Hepatocellular necrosis, hepatomegaly, fatty degeneration
Metabolic	Metabolic acidosis (elevated anionic gap)
Neurologic	Euphoria, stupor, agitation, delirium, coma; slurred speech; hallucinations, blurred vision; ataxia and difficult ambulation; tremor, and choreiform movements; depressed or hyperactive reflexes; EEG changes
Renal	Tubular acidosis, acute tubular necrosis
Respiratory	Cough (may be bloody), shortness of breath, dyspnea, pneumonitis, pulmonary edema, hemorrhagic conditions
Skin	Irritation, blistering, transient cyanosis

From ref. 8.

ing complications are CNS depression and chemical-induced pneumonitis.

CNS symptoms may include lethargy, generalized weakness, dizziness, mental confusion, irritability, convulsions, and coma (26). Intense CNS involvement is not usually significant. Although CNS symptoms were reported by Press (18) to be in the order of 91% of poisoned persons, most patients were only lethargic. Another 5% were semicomatose, 3% comatose, and 1% experienced seizures. CNS symptoms are more likely to occur with the highly volatile aromatic hydrocarbons (5).

Pulmonary toxicity is associated with aspiration and results in severe chemical pneumonitis. Initially, there is a burning sensation in the mouth and throat which causes the victim to gag, choke, cough, and gasp for air. Signs and symptoms of pulmonary toxicity following aspiration usually progress the first 24 hr, reach a plateau, and then subside between the second and fifth day (6).

Chest roentgenograms will show abnormalities within 30 min of aspiration, and almost all patients with lung involvement have positive signs of chemical pneumonitis within 12 hr (6).

As the hydrocarbon enters the lung, it causes intense local irritation resulting in inflammation, edema, hemorrhagic bronchopneumonia, and atelectasis (5). Postmortem examination of the lung reveals interstitial inflammation, hyperemia, vascular thrombosis, intraalveolar hemorrhage, bronchial and bronchiolar epithelial necrosis, and polymorphonuclear exudation (26).

A retrospective study of 950 children who ingested a petroleum distillate between 1969 and 1979 revealed the extent and outcome of the hydrocarbon ingestion problem (1). Eight hundred were asymptomatic at the time of examination and remained so for a 6- to 8-hr observation period. None exhibited abnormal chest films and all were treated as outpatients. The other 150 displayed symptoms of pneumonitis and were admitted for treatment.

The quantity of poison could be estimated in only 138 patients. In 67% of these persons the quantity was believed to be less than 30 ml.

Spontaneous vomiting occurred in 39% of those 150 patients who were hospitalized.

Vomiting occurred more often when the ingested substance was furniture polish, rather than gasoline, paint thinner, kerosene, or lighter fluid, but these differences were not significant. Furniture polish and lighter fluid caused more symptoms and roentgenographic evidence of pneumonitis in hospitalized children.

A definite correlation was shown between the presence of fever at or above 38°C and the observation of roentgenographic-detected damage. There was no correlation between the degree of fever and extent of pulmonary damage, however.

One hundred thirty-six (of the 150) children experienced no progressive pulmonary damage and most were discharged within 72 hr of ingestion. Fourteen experienced progressive respiratory symptoms. Two died of respiratory failure, one developed secondary pneumonia due to *Staphylococcus aureus*, and four required ventilatory support.

TREATMENT OF HYDROCARBON INGESTION

Many of the theories and procedures that are reported for managing hydrocarbon poisoning are based on the results of animal studies and, thus, they cannot always be directly related to clinical intoxication. Additionally, numerous hypotheses exist as to the correct method of antidoting hydrocarbon ingestion, and not everyone is in agreement. The conclusion is that there are no absolute procedures that should always be followed, and whereas most theories are at least partially correct, there are also some others that are partially incorrect.

One of the early determinations that must be made is to identify the specific hydrocarbon ingested and determine its potential for aspiration and systemic toxicity. As we pointed out earlier, not all hydrocarbons have the same potential for producing these specific toxic effects, and knowing the identity of the specific poison may help to determine what supplemental therapy must be used.

The victim of a liquid hydrocarbon ingestion should be examined by qualified emergency personnel as soon as possible. Consideration must be given to the degree of respiratory distress, extent of CNS symptoms, and radiographic evidence of hydrocarbon-induced pneumonitis before specific treatment can be suggested.

One of the overriding questions confronting an emergency-room attendant is whether the ingested hydrocarbon should be removed from the stomach. This question has been debated over the years and is still one of the most controversial subjects in clinical toxicology. There are many ways to examine the problem.

For example, if the quantity of hydrocarbon ingested is sufficient to cause intense CNS depression, the patient may be better off if the substance is removed. On the other hand, if the hydrocarbon substance is removed, by emesis or gastric lavage, and some of it should find its way into the trachea which would increase the risk of pulmonary complications, the patient may be better off to risk absorption and take his chance with the former problem. CNS sedation is usually easier to manage medically than most pulmonary complications.

The following guidelines can be used to determine the necessity of gastric emptying (8,26). It is indicated for hydrocarbon ingestions containing any quantity of aromatic hydrocarbons (benzene, toluene), halogenated hydrocarbons, heavy metals, camphor, or pesticides. For hydrocarbons such as naphtha, gasoline, kerosene, and turpentine, gastric evacuation is recommended only when the amount ingested exceeds 1 ml/kg. Thus, an average 70-kg man would need to swallow more than 70 ml (2.3 oz) before it would be removed. Gastric emptying is not indicated in those individuals who have spontaneously vomited, or have ingested a nonvolatile hydrocarbon (e.g., lubricating oil, mineral seal oil), and, of course, for those persons without a gag reflex or who are comatose or convulsing.

The next dilemma is: When the decision to empty the stomach has been made, should emesis be induced or gastric lavage be performed?

The present consensus is that emesis is preferred over gastric lavage.

Ng et al. (17) investigated this controversy in a retrospective study of 255 victims of petroleum distillate or turpentine poisoning. Twenty-nine percent of these victims received syrup of ipecac to induce vomiting and 16% received gastric lavage. On careful follow-up of those patients treated with ipecac syrup, 19% of the group were unchanged or worse than at the time of initial observation. This was contrasted with 39% of patients in the group that received gastric lavage and had worsened. The conclusion was that pneumonitis was more significant when gastric lavage was instituted to remove the poison from the stomach. Therefore, most clinicians believe that gastric lavage should be reserved only for the drowsy or stuporous patient with proven recent ingestion of hydrocarbon substance in excess of 30 ml, or if the hydrocarbon was the vehicle for a more toxic substance (e.g., a pesticide, heavy metal, etc.). If the removal of the hydrocarbon is indicated and there is no gag reflex present, gastric lavage is indicated, but the airway must first be protected.

In the past, numerous attempts have been made to reduce absorption of ingested hydrocarbon by giving the patient doses of activated charcoal or various oily substances. For the former, activated charcoal has not been shown to significantly affect the systemic absorption of hydrocarbons. Various oils of mineral and vegetable sources have been used to increase the viscosity of ingested hydrocarbons, and thus decrease the absorption as well as reduce the chance for aspiration during the act of vomiting. Some authorities advocate that oils also act as demulcents and cathartics and, therefore, should be beneficial.

However, in most studies where oils have been given, they have not shown clinical significance in reducing hydrocarbon absorption, and most emergency care personnel do not recommend their use. In fact, oil may actually enhance hydrocarbon absorption (Fig. 1). Gerarde (7) demonstrated that rats dosed with kerosene by intragastric intubation had higher blood levels

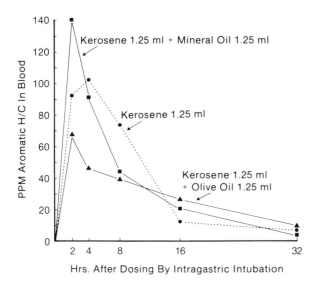

FIG. 1. Effect of olive oil and mineral oil on kerosene absorption. (From ref. 7.)

when mineral oil was given than when it was withheld.

Not all hydrocarbon substances are absorbed from the gastrointestinal tract. Whereas mineral seal oil, for example, is quite toxic if aspirated, there is no evidence it is significantly absorbed (20). Thus, there is little value in risking damage to the lungs by inducing emesis or lavage.

There is also the chance that even greater pulmonary damage will occur should the added oil be aspirated during emesis. Since complications resulting from systemic absorption are minor compared to those of pulmonary aspiration, any attempt to reduce absorption, in an otherwise healthy patient, is probably not warranted.

Much of the treatment for hydrocarbon ingestion is symptomatic and largely supportive. This includes providing oxygen when needed, placing the patient in a croup tent, providing intravenous fluids, controlling fever with antipyretics, and assuring careful monitoring by qualified medical personnel.

Glucocorticoid and antibiotic usage have been advocated in past years, but neither is considered beneficial. Antibiotics are indicated if infections occur, but should only be given at that time. Most pulmonary complications are nonbacterial (3). Glucocorticosteroids may actually increase the patient's chance of developing pulmonary bacterial infections by lowering the immune system response (9,24). An intermediate positive pressure breathing device (IPPB) may be employed, but because of the extremely delicate nature of the distal alveoli and airways during hydrocarbon poisoning, this may worsen the condition (8,12).

SUMMARY

Numerous products in the home are composed of hydrocarbon-containing substances. Many of these are not generally recognized as the extremely potent poisons they really are and, consequently, they are not stored or used properly. A good example is the red, or lemon-scented furniture polish product that we leave carelessly unattended. The suggestions outlined in this chapter on antidoting any ingested hydrocarbon poison must be adhered to.

Case Studies

CASE STUDIES: HYDROCARBON INTOXICATION

History: Case 1

A 19-month-old male was admitted to an emergency facility 24 hr following the ingestion of an unknown quantity of kerosene. The baby was given castor oil at home prior to losing consciousness.

On admission, the child was lavaged. His respirations were rapid (rate not reported), but not grunting. He had a temperature of 101°F, and pulse rate of 104 beats/min. He soon regained consciousness.

On roentgenologic examination, the medial aspect of both lower lung fields showed numerous coarse mottled densities. WBC count was 11,500 and the differential was normal. The child recovered in several days without additional treatment and with no apparent sequellae. (See ref. 14.)

History: Case 2

In a suicide attempt, a 40-year-old male injected himself intravenously with 3 ml of charcoal lighter fluid. He began complaining of burning chest pains and dyspnea about 2 to 3 hr later. He appeared at the emergency department the following morning with severe pleuritic chest pain, epigastric discomfort, and shortness of breath.

The following represent the clinical course:

Hospital admission	24 Hr later
Temperature: 38.1°C	Temperature: 38.1°C
Blood pressure: 100/58 mm Hg	Respiration rate: 30–60/min
Respiratory rate: 32/min	Bloody sputum: gram stain, numerous polys
Pulse rate: 100/min	Treatment: methylprednisolone
Chest examination: tachypnea, bibasilar rales	
Chest roentgenogram: diffuse fluffy infiltrates	

Radiographic studies of the lungs made between the 4th and 12th days showed steady improvement in pulmonary pathology. Repeated studies at 6, 12, and 18 months showed no residual abnormalities. (See ref. 22.)

Discussion

1. What is the significance of the production of a bloody pneumonitis? Would the same kind of pulmonary pathology be observed if the hydrocarbon was ingested (assuming greater quantities were ingested, of course)?

2. Both cases involved the production of a low-grade fever. Why were antibiotics not given? Are they indicated and, if so, what would be the antimicrobial therapy preferred?

3. In Case 1, the baby was given castor oil at home. Comment, please!

4. Where would the victim in Case 2 have found naphtha (e.g., what types of products contain this substance)?

Review Questions

1. List the following hydrocarbon substances in decreasing order of likelihood for causing symptoms of pulmonary damage: turpentine, mineral seal oil, gasoline, mineral spirit.

2. Which of the following is a true statement?
   A. Hydrocarbon substances that have a low viscosity are most likely to be aspirated.
   B. Glucocorticoids have been shown to reduce pulmonary complications of aspirated hydrocarbon substances.
   C. Poisoning by ingestion of turpentine should be antidoted similarly as for kerosene.
   D. CNS depression is the most severe and potentially dangerous symptom of hydrocarbon intoxication.

3. A distinction must be made between the incidence of poisoning by hydrocarbon substances and the severity of intoxication. Discuss these points.

4. The decision whether or not to remove ingested petroleum distillate from the stomach may be based on the quantity of substance swallowed. What is the rule of thumb for making the decision to go ahead with emesis?

5. Describe the relationship between a hydrocarbon compound's surface tension and its potential for aspiration.

6. When the decision has been made to remove gasoline from the stomach of a conscious, noncombative patient, which is the preferred method?
   A. Lavage
   B. Emesis

7. What characteristic of petroleum distillates is closely associated with great risk for CNS toxicity?

8. Discuss the use of intermittent positive pressure breathing devices in treating hydrocarbon poisoning.

9. Petroleum distillates absorbed into the systemic circulation cause a high incidence of pulmonary pathology.
   A. True
   B. False

10. Discuss the reasons why the quantity of gasoline that actually enters the lungs during aspiration is probably quite small.

11. Why is it stated that a victim of poisoning by certain pesticide products should be antidoted for petroleum distillate toxicity rather than the pesticide, per se?

12. Which of the following has proven antidotal activity in reducing the toxicity of petroleum distillates: antipyretics (I), mineral oil (II), or activated charcoal (III)?
    A. I only
    B. III only
    C. I and II only
    D. I and III only

13. Damage to the CNS by ingested hydrocarbons may be primary or secondary. What does this mean?

14. Antibiotics are sometimes indicated as part of the treatment for hydrocarbon poisoning. What is the indication for antiinfective therapy?

References

1. Anas, N., Namasonthi, V., and Ginsburg, C. M. (1981): Criteria for hospitalizing children who have ingested products containing hydrocarbons. *JAMA*, 246:840–843.
2. Beamon, R. F., Siegel, C. J., Landers, G., and Green, V. (1976): Hydrocarbon ingestion in children: A six-year retrospective study. *J. Am. Coll. Emerg. Phys.*, 5:771–775.
3. Brown, J., Burke, B., and Dajani, A. S. (1974): Experimental kerosene pneumonia: Evaluation of some therapeutic regimens. *J. Pediatr.*, 84:396–401.
4. Couleton, J. L., Hirsch, W., Brillman, J., Sanandria, J., Welty, T. K., Colaiaco, P., Koros, A., and Lober, A. (1983): Gasoline sniffing and lead toxicity in Navajo adolescents. *Pediatrics*, 71:113–117.
5. Eade, N. R., Taussig, L. M., and Marks, M. I. (1974): Hydrocarbon pneumonitis. *Pediatrics*, 54:351–356.
6. Foley, J. C., Dreyer, N. B., Soule, A. B., and Woll, E. (1954): Kerosene poisoning in young children. *Radiology*, 62:817–829.
7. Gerarde, H. W. (1959): Toxicological studies on hydrocarbons. V. Kerosine. *Toxicol. Appl. Pharmacol.*, 1:462–474.
8. Goldfrank, L., Kirstein, R., and Bresnitz, E. (1979): Gasoline and other hydrocarbons. *Hosp. Physician*, September, pp. 32–79.
9. Hardman, G., Tolson, R., and Haghdassarian, O. (1960): Prednisone in the management of kerosene pneumonia. *Indian Practitioner*, 13:615.
10. Huxtable, K. A., Bolande, R. P., and Klaus, M. (1964): Experimental furniture polish pneumonia in rats. *Pediatrics*, 34:228–230.
11. Jones, O. V., and Work, C. E. (1961): Volume of a swallow. *Am. J. Dis. Child.*, 102:427.
12. Karlson, K. H. (1982): Hydrocarbon poisoning in children. *South. Med. J.*, 75:839–840.
13. Kovanen, J., Somer, H., and Schroeder, P. (1983): Acute myopathy associated with gasoline sniffing. *Neurology*, 33:629–631.
14. Lesser, L. I., Weens, H. S., and McKey, J. D. (1943): Pulmonary manifestations following ingestion of kerosene. *J. Pediatr.*, 23:352–364.
15. Mann, M. D., Pirie, D. J., and Wolfsdorf, J. (1977): Kerosene absorption in primates. *J. Pediatr.*, 91:495.
16. Moriarty, R. W. (1979): Petroleum distillate poisonings. *Drug Therapy*, 9:135–139.
17. Ng, R. C., Darwish, H., and Stewart, D. A. (1974): Emergency treatment of petroleum distillate and turpentine ingestion. *CMA Journal*, 111:537–538.
18. Press, E. (1962): Cooperative kerosene poisoning study: Evaluation of gastric lavage and other factors in the treatment of accidental ingestion of petroleum distillate products. *Pediatrics*, 29:648–674.
19. Ross, C. A. (1982): Gasoline sniffing and lead encephalopathy. *CMA Journal*, 127:195–197.
20. Rumack, B. H. (1977): Hydrocarbon ingestions in perspective. *J. Am. Coll. Emerg. Phys.*, 6:172–173.
21. US Dept HEW (1978): Tabulations of 1976 case reports. Bulletin, National Clearinghouse for Poison Control Centers, Public Health Service, Bethesda, Maryland.
22. Vaziri, N. D., Smith, P. J., and Wilson, A. F. (1980): Toxicity with intravenous injection of nephtha in man. *Clin. Toxicol.*, 16:335–343.
23. Wolfe, B. M., Brodeur, A. E., and Shields, J. B. (1970): The role of gastrointestinal absorption of kerosene in producing pneumonitis in dogs. *J. Pediatr.*, 76:867.
24. Wolfe, J. E., Bone, R. C., and Ruth, W. E. (1977): Effects of corticosteroids in the treatment of patients with gastric aspiration. *Am. J. Med.*, 63:719–722.
25. Wolfsdorf, V., and Kundig, H. (1972): Kerosene poisoning in primates. *S. Afr. Med. J.*, 46:619.
26. Zieserl, E. (1979): Hydrocarbon ingestion and poisoning. *Compr. Ther.*, 5:35–42.

Corrosives

8

The category of corrosive substances is broad in nature. It includes acids (hydrochloric, sulfuric, oxalic, phenol, etc.) and alkali (potassium hydroxide, sodium hydroxide, sodium phosphate, potassium permanganate, etc.) per se, and a large variety of miscellaneous products found in the home and work place (creosote, electric dishwasher detergents, hydrogen fluoride, toilet bowl cleaners, etc.). Their chemical and physical properties vary widely, but the expected outcome following any toxic emergency is similar, regardless of the substance ingested. They all produce considerable tissue damage, but the site at which the damage occurs and the specific form of damage differ, depending on the corrosive. Table 1 lists some common acidic and alkaline corrosive products.

Most households contain a wide variety of corrosive substances that invite curious children to examine, or adults to use inappropriately. The toxic potential of most of these substances is obvious to adults, and they are avoided. All of them are extremely irritating to mucous membranes, and thus massive intentional ingestions are rare. On the other hand, even small quantities (in the range of one milliliter of liquid or a single granule of a solid) can be fatal to an adult, and especially a child, within a short period of time. Children have been known to suffer intense injury from these small quantities that required many years to medically and surgically correct. These injuries occurred, for example, when they drank the remaining few drops of a liquid corrosive from an otherwise appar-

TABLE 1. *Examples of common acids and alkalis*

Acid
  Hydrochloric acid
    Metal cleaners
    Muriatic acid
    Swimming pool cleaners
    Toilet bowl cleaners
  Sulfuric acid
    Battery acid
    Toilet bowl and drain cleaners
Alkali
  Sodium or potassium hydroxide
    Clinitest® tablets
    Detergents
    Drano® crystals
    Drain pipe and toilet bowl cleaners
    Lye
    Paint removers
    Washing powders
Others
  Ammonia (NH₄OH) solutions (hair products,
    jewelry cleaners, household cleaners)
  Electric dishwashing granules
  Potassium permanganate
  Sodium carbonate (nonphosphate) detergents
  Sodium hypochlorite (bleach)

From ref. 8.

ently empty container that had been discarded in the wastebasket (12).

Many other corrosive substances are not generally recognized as being dangerous, so few special precautions are taken to keep them away from an inquisitive child's reach, or to make sure that adults use them properly. For example, rust removers (oxalic acid), electric dishwasher detergents, and citrus-scented bowl cleaners fall into this category.

The first literature citation describing toxicologic damage from ingestion of a corrosive substance dates back to 1828 and involved sulfuric acid (15). The incidence of poisoning with these items has continued to increase over the years due to a great surge in production of corrosive substances. Tissue damage from corrosives is listed among the major types of poisoning emergencies that occur in the home.

It has been variously reported that 1.7 to 9.6% of all accidental ingestions by children involve alkali or acids (17). The major reason for the incidence of corrosive poisonings among children is that too many of these toxic substances are stored in old, unmarked beverage containers (23). Among adults, corrosive poisonings are often related to suicide attempts (3).

Traditionally the term *corrosive* denotes an *acidic* substance capable of inflicting tissue injury. *Caustic* describes an *alkaline* substance having similar properties.

The Federal Hazardous Substance Act of 1967 specifically defined the term corrosive as any substance that, in contact with living tissue, will cause destruction of tissue by chemical action (10). This definition does not differentiate acids from bases. Throughout this chapter and book, the term corrosive is used to encompass both extremes of pH, except where specifically indicated.

ACIDS

Strong acids are defined as substances with a pH below 2. However, some substances (e.g., lemon juice, carbonated beverages, etc.) can have a strongly acidic pH but not be corrosive.

Included under this topic is a wide variety of inorganic (sulfuric, hydrochloric-muriatic, nitric, phosphoric, etc.) and organic (oxalic, tartaric, acetic, etc.) acids. Even though acids can produce similar tissue damage, but differing in intensity, and even though all can cause systemic problems, not all are common causes of poisoning (e.g., nitric acid, phosphoric acid), and not all are sufficiently corrosive to be of major toxicological concern (e.g., acetic acid, tartaric acid).

Corrosive damage is caused by direct chemical action on the involved tissue. The resulting lesion represents a form of *coagulative necrosis*, meaning that the acid denatures all tissue protein to form an acid proteinate. As a result, both structural and enzymatic proteins are denatured, and cell lysis is blocked. Therefore, cell morphology is not greatly interrupted. In addition, a firm scab (eschar) is formed which delays further corrosive damage and helps reduce systemic absorption. Thus, damage, especially with small quantities of acid, is frequently limited to local sites of injury to the skin or the gastrointestinal tract, rather than to systemic responses.

Following acid ingestion, an intense corrosive damage to the oral mucosa and esophagus may be seen, but most significant damage is limited to the stomach (Table 2). The involved areas frequently appear brown or black (except for picric and nitric acids which stain tissue yellow). Precipitated blood may be found in the stomach and is described as having a "coffee-grounds" consistency. Damaged gastric glands are usually not regenerated, but are replaced by a thin epithelial layer. Gastric motility is also disrupted (15).

Ingested acid normally passes through the esophagus quickly and, therefore, causes little damage to this structure. Studies have shown that esophageal damage occurs in as few as 6 to 20% of all acid ingestions (3,6). This is not to imply that severe damage could not result if acid were left in contact with the esophageal tissue. A 9% sulfuric acid solution for 30 sec caused coagulative necrosis in one study (1). Therefore, esophageal damage is usually minimal and is a function of the volume ingested, acid strength, and time of contact. Thus, emetics are contraindicated in acid ingestions, since they would increase the contact time.

Strong mineral acids, such as sulfuric, are much more likely to cause gastric necrosis and perforation than weaker ones such as hydrochloric. However, chronic gastric problems are reported more frequently following hydrochloric acid ingestion, rather than sulfuric acid. This may be due to the severity of damage that oc-curs from sulfuric acid ingestion. Victims of the latter are more likely to die shortly after ingestion.

Table 3 lists case reports in the English language that describe toxic events following acid ingestion, from 1930 to 1979. From the table it can be seen that the premorbid condition of the stomach is a fairly good predictor of the gastric site of toxic injury. In patients with a full stomach before acid ingestion, the damage was mainly confined to pyloric and lesser curvature regions. For those victims with a fluid-filled stomach, damage was proximal and generalized. For fasting persons, acid ingestion caused antral damage as well as a wide variety of other involvements.

Damage to the small intestine, as a result of acid ingestion, is rare. This most likely relates to pylorospasm induced by the acid which limits its entry into the duodenum.

Penner (15) has written an excellent review of the pathogenesis of acid toxicity. For further information this source should be consulted. Table 4 lists major characteristics that have been reported for acid and base poisonings, according to the route of exposure.

Management of Acid Poisoning

Poisoning by acid, locally or systemically, should be considered a medical emergency and treatment must be initiated at once. Unfortunately, even though reports of acid ingestion and resultant toxicity continue to appear in the literature, there are still too few good clinical studies that have related pathogenesis to the best therapeutic management. The rules of treatment presented in this chapter have been established based on clinical experience; they do not always receive universal acceptance.

Skin Contamination

Contamination of the skin or eye with acid must be given immediate attention. The area should be thoroughly washed with large quantities of lukewarm water. A 15 to 20 min wash is necessary to completely neutralize and remove all residual traces of the contaminant.

TABLE 2. *Sites and types of damage following ingestion of a corrosive[a]*

Corrosive type	Site of injury	Type of injury
Acid	Stomach	Coagulative necrosis
Base	Esophagus	Liquefactive necrosis

[a]Tissue damage by corrosives is a function of numerous factors (see text). The information presented in this table represents the classic situation, but may vary depending on these factors.

TABLE 3. *Reported cases of acid ingestion*[a]

Report	Acid	Premorbid state of stomach	Almost entire stomach	Proximal body	Lesser curvature	Antrum	Pylorus	Associated injuries
1.	HNO	Full			x		x	
	H_2SO_4	Full			x		x	
	H_2SO_4	Full			x		x	
2.	HCl	Unknown				x		
3.	HCl	Unknown			x	x		
4.	H_2SO_4	Unknown				x		
5.	H_2SO_4	Unknown				x	x	
6.	HNO_3	Unknown					x	Subsequent gastric carcinoma; duodenal involvement
7.	HCl	Probably fluid-filled		x				
8.	HCl	Fluid-filled	x					
9.	HCl	Unknown		x				
10.	HCl	Empty	Some	Slight	x	x	x	
11.	HCl	Unknown				x	x	
12.	HCl	4 hr postprandial	x					Esophagus
13.	HCl	Full				x	x	
14.	HCl	Empty				x		
15.	HCl	Probably full			x	x		
16.	HCl	Unknown		x		x		
	HCl	Unknown				x		
17.	HCl	Unknown		x	x	x	x	
	HCl	Unknown			x	x		
	HCl	Unknown				x	x	
	HCl	Unknown	x		x			Esophagus
18.	HCl	Empty			x	x	x	Duodenum
19.	HCl	Empty	x					
20.	HCl	Unknown	x					Extensive necrotizing gastritis and proximal enteritis
21.	HCl	Unknown				x	x	
22.	HCl	Unknown			x	x		
23.	HCl	Unknown			x	x		
24.	H_2SO_4	Unknown					x	Esophagus
25.	H_2SO_4	Empty	Not clear	x		x	x	Duodenum, jejunum, proximal ileum
	H_2SO_4	Probably empty				x		Esophagus
	HCl	Unknown	x				x	Esophagus
	NH_4Cl Phenol	Unknown	Not clear			x		Duodenum, jejunum, proximal ileum
26.	Unknown acid	Fluid-filled	x			x	x	Duodenum
27.	H_2SO_4	Unknown				x	x	
	HCl	Unknown			x	x	x	Mild esophagitis
	HCl	Unknown	Some			x	x	Duodenum
28.	HCl	Unknown				x	x	
	HCl	Unknown				x	x	
	HCl	Unknown				x		
29.	H_2SO_4	Unknown	x					Duodenum
	H_2SO_4	Unknown	x					
	H_2SO_4	Unknown				x		Esophagus
30.	H_2SO_4	Unknown	x					
	H_2SO_4	Unknown	x					Pneumonitis, duodenum
	H_2SO_4	Unknown				x	x	Distal esophagus
31.	H_2SO_4	Unknown	x			x	x	Minor esophageal
32.	H_2SO_4	Unknown				x	x	Esophagus, duodenum

[a]Reported for the period 1930–1979.
From ref. 15.

TABLE 4. *Clinical manifestations of corrosive toxicity*

Acute poisoning	
Route of exposure	Signs and symptoms
Ingestion	Severe burning pain in mouth, throat, and abdomen
	Vomiting (possibly blood-tinged)
	Diarrhea (bloody, mucoid)
	Stains around mouth
	Dysphagia, drooling
	Hypotension
Inhalation	Bronchial irritation
	Pulmonary edema
	Frothy sputum
	Moist rales
	Hypotension
	Hemoptysis
	Dyspnea
Dermal	Staining of skin
	Burning pain
Ocular	Conjunctivitis
	Corneal destruction
	Pain, lacrimation
	Photophobia

Contaminated clothing and jewelry should be removed from the skin, and contact lenses, if present, should be removed from the eye to avoid prolonged contact of acid with the area.

A mild soap solution may be used for washing the skin and as an aid in neutralizing the acid, but should not be placed into the eye. After washing, no cream, ointment, or dressing of any kind should ever be applied to the affected area. These may cause further tissue damage to an already damaged skin or eye, and make it difficult for emergency room personnel to remove them without causing additional irritation and intense pain.

Systemic Ingestion

Management of ingested acid is outlined in Fig. 1. Initial treatment primarily involves dilution with either water or milk. However, any reported advantage of milk over water is probably not significant, and water should always be the first choice. Under no circumstances should carbonated beverages ever be used, be-cause large quantities of carbon dioxide gas are released which quickly distend the stomach wall. This distension imposes a greater chance for perforation of already weakened tissues, and may hasten the time for gastric emptying. Additionally, this reaction is exothermic and heat released may cause further injury to the stomach. The clinical significance of this reaction is unknown at this time (14).

Frequently when managing a victim of acid ingestion, the corrosive action is treated by dilution, but damage due to exothermic heat production is ignored. This results in the following dilemma: "To dilute (neutralize) or not dilute—that is the question!" The amount of heat released when strong acids come in contact with water or antacids is tremendous, and must always be considered when contemplating dilution of ingested acids.

For example, a 55-ml quantity of sulfuric acid, 91.6% by weight, mixed with 54 ml water will result almost instantaneously in a solution with a temperature of 79°C. If the 55-ml sample of acid is diluted with water to 1000 ml, the temperature still rises to 14°C (15). From basic chemistry we can recall that when water is added to sulfuric acid (as opposed to the reverse) it results in an explosive release of steam and heat. The resulting diluted solution still has a pH of zero and is highly corrosive.

Mixed with antacids, heat also forms. The heat of neutralization of 1 mole sulfuric acid with magnesium hydroxide suspension (80 mg/ml) is approximately 40 kcal. Approximately 730 ml of anatacid would be required to neutralize the acid, and final temperature of the mixture would be about 62°C (15).

Emesis must be avoided to prevent recurrent damage to a possibly already damaged esophagus. If a large quantity of acid has been swallowed, gastric lavage should be considered (15). Caution must be exercised so that the lavage tube does not cause perforation. Sometimes lubricating the tube with glycerin is helpful in preventing perforation.

When lavage is planned, it is best to perform it as soon as the diagnosis of acid ingestion has

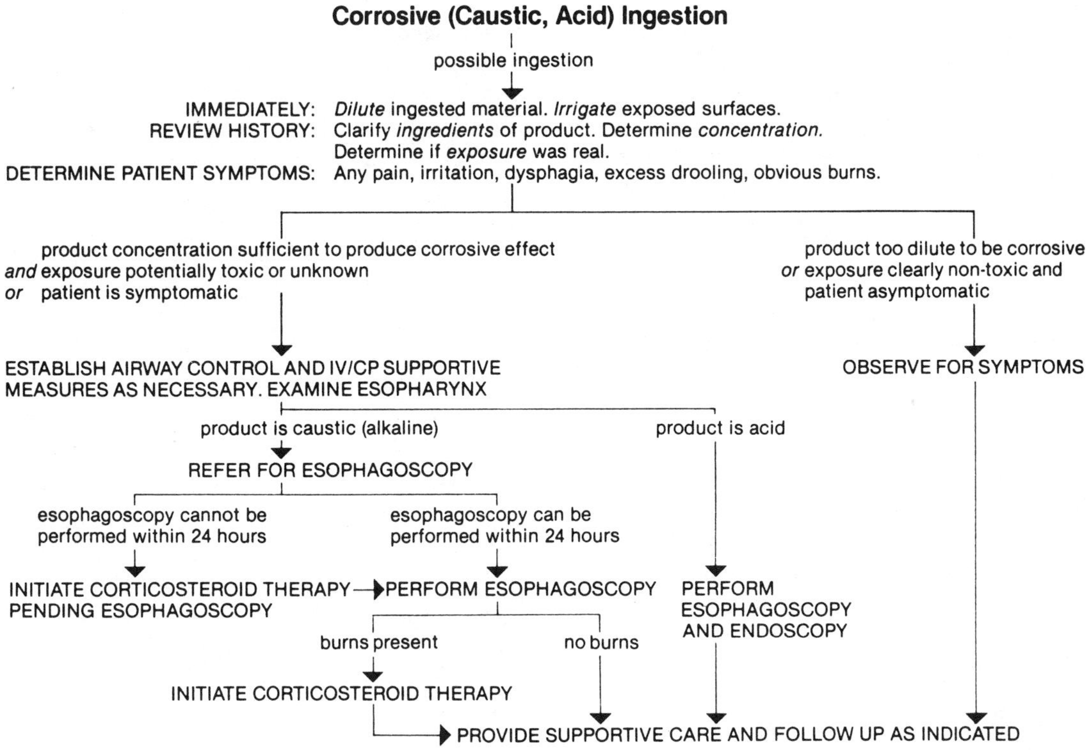

Corrosive (Caustic, Acid) Ingestion

possible ingestion

IMMEDIATELY: *Dilute* ingested material. *Irrigate* exposed surfaces.
REVIEW HISTORY: Clarify *ingredients* of product. Determine *concentration*.
Determine if *exposure* was real.
DETERMINE PATIENT SYMPTOMS: Any pain, irritation, dysphagia, excess drooling, obvious burns.

product concentration sufficient to produce corrosive effect
and exposure potentially toxic or unknown
or patient is symptomatic

product too dilute to be corrosive
or exposure clearly non-toxic and
patient asymptomatic

ESTABLISH AIRWAY CONTROL AND IV/CP SUPPORTIVE
MEASURES AS NECESSARY. EXAMINE ESOPHARYNX

OBSERVE FOR SYMPTOMS

product is caustic (alkaline)   product is acid

REFER FOR ESOPHAGOSCOPY

esophagoscopy cannot be   esophagoscopy can be
performed within 24 hours   performed within 24 hours

INITIATE CORTICOSTEROID THERAPY→PERFORM ESOPHAGOSCOPY   PERFORM
PENDING ESOPHAGOSCOPY   ESOPHAGOSCOPY
                                                                 AND ENDOSCOPY

burns present   no burns

INITIATE CORTICOSTEROID THERAPY

PROVIDE SUPPORTIVE CARE AND FOLLOW UP AS INDICATED

FIG. 1. Flow chart illustrating the steps involved in assessment and management of a victim of corrosive ingestion. (Reproduced with permission of The Soap and Detergent Association.)

been confirmed. First, the acid is suctioned out of the stomach as completely as possible. This will reduce the amount of heat produced. Cold water or milk can then be used as the lavage fluid, followed by antacid washes. The tube should be repositioned frequently to assure that all traces of acid have been removed.

Surgical resection of damaged tissue is sometimes advised, but has not proven to be beneficial. It is not always possible to easily identify the area of damage, and after resection, leaking may occur at anastomoses. When tissue has been damaged beyond repair, it is usually removed surgically.

The remaining treatment is largely supportive. Acids, unlike alkali, do not produce their entire range of toxic damage immediately and, in fact, injury may continue to develop over 90 or more minutes (16). Thus, the patient must be closely monitored over this period and treat-

ment continued, even in the absence of perceptible or worsening symptoms.

Hydrogen fluoride causes damage of a nature that differs from other acids just considered, and therefore it is described separately.

Hydrogen fluoride is a widely used industrial compound that exists as a colorless, volatile liquid which is extremely corrosive. Its commercial uses, besides etching glass and cleaning metal, include production of various synthetic chemicals, and it is a fuel source in certain types of rockets. Industrial smoke often contains high levels of hydrogen fluoride because it is evolved from burning coal.

Hydrogen fluoride causes deep corrosive lesions on the skin or tissues. It has a high affinity for water and, consequently, rapidly hydrolyzes to hydrochloric acid even in the air.

Most deaths have been attributed to pulmonary complications following breathing of hydrogen fluoride gas. On the other hand, systemic absorption can occur through the skin. This can result in acute fluoride poisoning that primarily involves the gastrointestinal tract, brain, kidney, and liver. Chronic exposure has produced skeletal fluorosis (i.e., osteosclerosis, periosteal appositions of bone, and calcification of ligaments and joints) (5). Thus, fluoride poisoning leads to hypocalcemia and its associated sequela, and to hypomagnesemia. Intoxication by sodium fluoride used as an insecticide is discussed in more depth in Chapter 9.

ALKALI

Alkaline substances may be defined as chemicals that have a pH of 11.5 or higher. Careful examination of the label of any substance known to be alkaline is sometimes misleading when trying to determine the degree of alkalinity. For example, a reported pH value of a product intended to be diluted before use may refer either to the concentrated or to the diluted form. So the importance of a principle previously discussed once again becomes relevant. That is, always read the label carefully.

One way to establish the degree of alkalinity is to report the potency as a percent of sodium hydroxide. The majority of household alkaline products contain this information, and a concentration of sodium hydroxide greater than 1% can cause tissue damage (14). The degree of injury is related to the quantity, concentration, length of exposure, and type of alkali.

In the United States the greatest number of injuries from corrosive substances involves ingestion of alkali, rather than acids. The reason is probably related to the wider availability of alkaline household products. Also, some people may not recognize the extreme toxic potential of many alkali products. While the term "acid" is a common household term, "alkali" or "base" is less readily recognized. Therefore, many alkaline substances, such as dishwasher detergents, nonphosphate detergents, etc., are stored in areas where children have easy access to them.

Most damage from ingested alkali occurs primarily to the esophagus (Table 2), with gastric involvement reported in about 20% of cases. Seventy-five percent of all caustic injury to the esophagus, in children under 5 years, is from sodium hydroxide. Eighty-three percent of these cases involve children under 3 years, and 62% are boys (2). Gastric acid, by the way, is not strong enough or present in sufficient quantity to neutralize even small quantities of strong alkali.

The physical form of an alkali substance may help to ascertain the site of caustic damage. For example, solid crystalline forms are not easily swallowed, but are not readily spit out, either. So they frequently adhere to the glossopharyngeal, palatal, and proximal esophageal mucosa to cause deep, irregular painful burns (7). Because of this adherence proximally, less damage is apt to occur at more distant sites.

Liquid alkaline substances, on the other hand, because they freely pass through the esophagus, generally cause more diffuse damage primarily to the esophagus, but will also damage the stomach (11).

Oral caustic burns cause discomfort, but despite a lack of dysphagia, esophageal injury may be present and emergency procedures must still be initiated.

Examining the mouth of a child often lends support to determine if an alkali substance was ingested. Other times, a probable diagnosis can only be made from the child's obvious distress, associated with the discovery of an overturned or partially emptied alkaline product container.

Tissue damage from alkali ingestion is a form of *liquefactive necrosis* which destroys not only the surface epithelium, but also the full tissue thickness (7). Consequently, systemic complications are common with alkali intoxication.

Esophageal damage following alkali injury occurs in stages (21). Initially, in the acute phase which manifests within 3 to 5 days, intramucosal or transmural damage involving the periesophageal tissues and structures in the mediastinum are seen. Inflammation, edema, and congestion occur throughout the entire wall of the esophagus. In intense cases, the esophagus may perforate.

The second stage occurs over the next 5 to 12 days and is characterized by liquefactive necrosis resulting in intense inflammation and edema. This is the point at which the esophageal wall is most susceptible to ulceration, bleeding, and perforation. To illustrate the intense potential for damage, a 10-sec exposure of rabbit esophagus to 7 N (22.5%) sodium hydroxide produces necrosis to all layers of the tissue. This phase is also associated with the deposition of fresh granulation tissue which eventually is replaced by collagen fibers.

Following the acute stage, healing and scarring begin. After a period, usually longer than 3 to 4 weeks, contraction and stricture are seen. Esophageal strictures are the most frequently observed complication of alkali ingestion. The usual incidence of strictures in granular or solid lye ingestions is 10 to 25% compared to approximately 100% for liquid lye (2,7).

Again, the clinical manifestations of corrosive exposures are listed in Table 4.

Management of Alkali Poisoning

Treatment of poisoning by alkali is largely similar to that of acid ingestion, and it is often just as abstract.

Skin Contamination

Skin and eye contamination should be immediately and thoroughly washed with lukewarm water for at least 15 to 20 min. All contaminated clothing and jewelry should be removed from the skin, and contact lenses, if present, removed from the eye. As with acids, no medicament should be placed on the lesion. Strong soap, of course, should not be used during or after the rinsing process.

Systemic Ingestion

Ingestion of even a single granule of solid material or a milliliter or more of a liquid caustic warrants emergency consultation by qualified medical personnel. The extent of damage cannot be estimated from presenting symptoms. If a victim displays burns around the mouth and lips, then moderate-to-severe toxicity may be suspected. However, despite an absence of observable burns in or around the mouth, severe esophageal damage may still be present. Reflex swallowing of irritating substances is so quick, the substance may be present in the mouth only for a short period.

As with acid ingestions, the treatment regimen for alkali ingestion is not standardized and there are many precautions that must be kept in mind. For example, administering an emetic is contraindicated, especially for alkali poisoning, since the primary site of toxic action is the esophagus. The risk here is twofold. First, this reexposes the esophagus to the corrosive and, second, there is the possibility of aspirating the contents to cause severe edema, inflammation, and ulceration of the glottis, and aspiration pneumonitis.

Gastric lavage is also not readily recommended for alkali ingestions, but is occasionally performed for large volumes of acid (15). Also, there is no great advantage in the use of activated charcoal, since caustics adsorb poorly to it and it interferes with the endoscopy procedure used to determine the extent of injury (8).

As a means of terminating exposure, the question of dilution or neutralization following an alkali ingestion has once again been proposed. The general recommendation is to dilute it with one or two glassfuls of milk or water. The objective is to minimize damage to the mouth, esophagus, and stomach.

Those who disagree with this approach contend that damage is instantaneous, and the resulting exothermic reaction only increases the risk of further damage and vomiting (8,15). Also, in the case of a small child, it is difficult to persuade them to drink *anything* after the ingestion of a corrosive, because of the pain and tenderness experienced. In any case, neutralization is contraindicated.

The neutralization/dilution question has been examined by Rumack and Burrington (18). In a series of *in vitro* experiments, a weighed quantity of Crystal Drano®, or a Clinitest® tablet (Table 5) was exposed to water, milk, lemon juice, and vinegar. The resulting temperature

TABLE 5. *Composition of Drano® crystals and Clinitest® tablets*

Drano® crystals	
Sodium hydroxide	54.2%
Sodium nitrate	30.45%
Aluminum shavings	4.10%
Inert substances	11.25%
Clinitest® tablets	
Sodium hydroxide	232.5 mg
Sodium carbonate	80.0 mg
Copper sulfate	20.0 mg
Citric acid	300.0 mg

was determined and plotted as shown in Figs. 2 and 3.

We can see from the figures that the choice of diluent does make a difference in the amount of heat formed and its rate of formation. Milk appears to be the diluent of choice for Clinitest® tablets. Heat production was slower when milk was added to Drano®. It is difficult to state with certainty that milk should be used to dilute Drano® crystals, since the temperature at the end of 2 min is the same as with the other diluents. However, the delayed formation of heat over the 2-min period could possibly be an advantage when lavage was being performed. If a milk solution were instilled and quickly removed, and the process were repeated as discussed above, heat-induced tissue damage should be minimized.

Lesions may develop for 24 or more hours following ingestion, so the patient must be observed closely for several days following the ingestion.

If swallowing is possible, dairy products such as ice cream and milk are allowable. As long as the individual can swallow, all medications and clear liquids can be given orally and the diet increased progressively, as tolerated.

Whenever surgery is indicated it must be done quickly. Early indications for surgery include mediastinal drainage following acute perforation, tracheostomy for laryngeal edema and respiratory distress, or a gastrostomy for feeding in acute severe injuries or extensive chronic strictures (2). Occasionally the esophagus will require reconstruction and in this case, surgery is indicated.

Steroids and Antibiotics

Glucocorticoid steroids are usually administered to reduce fibrosis and esophageal rupture following alkali ingestion. The value of steroids following an acid ingestion is questionable since esophageal stricture is less common (15). Experimentally, using corticosteroids within the first 24 to 48 hr following caustic damage results in a lessened degree of stricture (8,22). Steroids are probably most effective in preventing stricture in cases of second degree burns, are less effective in reducing damage in first

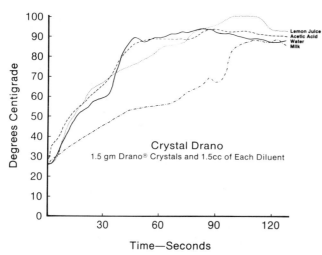

FIG. 2. The heat of reaction that occurs when various diluents are added to Crystal Drano®. (From ref. 18.)

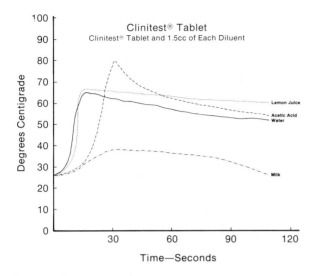

100
90
80
70
60
50
40
30
20
10
0

Clinitest® Tablet
Clinitest® Tablet and 1.5cc of Each Diluent

Degrees Centigrade

Lemon Juice
Acetic Acid
Water
Milk

30   60   90   120

Time—Seconds

FIG. 3. The heat of reaction that occurs when various diluents are added to Clinitest® tablets. (From ref. 18.)

degree burns of the esophagus, and are questionable in treating third degree burns (21,22). On the other hand, there is the possibility of an increased incidence of infection because of steroid-induced reduction of resistance, and the delay of healing in cases of severe ulceration. Antibiotics are administered to reduce further complications from microbial invasion. Therapy with both agents must be started quickly to be effective.

Bougienage

Bougienage is a procedure whereby a bougie (dilator) is passed through the esophagus to increase its caliber following stricture. Increasing the size of the dilator over a period of time aids in eventual widening of the esophageal lumen. For severe stricture, bougienage may be required over many years or a lifetime.

A flow chart that lists important decisions that must be made, and procedures to follow in the treatment of corrosive poisonings is shown in Fig. 1. This figure may be helpful when reviewing the major treatment modalities discussed in this chapter.

SUMMARY

Know when to treat a poisoning event by a corrosive item. While many elements of acidic and alkaline poisonings are similar, others may

be different. Be able to distinguish between the two, but more importantly, know what to do in case of poisoning.

Case Studies

CASE STUDY: CORROSIVE ALKALI TABLET INGESTION

History

A 38-year-old diabetic female eventually sought medical attention after ingesting 75 Clinitest® tablets (see Table 5) approximately one week before. She was nauseated immediately following the ingestion and vomited everything she tried to eat or drink. Still, she did not seek immediate medical attention. Several days later, she was seen in the emergency room for hypoglycemic coma and severe abdominal cramping. It was not until then that the patient admitted to ingesting the Clinitest® tablets.

On examination with fiberoptic endoscopy, the distal half of the esophagus showed white plaques with erythematous mucosa and ulceration surrounding them.

The endoscope was not advanced into the stomach until a week later. At that time stricture of the distal esophagus and esophagitis were observed. Three weeks later, pathologic changes in the antral portion of the stomach included contraction and ulceration. Further studies revealed esophagitis and food retained in the stomach. The duodenum appeared normal.

Treatment. The constricted esophagus was dilated with Hurst bougies. Eventually a hemigastrectomy and gastroduodenotomy were performed. On examination of the removed tissue, a benign gastric ulcer with severe adjacent fibrosis and inflammation was noted. (See ref. 9.)

Discussion

1. Following ingestion of 75 Clinitest® tablets, why did not symptoms appear sooner? Why did this patient survive?

2. What was the purpose of the Hurst bougies?

3. The endoscopic examination was undertaken quite slowly (e.g., only the proximal half of the esophagus being examined initially, with the next portion not looked at until a week later). Discuss the reason for this delay.

4. Define the terms endoscopy, hemigastrectomy, and gastroduodenotomy.

CASE STUDY: TOXICITY TO ALKALINE BATTERY INGESTION

History

A 16-month-old female presented to an emergency facility as an alert, irritable, tachypneic child. Her vital signs included: temperature, 102.2°F; pulse rate, 172 beats/min; respirations, 52/min; and blood pressure, 118/80 mm Hg. She was estimated to be 10% dehydrated.

Previous to her admission, she had a vomiting episode and developed a fever. It was not until she became progressively irritable and developed abdominal distension and tachypnea that she was brought to the hospital.

During her examination, chest X-rays revealed a round, radiopaque foreign body lodged in the upper thoracic region. At this time, the parents remembered that a battery for their camera flash attachment had been missing for about 3 days. There was no other information the family could provide at this time.

Laboratory results were all within the normal physiological limits.

Treatment. Treatment of the child began with a thoracostomy which resulted in removing about 100 ml of a straw-colored fluid mixed with black particulate matter. Following an esophagoscopy, a flat alkaline camera battery measuring approximately 22 mm × 5 mm (about the size of three stacked quarters) was recovered. There were signs of necrosis around

the esophagus and it was felt the esophagus was probably perforated.

She was given clindamycin hydrochloride intravenously, and fluid replacement. She remained stable after the operation, but was sent back to the operating room to have the mediastinum drained and a feeding gastrostomy inserted.

Approximately 2 hr postoperative she died from cardiopulmonary arrest. A large amount of blood was removed from her stomach during resuscitation attempts. (See ref. 19.)

Discussion

1. The outstanding major point to be emphasized with regard to this case report is that an object, about the thickness of three stacked quarters was swallowed and caused the child to die, not from suffocation, but from esophageal perforation. A postmortem examination showed that death was due to massive hemorrhage caused by perforation. Why did this smooth, flat object lodge in the esophagus and not enter the stomach?

2. It is estimated that batteries contain a 45% potassium hydroxide solution which is on the order of 8 N KOH. Describe the type of corrosive injury that occurs with a caustic substance of this magnitude.

CASE STUDY: BATTERY ACID INGESTION

History

A 49-year-old male who owned an automotive garage ingested an undetermined quantity of battery acid (concentrated sulfuric acid). On admission to the emergency room he complained of burning in his mouth and dysphagia. Shortly thereafter, he vomited on his own. A frothy, blood-tinged secretion was observed in his mouth and pharynx. The mucosa of the hypopharynx was white in color and the uvula swollen. His abdomen was tender on touch; bowel sounds were minimal.

The following laboratory results were obtained:

WBC	= 24,000 mm^3
Hct	= 51%
PTT	= 100 sec
PT	= 40% (16.8 sec)
pH	= 7.32
P_{O_2}	= 79 mm Hg
P_{CO_2}	= 33 mm Hg

Abdominal roentgenography showed a large radiopaque mass in the region of the stomach.

Treatment. Treatment consisted of intravenous penicillin G potassium and hydrocortisone acetate. Approximately 12 hr post-admission, the patient experienced respiratory problems and a tracheostomy was performed. A gastrostomy was planned. However, on close examination, blood was found in the abdominal cavity. A gastrectomy was therefore performed.

Three days later, the patient was readmitted to surgery for further examination and possible reassessment of his condition. At that time, 1,500 ml of fresh blood was found in the abdominal cavity. A gangrenous portion of the ileum was removed.

The patient was followed closely and on the 11th hospital day, upper gastrointestinal bleeding from an erythematous esophagus developed. There was no esophageal stricture. By the 16th hospital day, he was drinking fluids. Six months later the patient showed complete recovery, weight gain, and no signs of esophageal stricture. (See ref. 4.)

Discussion

1. Did the ingestion of battery acid produce the expected type of injury?

2. What was the purpose of treating this patient with an antibiotic and a steroid?

3. Although a gastrostomy was originally planned, a gastrectomy was performed. Of what value would this latter procedure be?

CASE STUDIES: EYE INJURIES FROM BATTERY EXPLOSION

History: Case 1

A 22-year-old male was improperly using the jumper cables when trying to jump-start his friend's car. Because of this, the battery exploded and some of the battery acid came into contact with his left eye. He was not wearing glasses at the time. His visual acuity before the accident was 20/70 in the left eye.

The acid caused a mild conjunctival hyperemia, and a 5-mm perforating corneal laceration. The fundus was edematous and a subcapsular cataract had begun to form.

The lesion was surgically repaired and he recovered without apparent permanent eye damage. (See ref. 13.)

History: Case 2

A 27-year-old male was repairing a loose positive terminal connection in a battery. He accidentally touched the handle of his pliers with the negative ground cable, causing a spark that ignited the battery. He was not wearing glasses, and acid splashed into his eyes. There was a mild to moderate degree of hyperemia of both conjunctivae. Also, there were areas of ischemic conjunctival necrosis. Both corneas had epithelial abrasions, and some corneal tissue sloughed off. It did regenerate. Lenses were clear. The fundus of the right eye showed macular edema. (See ref. 13.)

History: Case 3

A 24-year-old male suffered eye damage after using a cigarette lighter while checking the fluid level of his dead car battery. He also was not wearing any eye glasses at the time of the accident.

On examination, the right eye showed mild conjunctival hyperemia, a corneal abrasion, and an edematous fundus. There was a tear in the retina which was surgically repaired. The left eye was normal. Vision returned to normal in the right eye in less than a month. (See ref. 13.)

Discussion

1. What were the areas of the eye most commonly involved in these case studies?

2. From the discussion in this chapter, what is the best initial method to treat these types of eye injuries?

3. What was the nature of the acid that caused eye damage to these victims?

CASE STUDY: POISONING BY HYDROFLUORIC ACID

History

A petroleum refinery operator was working in an alkylation unit of the plant. This unit used hydrofluoric acid as a catalyst to produce high octane gasoline components. At the time of the accident, the unit was shut down and neutralization of the hydrofluoric acid was almost completed.

The operator attempted to remove a plug and was splashed in the face with anhydrous hydrofluoric acid. He was wearing protective clothing which consisted of a hard hat with safety visor, neoprene boots, gloves, and jacket. After a few minutes he was washed with water, and a magnesium oxide preparation was applied to the exposed area.

The patient was quickly transported to an emergency facility, arriving with stable vital signs: blood pressure 130/88 mm Hg, pulse 88 beats/min, respirations 32/min. There were third degree burns throughout the lower quarter of his forehead, both eyelids, and cheeks, nose, and upper lip. Some keratoconjunctivitis was reported, but no corneal damage. Also, dysphagia was evident, but breath sounds were clear.

Treatment. His treatment consisted of injecting the burn area with 40 ml of 10% calcium gluconate, and intubation of the airway to assess respiratory function. The ECG showed a widening of the QT interval. Morphine 10 mg s.c. was given for pain; a local anesthetic product was instilled into the eyes to reduce irritation.

The following laboratory findings were obtained:

pH	= 7.21
Po_2	= 68 mm Hg
Pco_2	= 38 mm Hg
HCO_3	= 15 mEq/L
O_2 saturation	= 88%
Serum Ca^{2+}	= 3.5 mg%

The patient was later taken to the operating room for a tangential excision of the eschar and debridement of the burn area. He progressed satisfactorily. In the recovery room, however, he developed ventricular fibrillation, which was converted, but he subsequently died from a series of arrhythmias resulting in asystole. (See ref. 20.)

Discussion

1. How does hydrofluoric acid manifest its systemic toxic action?

2. Why were serum calcium levels so low? What was the relationship between the calcium level and the cause of death?

3. Usually, tetany is a clinical manifestation of hypocalcemia but, in this patient, what was the sign that indicated a decreased serum calcium level?

Review Questions

1. Cite the pros and cons (if any) of diluting ingested acids and bases (a) with water, (b) with milk, and (c) with carbonated beverages.

2. What is a bougie? When would it be used?

3. A particular danger exists when ingested acid or base is "neutralized" *in vivo* with another chemical agent. Describe the potential problem.

4. Describe the toxic reaction expected from ingesting Clinitest® tablets.

5. Ingested acids and bases cause tissue necrosis that differs from each other by its site and description of damage. Fill in the blanks:

	Site of damage	Type of necrosis
Acid	_____	_____
Base	_____	_____

6. Electric dishwasher detergents are highly:
   A. Acidic
   B. Alkaline

7. Poisoning by a "rust remover" will most likely involve which of the following substances?
   A. Hydrochloric acid
   B. Sulfuric acid
   C. Oxalic acid
   D. Ascorbic acid

8. Picric and nitric acid burns to the skin will appear as what color?
   A. Black/brown
   B. Blue/purple
   C. Red
   D. Yellow

9. What is the corrosive constituent of Drano® crystals?

10. Strong acids and alkali can be distinguished or defined based on their pH value. What is this numerical value for each substance?

11. A patient presents at the emergency room with fine material in the stomach that is described as "coffee-grounds" in consistency. What is the most likely source of this material?

12. It is often stated that no creams or ointments should be placed on skin that has been severely damaged by an acid or alkali, if the victim is to be transported to a physician. Why is this so?

13. Outline the procedure for treating acid or alkali burns to the eye.

14. Strongly acidic substances are all strongly corrosive.
    A. True
    B. False

15. Compare and contrast use of the terms "caustic" and "corrosive."

16. To which of the following blood electrolytes

does sodium fluoride react to cause major deficiency problems?

A. Potassium
B. Manganese
C. Chloride
D. Calcium

17. Corticosteroids and antibiotics are often given following ingestion of corrosive substances. Why?

18. Poisoning by muriatic acid indicates that treatment is required for which of the following acids:

A. Hydrochloric
B. Sulfuric
C. Oxalic
D. Tartaric

19. In the United States, which is the more common cause of poisoning?

A. Acids
B. Alkali

References

1. Ashcraft, K. W., and Padula, R. T. (1974): The effect of dilute corrosives on the stomach. *Pediatrics*, 53:226–232.
2. Buntain, W. L., and Cain, W. C. (1981): Caustic injuries to the esophagus: A pediatric overview. *South. Med. J.*, 74:590.
3. Cello, J. P., Fogel, R. P., and Boland, C. R. (1980): Liquid caustic ingestion. *Arch. Intern. Med.*, 140:501–504.
4. Chodak, G. W., and Passaro, E. (1978): Acid ingestion. Need for gastric resection. *JAMA*, 239:225–226.
5. Hodge, H. C., and Smith, F. A. (1965): *Fluorine Chemistry*, Vol. IV. Academic Press, New York.
6. Hodgson, J. H. (1958): Corrosive stricture of the stomach: Case report and review of the literature. *Br. J. Surg.*, 44:358–361.
7. Kirsh, M. M., and Ritter, F. (1976): Caustic ingestion and subsequent damage to the oropharyngeal and digestive passages. *Ann. Thorac. Surg.*, 21:74–82.
8. Knopp, R. (1979): Caustic ingestions. *J. Am. Coll. Emerg. Phys.*, 8:329–336.
9. Lowe, J. E., Graham, D. Y., Boisaubin, E. V., and Lanza, F. L. (1979): Corrosive injury to the stomach: The natural history and role of fiberoptic endoscopy. *Am. J. Surg.*, 137:803–806.
10. McCutcheon, R. S. (1980): Toxicology and the law. In: *Toxicology—The Basic Science of Poisons*, 2nd ed., edited by J. Doull, C. D. Klaassen, and M. O. Amdur, pp. 727–733. Macmillan, New York.
11. Messersmith, J. K., Oglesby, J. E. and Mahoney, W. D. (1970): Gastric erosion from alkali ingestion. *Am. J. Surg.*, 119:740–741.
12. Middelkamp, J. N., Ferguson, T. B., and Roper, C. L. (1969): Ingestion of liquid drain cleaner. *Gen. Pract.*, 40:86–89.
13. Minatoya, H. K. (1978): Eye injury from exploding car batteries. *Arch. Ophthalmol.*, 96:477–481.
14. Moriarty, R. W. (1979): Corrosive chemicals: Acids and alkalis. *Drug Ther.*, 9:89–99.
15. Penner, G. E. (1980): Acid ingestion: Toxicology and treatment. *Ann. Emerg. Med.*, 9:374–379.
16. Ritter, F. N., Newman, M. H., and Newman, D. E. (1968): A clinical and experimental study of corrosive burns of the stomach. *Ann. Otol. Rhinol. Laryngol.*, 77:830–841.
17. Roy, C. C., Silverman, A., and Cozzetto, F. J. (1975): *Pediatric Clinical Gastroenterology*. Mosby, St. Louis, Missouri.
18. Rumack, B. H., and Burrington, J. D. (1977): Caustic ingestions: A rational look at diluents. *Clin. Toxicol.*, 11:27–34.
19. Shabino, C. L., and Feinberg, A. N. (1979): Esophageal perforation secondary to alkaline battery ingestion. *J. Am. Coll. Emerg. Phys.*, 8:360–362.
20. Tepperman, P. B. (1980): Fatality due to acute systemic fluoride poisoning following a hydrofluoric acid skin burn. *J. Occupational Med.*, 22:691–692.
21. Tewfik, T. L., and Schloss, M. D. (1980): Ingestion of lye and other corrosive agents—a study of 86 infant and child cases. *J. Otolaryngol.*, 9:72–77.
22. Webb, W. R., Kontras, P., and Ecker, R. R. (1970): An evaluation of steroids in caustic burns of the esophagus. *Ann. Thorac. Surg.*, 9:95–98.
23. Winther, L. K. (1978): Accidental corrosive burns of the esophagus. *J. Laryngol. Otol.*, 92:693.

Pesticides

9

Mankind has long felt an obsession to rid his environment of pests. First of all, they are devastating to crops and food supplies and, second, life is basically more enjoyable without them. Indeed, the Old Testament makes several references to widespread destruction of early Egypt caused by insects, especially the locust. Still, today, even with very effective insecticides available for locusts, there is a vast amount of damage to food supplies in the Near East and Africa.

Pesticides are compounds that are designed to kill various pests (both plants and animals) that interfere with man's comfort, health, or economic well-being. They are widely used, in one form or another, in most countries around the world to protect agricultural and horticultural crops against damage. They are also employed at home and work to assure a pest-free environment. Overall, pesticides account for a small, but significant, number of human poisonings. Deaths reported from exposure are relatively rare, although it is estimated that for each death there are another 100 nonfatal poisonings (17).

Insecticides are the most commonly encountered *pesticides* in developing countries, while *herbicides* are more commonly encountered in developed countries. The United States is still the largest user of pesticides. A recent assessment of use, based on retail sales, showed the following data: United States, 45%; Western Europe, 25%; Japan, 12%; remaining countries combined, 18% (8). If all pesticidal products in current use around the world were grouped together, their number would total in the tens of thousands, and their discussion would comprise a major part of this book. More realistically, however, if we consider just those pesticides that are the more common cause of acute intoxication in America and, except for a few examples, omit those from our discussion that cause their major impact on the ecological system through chronic poisoning, the list narrows considerably. Thus, we will only consider a few selected insecticides and herbicides as being examples of those pesticides that are most generally encountered in poisoning cases, or at least

those that have the greatest potential for poisoning. These pesticides may also be categorized together to make their study more feasible.

It should not be forgotten that many of the poisons discussed elsewhere in this book have been used at one time or another for killing various pests and, indeed, some are still used. For example, arsenic is an effective and widely used herbicide, as are certain other heavy metals (i.e., mercury, copper). Hydrogen cyanide is used as a fumigant to control insects and certain rodents. Creosote (a petroleum product) protects wood against insect damage. Lime (an alkali) protects against fungus. These are only a few examples, but they illustrate the wide variety of substances used.

In most instances, a solid understanding of the medical problems and complications encountered with the pesticides discussed in this chapter, as well as the principles that govern their antidoting, will be sufficient to provide a good understanding of most other pesticidal chemicals as well.

Most poisoning by pesticides occur as a result of misuse or accidental exposure. At home, poisoning usually occurs by oral ingestion; at work, exposure is most frequently dermal exposure or inhalation (45).

INSECTICIDES

Organophosphorus Compounds

More than 50,000 organophosphate compounds have been synthesized and tested for insecticidal activity. However, the number actually employed for this purpose today probably does not exceed three dozen. In addition to organophosphate insecticides, several medical uses are known for these compounds, all of which produce similar toxic effects if ingested. The same basic principles for handling their toxicity apply.

For example, physostigmine (eserine), edrophonium, and neostigmine are employed for their cholinomimetic (acetylcholine-like) activity. They are used in the diagnosis or treatment of a variety of neuromuscular disorders, including myasthenia gravis. Physostigmine is also an important antidote for treating toxic ingestions of anticholinergic substances (e.g., tricyclic antidepressants, atropine, jimson weed, etc.) and is discussed in subsequent chapters. Physostigmine, echothiophate iodide, and other organophosphorous drugs are also instilled directly into glaucomatous eyes to reduce intraocular pressure.

Discovery of Organophosphorus Compounds

The organophosphorus compounds were first synthesized in Germany during the early days of World War II. Their use as nerve gases in chemical warfare was quickly recognized, as was their potential utility as insecticides. Early syntheses included compounds such as tetraethyl pyrophosphate (TEPP), parathion, and schradan which were extremely effective insecticides, but also quite toxic to mammals. Research continued toward development of additional compounds that maintained insecticide potency with less risk to humans (e.g., malathion), but it must be strongly emphasized that all organophosphate insecticides are potentially toxic. The chemical structures of a few examples are shown in Fig. 1.

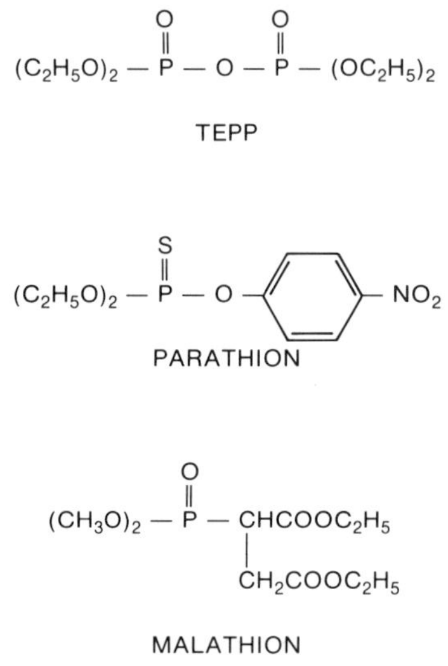

$$(C_2H_5O)_2 - \overset{\overset{\displaystyle O}{\|}}{P} - O - \overset{\overset{\displaystyle O}{\|}}{P} - (OC_2H_5)_2$$

TEPP

$$(C_2H_5O)_2 - \overset{\overset{\displaystyle S}{\|}}{P} - O - \langle\!\!\langle\ \rangle\!\!\rangle - NO_2$$

PARATHION

$$(CH_3O)_2 - \overset{\overset{\displaystyle O}{\|}}{P} - \underset{\underset{\displaystyle CH_2COOC_2H_5}{|}}{CHCOOC_2H_5}$$

MALATHION

FIG. 1. Structural formulae for representative organophosphorus insecticides.

Mechanism of Organophosphorus Compound Toxicity

The organophosphorus insecticides are among the most toxic of all substances that cause poisoning in humans, and are the most frequently encountered insecticide poison (36). Ingestion of as little as several milligrams may be lethal. However, most require a higher quantity to kill an adult (Table 1).

Organophosphate insecticides inhibit the action of pseudocholinesterase in the plasma and acetylcholinesterase in RBCs and at synapses. These enzymes normally hydrolyze acetylcholine to terminate its actions. When the enzymes are inhibited, however, acetylcholine levels increase and bind to muscarinic and nicotinic receptors in both the central and peripheral nervous systems. Because of the widespread distribution of neurons responding to acetylcholine activation (Fig. 2), organophosphorus poisoning induces a large variety of toxic symptoms that affect nearly the entire body.

Recall that acetylcholine is the excitatory chemical mediator released by nerve impulses in both the sympathetic and parasympathetic portions of the autonomic nervous system (32). These impulses stimulate the neuromuscular junction of skeletal muscle and neurons within the CNS. Generally, intoxication by low (nonlethal) doses of an organophosphorus compound

TABLE 1. *Organophosphate insecticide human LD_{50} values*

Compound	LD_{50} (mg/kg)
Akton	146
Coroxon	12
Diazinon	100
Dichlorvos	56
Ethion	27
Malathion	1,375
Mecarbam	36
Methyl parathion	10
Parathion	3
Sevin	274
Systox	2.5
TEPP (tetraethyl pyrophosphate)	1

From ref. 11.

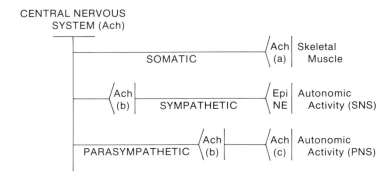

FIG. 2. Distribution of acetylcholine (Ach) throughout the body. Location includes the CNS, neuromuscular junctions (a), autonomic ganglia (b), and muscarinic sites (c).

will manifest primarily with symptoms attributed to stimulation of muscarinic (postganglionic, parasympathetic) sites. With larger doses, however, nicotinic sites (autonomic ganglia) and central muscarinic receptors are also stimulated.

Enzyme inhibition occurs because the organophosphorus compound phosphorylates the enzyme and, thereby, forms a stable complex. Those compounds with ethyl or methyl groups as their alkyl substituents form enzyme-chemical complexes that may allow spontaneous regeneration of enzyme within several hours. Compounds with secondary or tertiary alkyl groups, however, form enzyme-chemical complexes that are much more stable and are generally irreversible (40). Generally, 1 to 4 weeks is required for plasma pseudocholinesterase and 4 weeks to several months for RBC and synaptic cholinesterase activity to return to normal (1).

A separate group of organophosphate compounds, the carbamate insecticides, have a similar mechanism of toxic action (36,40). Poisoning by a carbamate insecticide is generally less severe, with signs and symptoms usually limited to muscarinic effects. Extremely large doses are needed to impart nicotinic effects, except for the insecticide, temik, which is extremely toxic and limited in use to greenhouse applications. All carbamate insecticides form phosphorylated enzyme complexes that are weak and rapidly reversible. Thus, survival from poisoning by one of these is more assured.

TABLE 2. *Signs and symptoms of organophosphate poisoning*

Muscarinic
  SLUD: *s*alivation, *l*acrimation, *u*rination, *d*iarrhea (or *d*efecation)
  Abdominal cramping
  Nausea and vomiting
  Bradycardia and heart block
  Tightness in chest; wheezing
  Miosis
  Tenesmus
  Sweating

Nicotinic
  Fatigue; weakness
  Twitching and fasciculations; tremor
  Paralysis
  Dyspnea
  Pallor
  Tachycardia (from ganglionic stimulation); hypertension

Central nervous system
  Anxiety, restlessness, insomnia, nightmares, confusion; neurosis
  Headache
  Ataxia
  Confusion
  Emotional instability
  Giddiness
  Slurred speech
  Generalized weakness
  Convulsions
  Depressed respiration and cardiovascular functions
  Cheyne-Stokes respiration
  Coma

Characteristics of Organophosphate Poisoning

As shown in Table 2, poisoning by organophosphorus compounds may inflict a large variety of toxic actions. Each of these signs and symptoms is attributed to persistent acetylcholine stimulation, or to depression which follows stimulation.

Early signs and symptoms that denote intoxication and are strongly suggestive of organophosphate poisoning include miosis (pinpoint pupils) and blurred vision, and a response termed the SLUD syndrome. SLUD refers to *s*alivation, *l*acrimation, *u*rination, and *d*iarrhea. Each of these effects is due to stimulation of muscarinic receptors in the eye and smooth muscle as acetylcholine levels increase. Additionally, browache, wheezing, and a feeling of tightness in the chest may be felt early or with low doses.

As poisoning continues, or with larger doses, nicotinic and central stimulation dominate most of the muscarinic effects, and the additional clinical manifestations of organophosphate poisoning symptoms shown in Table 2 are experienced. For example, the usual muscarinic effect of acetylcholine is bradycardia. When adrenergic ganglia (nicotinic response) are stimulated, bradycardia may be reversed and tachycardia will be the major effect.

Stimulation at the nicotinic and central receptors is largely a persistent depolarization which is then followed by depression. In other words, massive acetylcholine-induced activation of receptors cause their depolarization (and, hence, stimulation), but because this transmitter attack is persistent (no acetylcholinesterase to remove the acetylcholine) the nerve fibers cannot become repolarized. Shortly, depression of responses follows stimulation.

Organophosphate insecticides may be absorbed from all routes of exposure. Following poisoning by inhalation of vapors, symptoms may manifest within minutes. Oral ingestion or subcutaneous absorption generally requires a longer period to cause symptoms. Most occupational exposures occur by the dermal and inhalational routes. Nonoccupational poisoning is most frequently encountered by ingestion.

Limited exposures may cause localized effects. For example, percutaneous absorption of an organophosphorus compound over a small confined area may cause intense sweating and twitching of the muscles in that area only. A vapor that comes in contact with the eye may cause only miosis or blurred vision. Brief inhalation of a small concentration may cause only wheezing and coughing.

An uncommon sequela of poisoning by a few organophosphate insecticides that occurs in a few rare instances is termed *delayed neurotoxic effects*. This results from phosphorylation of neuronal protein (36).

Onset of symptoms may be delayed for days to weeks. They typically begin in the distal portions of the lower limbs as ataxia, and progress to generalized muscular weakness and flaccidity of the legs. Some victims lose complete control of their legs and arms. Symptoms usually reach their peak in a few weeks and then subside, although complete recovery is not always achieved. The effect is not related to inhibition of acetylcholinesterase enzyme, and it is not treatable with atropine or pralidoxime. A single acute exposure to a massive dose may cause onset of symptoms in minutes or may be delayed for up to 12 hr, although this is rare. Death is usually due to respiratory failure, accompanied by cardiovascular failure.

Differences in the onset of toxic symptoms of central origin may be explained by one or more mechanisms. The first parameter is the lipid solubility of the organophosphate. The degree of lipid solubility, of course, would be directly proportional to the ability of the compound to penetrate the blood-brain barrier and enter the CNS. Another reason for a delayed onset relates to the metabolic activation of certain compounds. A common example is the hepatic conversion of parathion to paraoxon which is a stronger cholinesterase inhibitor than parathion. This conversion must occur before toxic activity is manifest.

Another consideration is the phenomenon referred to as *enzyme aging*. Enzyme aging is a process whereby, once phosphorylation occurs, additional chemical changes (e.g., loss of an alkyl or alkoxy group) also occur to strengthen the phosphorylated complex even more. Aging occurs more readily with organophosphate poisons that contain tertiary alkoxy groups. The process may begin within minutes to hours after the complex forms. Once it occurs, the enzyme complex is then resistant to reactivation by pralidoxime.

Treatment of Organophosphate Poisoning

Treatment of organophosphate poisoning should begin immediately, once a probable diagnosis is made. Hesitation for a few minutes following a severe exposure will greatly decrease the victim's chance for surviving a potentially lethal dose. A presumptive diagnosis can usually be readily made based on the patient's exposure history coupled with the presenting signs and symptoms which are characteristic and unrelenting.

' In severe intoxication, or following chronic exposure where organophosphorus poisoning is suspected, plasma pseudocholinesterase and erythrocytic acetylcholinesterase activity should be measured. Erythrocyte enzyme levels closely correlate to levels of enzyme in the CNS, so this extrapolation can be made (36). Although normal acetylcholinesterase activity varies widely among different people, it will be significantly depressed well below the low end of the normal range when poisoning has occurred and symptoms are present.

For mild-to-moderate exposures, atropine sulfate, at doses of 1 to 2 mg i.v., should be given as needed, usually every hour up to 25 to 50 mg daily (12). Atropine blocks peripheral muscarinic effects and many of the central muscarinic actions. It will not reverse the neuromuscular paralysis seen in massive exposure.

For acute exposures of large quantities of organophosphates, or following chronic poisoning when symptoms are severe, vigorous antidoting measures are, indeed, indicated. To begin with, atropine sulfate is given at a dose of up to 2 to 4 mg i.v. If the victim develops tachycardia, dry mouth, or any other anticholinergic symptom, it is unlikely the poisoning is related to an organophosphate or carbamate insecticide. If the cholinergic symptoms (e.g., bradycardia, salivation, abdominal cramps) then reappear, atropine should be given every 5 to 10 min, or until symptoms of atropine toxicity appear. Atropine doses are discussed here to give some

idea of the importance for quick treatment. Normal therapeutic doses of atropine needed to achieve an antimuscarinic action are as low as 0.4 mg every 4 hr.

Pralidoxime (2-PAM) is a specific antidote for organophosphate poisoning. It is commercially available as the chlorine salt, packaged in 1-g ampules (Fig. 3). Its action is to regenerate acetylcholinesterase and, thus, promote hydrolysis of accumulated acetylcholine. 2-PAM does this by combining directly with the organophosphate portion of the phosphorylated enzyme complex, thereby releasing it from its enzyme substrate. It is normally administered in a 1-g dose which may be repeated after 20 min, if muscular weakness is not reversed.

2-PAM is a quaternary amine and does not readily penetrate into the CNS. It is, therefore, without significant effect on brain acetylcholinesterase enzyme inhibition. It also has little effect on the autonomic muscarinic sites. Its greatest affinity for phosphorylated enzyme is at the neuromuscular junction and, hence, most of its beneficial actions are directed toward reestablishing skeletal muscle activity. Skeletal muscle normally begins to respond by reactivation of enzyme within several minutes of 2-PAM administration. Because of these site limitations for 2-PAM, atropine must also be given if the patient is to be successfully antidoted (Table 3).

TABLE 3. *Reduction of toxicity of sarin in mice by atropine and pralidoxime[a]*

Treatment	LD$_{50}$ (μg/kg)
None	14.5
Atropine	38.0
Pralidoxime	18.4
Atropine and pralidoxime (5 mg/kg)	365
Atropine and pralidoxime (10 mg/kg)	1,321

[a]Neither atropine nor pralidoxime alone significantly reduced toxicity of this organophosphorus compound. However, when the two antidotes were combined, the LD$_{50}$ dose of sarin was greatly increased.
From ref. 38.

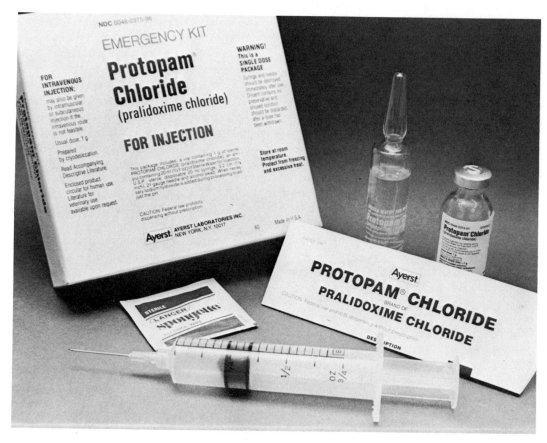

FIG. 3.   Pralidoxime chloride (2-PAM) antidote for organophosphorus poisoning. (Photograph courtesy of Ayerst Laboratories, Inc.)

Contaminated clothing and contact lenses should be removed, as quickly as possible, to prevent further absorption. The skin should be washed with soap, as this helps remove the poison and hydrolyze it to a less toxic form. The eyes should be rinsed with lukewarm water for 15 to 20 min, if exposure has occurred.

Other symptoms (e.g., convulsions, shock, etc.) should be treated as required and additional general supportive measures given. Cyanosis must be reversed with continued respiratory assistance.

2-PAM has significant neuromuscular blocking activity because it has acetylcholinesterase inhibitory actions of its own. In high doses it can block the neuromuscular junction by inhibiting acetylcholinesterase. These effects are not usually seen at the usual therapeutic doses of 1 to 2 g i.v. But because of them, 2-PAM is contraindicated in treating poisoning by carbaryl, a carbamate acetyl cholinesterase inhibitor. The reversal process is so quick and complete that adding another enzyme inhibitor (albeit a weak and short-acting one) may further potentiate toxicity. The same contraindication also holds (for the same reasoning) for treating overdoses of the drugs physostigmine and neostigmine, both of which are reversible acetylcholinesterase inhibitors.

Chlorinated Hydrocarbons

The chlorinated hydrocarbons consist of a group of compounds shown in Table 4. Of these, DDT (chlorophenothane, dichloro-diphenyl-trichloroethane) is the best known, and is used

TABLE 4. *Chlorinated hydrocarbon insecticides*

Group	Compounds
Cyclodienes	Aldrin, chlordane, dieldrin, heptachlor, endrin, toxaphene, kepone, mirex
Hexachlorocyclohexanes	Lindane
Chlorinated ethane derivatives	DDT

as a basis of comparison for all other chlorinated hydrocarbon insecticides. It is also the prototype for our discussion, since most research on the chlorinated hydrocarbons has been conducted with it. One of the chlorinated hydrocarbon insecticides, lindane (γ-benzene hexachloride, Kwell®, etc.) is used exclusively for direct application to the skin as a pediculicide and scabicide.

Discovery of Chlorinated Hydrocarbons

DDT was synthesized as early as 1874, but its activity as an insecticide was not discovered until the early 1940s. Its insecticidal potency quickly became apparent as reports began to filter in that it was effective in controlling insecticidal pests when applied over large areas. Many diseases carried by various insects were literally eliminated from those areas. It has been stated that DDT helped the Western allies win World War II, since it permitted western soldiers to survive for prolonged periods in areas of the world where they had been previously unable to do so, because of prevalent disease conditions. It was widely used throughout the war by applying the powder directly to the body as an ectoparasiticide (34).

The chlorinated hydrocarbon insecticides, as a class, have a low solubility in water. Hence, they are not biodegradable and persist for prolonged periods in the environment. The half-life for DDT and its derivatives is nearly 10 years. What at one time was generally lauded as an advantage has now, however, caused the

chlorinated hydrocarbons as a class to fall into disfavor. These compounds are extremely lipid-soluble and, therefore, accumulate in body adipose tissues and are implicated as the cause of a wide variety of toxic effects which are species-dependent. Following cessation of exposure, the rate for elimination of stored DDT from the body is only 1% per day.

On the other hand, chlorinated hydrocarbon insecticides are relatively safe and nontoxic when compared on a milligram-to-milligram basis to the organophosphorus compounds. Acute poisoning and death are rare. Part of this relative safety is no doubt due to their lipid solubility and storage in adipose tissue. This helps keep them out of the brain, where the toxic damage would be greatest. The fact that these compounds are highly lipid-soluble also accounts for its selective toxicity to insects. They can easily penetrate the exoskeleton of insects, but percutaneous absorption in mammals is relatively poor. To illustrate, the oral LD_{50} for DDT in rats is approximately 118 mg/kg, whereas the dermal LD_{50} is 2,510 mg/kg.

Still, this can be stated only in the most general terms, for the toxic potential of this class of insecticides ranges from slightly toxic to highly toxic (Chapter 1). Even though DDT and the other chlorinated hydrocarbon insecticides are classified as neurotoxic, their exact mechanism of toxic action has not been completely elucidated. This is true despite having been in use and studied for more than four decades. It could well be that with continued scientific research an entirely new area of great toxicological concern will emerge regarding chronic exposure.

For example, kepone was at first thought to be a safe substitute for DDT. Its production was stepped up when DDT use was curtailed in the United States during the early 1970s. However, after a few short years, kepone use was also banned in the United States when it was shown to be extremely toxic to the workers who manufactured it. Mirex, another chlorinated hydrocarbon insecticide, is used in parts of the South to control the aggressive fire ant. It is chemically identical to kepone, except for one oxygen atom. Mirex use is now in jeopardy, because it is thought to be a carcinogen, at least in mice. DDT exposure over a prolonged period is also believed to be carcinogenic, but there is still debate on this issue.

It could be that an entirely new listing of toxic effects following chronic exposure will emerge with time. Every American born since the mid-1940s has been exposed to DDT and a wide variety of other chlorinated hydrocarbon substances. Each person is, therefore, believed to have a significant body burden of these substances accumulated in adipose tissue.

Mechanism of Chlorinated Hydrocarbon Toxicity

There is considerable controversy regarding the mechanism of toxicity for DDT. It is classified as a neurotoxin and the brain is its site of toxic action. The sensory and motor nerve fibers and the motor cortex are affected. On the other hand, following poisoning there is usually little or no pathologic change. In some animal studies, rats have developed histologic liver changes, but these have been reversible with cessation of exposure (27). A definite correlation between CNS levels and severity of toxic signs can be shown (9). DDT interferes with normal movement of sodium and potassium across neuronal membranes and, consequently, it interferes with normal electrical activity.

The number of clear-cut fatalities to chlorinated hydrocarbons is small although they still occasionally are reported. Ingestion of 10 mg/kg will usually cause toxic effects, with their onset appearing in several hours. It can cause acute poisoning, but victims usually survive if proper supportive therapy is applied. The estimated LD_{50} of DDT in man is 300 to 500 mg/kg. We should remember that there is always room for question regarding the actual cause of death from liquid preparations. In numerous instances of reported toxicity to DDT, one wonders if the fatalities were not due more to the product's solvent vehicle, in some cases kerosene, rather than to the insecticide.

Clinical Manifestations of Chlorinated Hydrocarbons

Clinically reported signs and symptoms for DDT are listed in Table 5. DDT, like other chlorinated hydrocarbons, sensitizes the myocardium to catecholamines. This may be why it causes ventricular fibrillation and death in animals that receive it intravenously.

DDT was banned from use for all but a few essential applications in the United States in 1972, and several other chlorinated hydrocarbon insecticides listed in Table 4 have largely replaced it. Methoxychlor causes similar signs and symptoms following poisoning, but it is generally less toxic. Toxaphene also causes similar effects, but is readily metabolized and quickly excreted. Recent evidence suggests that it may be carcinogenic. Aldrin, dieldrin, heptachlor, and chlordane are all more toxic than DDT. They frequently cause convulsions before the other, less serious, CNS stimulation effects are prominent. Thus, they have all been replaced, whenever appropriate, by other compounds such as pyrethrins and some of the organophosphate insecticides that have a wide safety margin.

Lindane is highly lipid-soluble and readily penetrates through the skin. Although systemic toxicity has occurred following topical use (28), most poisoning reports indicate that it was ingested.

Signs and symptoms of toxicity to lindane are largely identical to those of DDT, and include CNS stimulation and sensitization of the myocardium. Following acute exposure to large doses, violent convulsions are common. Fatty

TABLE 5. *Signs and symptoms of DDT intoxication*

Nausea, vomiting
Paresthesias of tongue, lips, and face
Restlessness
Apprehension, irritability
Tremor
Convulsions
Hypersusceptibility to stimuli
Coma
Respiratory failure
Death

changes can be seen in the liver, and the kidney tubules show degeneration.

Treatment of Chlorinated Hydrocarbon Poisoning

Treatment of chlorinated hydrocarbon poisoning is largely supportive. CNS depressants and anticonvulsants are necessary to control tremors and convulsions. Diazepam has largely replaced phenobarbital for treating tremors and convulsions because of its lower incidence and severity of respiratory depressant action. Calcium gluconate is occasionally given to reverse tremors. Oily cathartics are contraindicated since they may enhance absorption.

Insecticides From Botanical Origin

Pyrethrum (Pyrethrins)

Pyrethrum is obtained from the yellow flower *Chrysanthemum cinerariaefolium*. Its active principles include pyrethrin I and II and cinerin I and II. The pyrethrins are esters formed from two acids, chrysanthemic acid and pyrethric acid, and three alcohols, jasmolone, cinerolone, and pyrethrolone. Pyrethrins are incorporated into a large variety of household insecticidal products because of their rapid knock-down action and mammalian safety (36).

Severe poisoning from pyrethrins is rare, although injecting or inhaling a pyrethrin insecticide can cause nausea, vomiting, muscular paralysis, and death. Massive doses may induce CNS symptoms including excitation and convulsions that terminate in paralysis. Death occurs from respiratory failure (18).

Contact dermatitis is the most frequent adverse effect to pyrethrins and, in allergic individuals, asthma and rhinitis may occur. Pyrethrins are poorly absorbed across intact skin and, once absorbed by mammals, are rapidly broken down. The human fatal dose is reported at 50 g/70 kg (16). Most toxicity reports to pyrethrin-containing products are due to other ingredients in the preparation, usually a petroleum distillate solvent (3).

Commonly marketed products combine pyrethrins, 0.17 to 0.33% with piperonyl butoxide, 2 to 4% for use as a pediculicide. Piperonyl butoxide is a pharmacological synergist to pyrethrins. It interferes with the insect's ability to destory pyrethrins by oxidative degradation (5,42). Piperonyl butoxide is also poorly absorbed following cutaneous application to mammals and is relatively nontoxic. Its fatal human dose is reported at 11.5 g/kg (11).

Treatment is symptomatic. Poisoning by preparations containing a petroleum solvent must be antidoted for that substance. In severe intoxications, especially in individuals with a history of allergy, anaphylaxis must be treated with epinephrine.

Rotenone

Rotenone, an insecticide of botanical origin, has long been used to control a large variety of insect pests. For many centuries, plants containing rotenoids have been used as fish poisons. The poisonous substituents dissolved in the water were absorbed through the gills. Because in much of the early investigation of rotenone, one of the rotenoid poisons employed the substance obtained from plants of the genus *Derris*, the term "derris" persisted as a synonym for rotenone. Today, rotenone is still a widely used insecticide that is fairly safe to humans following exposure. The human lethal dose is reported at 100 to 200 g/kg orally.

Signs and symptoms of poisoning, when it occurs, include gastrointestinal irritation, nausea and vomiting, and respiratory depression. Death from massive exposure occurs from respiratory paralysis, although liver and kidney damage may be detected following chronic exposure.

The exact mechanism for rotenone-induced damage is elusive. It inhibits oxidative phosphorylation, which may be a factor (36).

Rotenone exposure by inhalation is considered to be of greater toxicologic concern than following oral administration. In the lungs, rotenone can cause intense respiratory stimulation, followed by depression and convulsions.

In the stomach, however, a significant amount of an ingested dose is frequently expelled because of its irritant gastrointestinal action, and thus its toxic potential from this route of exposure is less significant.

Treatment of rotenone poisoning includes supportive therapy and management of symptoms. There is no specific antidote.

Nicotine

Nicotine is extracted from tobacco and is a very potent contact insecticide against a large variety of insects. It is commercially available as Black Leaf-40®, a 40% solution of nicotine sulfate.

Nicotine stimulates the autonomic ganglia (both sympathetic and parasympathetic), the neuromuscular junctions, and certain neuronal pathways in the CNS. Its initial effects (Table 6) are stimulatory in nature, mimicking an acetylcholine overdose. For example, dizziness, miosis, vomiting, and the SLUD syndrome are encountered shortly after poisoning. These effects progress rapidly to persistent muscular weakness, tremors, then convulsions, and eventually to paralysis and CNS depression. Death occurs from respiratory failure, which follows both from paralysis of respiratory muscles and from blockade of central respiratory mechanisms.

Nicotine also causes release of catecholamines in several organs which mimics sympathetic stimulation.

Overall, clinical characterization of nicotine poisoning is quite complex, and the presenting symptoms following exposure may vary widely among different people. The ultimate response represents a summation of several opposing forces.

For example, nicotine may cause tachycardia by stimulating ganglia or blocking parasympathetic ganglia. It may induce bradycardia by blocking sympathetic ganglia or by stimulating the parasympathetic ganglia. It is difficult to predict, *a priori*, how an individual will respond.

Nicotine acts quickly, with death often occurring within minutes to a few hours. It readily penetrates the skin and is absorbed through inhalation of its vapors, while absorption from the gastrointestinal tract may be delayed because of reduced gastric emptying (40).

Nicotine-containing insecticide products should be quickly washed off the skin and all contaminated clothing removed. Ingested nicotine should be quickly removed from the stomach by active lavage or emesis. Activated charcoal, following this removal process, is recommended. Other treatment is purely symptomatic. Atropine sulfate is frequently given in maximally tolerated doses, but once symptoms of generalized depression occur, atropine therapy is without much benefit. An α-adrenergic blocking agent, such as phentolamine, may reverse severe hypertension and sympathetic stimulation in selected persons.

HERBICIDES

Chlorophenoxy Herbicides

Two substances, 2,4-dichlorophenoxyacetic acid (2,4-D) and 2,4,5-trichlorophenoxyacetic acid (2,4,5-T) and their esters and salts, are among the most widely used herbicides. They are used to control many broad-leaf woody plants growing along highways and other rights of way. In fact, they can quickly and completely defoliate an entire area of woody plants (36). They are also the subject of extensive contemporary public interest and concern stemming around a contaminant of 2,4,5-T called 2,3,4,8-tetrachlorodibenzo-p-dioxin (TCDD or dioxin), which

TABLE 6. *Progression of signs and symptoms in acute nicotine poisoning*

Nausea, vomiting, diarrhea
Salivation
Abdominal cramps
Cold sweat
Dizziness
Bradycardia
Hypotension
Dyspnea
Cardiovascular collapse
Convulsions
Death

is a potent teratogen and possible carcinogen (2,35,36).

Dioxin is also reported to be the most toxic man-made chemical known, with toxic doses for most animals being in the microgram range. Because of the widespread and sometimes careless use of 2,4,5-T, it is believed that hundreds of thousands of Americans, regrettably, may have been exposed to dioxin and, thus, they and their immediate offspring have been poisoned. The controversy over dioxin will undoubtedly continue for the next several decades. At present, the concentration of dioxin in 2,4,5-T is closely regulated at 0.1 ppm or less.

The acute human toxic dose of chlorphenoxy herbicides is approximately 3 to 4 g. One victim of poisoning did not survive a dose of at least 6.5 g of 2,4,5-T (27).

Whereas the compounds act as growth hormones in plants, they do not possess hormonal action in humans. Their mechanism of toxicity is, at present, unknown. Nonspecific liver and kidney changes can be seen following exposure (16). The substances do not accumulate in the body and the plasma half-life in animals is about 24 hr (15).

Signs and symptoms of toxicity are listed in Table 7. The principal findings of 2,4-D poisoning in animals and man include muscular weakness and hypotension. Death following a massive ingestion is believed to be due to ventricular fibrillation (21,36). A commonly reported form of severe dermatitis, called *chloracne*, may be due to dioxin.

Treatment of 2,4-D poisoning involves rapid removal of the substance from the gastrointestinal tract by emesis or gastric lavage, followed by a saline cathartic. The skin should be thoroughly scrubbed with soap and water, after removal of contaminated clothing. Specific symptoms are treated as needed; e.g., lidocaine for ventricular fibrillation and diazepam for convulsions. The pKa for 2,4-D is 2.6, so it will be excreted more efficiently in an alkaline urine. Sodium bicarbonate, 10 to 15 g/day, is given for this purpose.

Bipyridyl Compounds

Paraquat and diquat are the most familiar substances of this group. Both produce acute and chronic toxic effects that differ from one another. Paraquat is the better known herbicide and the more potentially toxic (22). Over the previous few years, hundreds of cases of toxicity have been reported (24,36), with an overall mortality rate for paraquat about 70% (22).

Both paraquat and diquat are rapidly acting herbicides that do not persist in the environment because they are quickly inactivated by the clay in soil.

Paraquat has also been the subject of considerable recent public interest and concern. It has been widely used to control illicit production of marijuana and heroin from plants growing in the back country areas of Mexico and selected areas in the southern states. Consequently, high concentrations of paraquat have been reported in some marijuana cigarettes. It is suggested that "scarring" of lung tissue could occur from smoking these cigarettes or ingesting baked goods made from the plant. There is little evidence at present to document this claim (23). However, common sense dictates that such "tainted" marijuana products should be avoided.

Pathologic changes to lung, kidney, liver, adrenals, and heart tissue may be noted following paraquat intoxication. This pathology is not dependent on exposure by any specific route, and thus subcutaneous injection of pure paraquat will induce the same pulmonary changes as those which occur following inhalation of smoke-borne particles.

The precise mechanism of toxicity is believed to be due to free radical formation (13,22). These react with cell constituents to cause their

TABLE 7. *Toxicity characteristics of acute chlorphenoxy herbicide poisoning*

Burning pain in the nose, eyes, throat, and bronchi
Vomiting, diarrhea
Abdominal pain
Lethargy
Weakness
Muscle twitching

biochemical destruction. Another thought is that paraquat is oxidized to form superoxide radicals which react with unsaturated lipids of cell membranes to cause their destruction (36).

Signs and symptoms of paraquat and diquat poisoning are listed in Table 8. The first symptoms include a burning sensation in the mouth and throat which may progress to ulceration 1 to 2 days later. However, the most significant toxic events are those on the lungs and are usually noted 5 to 30 days following ingestion (31). Massive doses may be fatal within 24 hr (22).

Paraquat causes widespread cellular proliferation leading to eventual pulmonary edema, hyaline membrane formation, and intense inflammation, and, in turn, to respiratory distress and death. Diquat differs from paraquat primarily in that it does not produce these specific pulmonary changes. The lung seems to selectively concentrate paraquat, but not diquat (39).

In animal studies where sublethal doses have been given, or when animals have initially survived potentially lethal doses, lesions in the lungs develop that eventually lead to fibrosis and death. In rats, proliferation of cells at first appears as fibroblasts arising from the adventitia of blood vessels and fibrous tissue around bronchi. The proliferating cells extend into the alveolar walls, causing hypertrophy of alveolar epithelial cells and subsequent thickening of the septa (19). A single exposure to paraquat is sufficient to induce these changes.

Another bipyridyl derivative, chlormequat, produces toxic effects primarily on the kidney. It could well be that with continued research,

diquat will also emerge as a source of selective toxicity on a different target system, but, at this time, this remains purely speculative.

Initial symptoms of poisoning such as gastrointestinal irritation may occur within hours, but the onset of respiratory problems and death may take several days. For example, a victim who ingested a small quantity (probably no more than several milliliters) of paraquat did not develop respiratory distress until 2 weeks later (36).

Both paraquat and diquat, which are weak bases, are only minimally absorbed from the stomach. This is contrasted to the weak acids, 2,4-D and 2,4,5-T, which are rapidly absorbed from that site. As it is quickly inactivated by the soil, paraquat is also rapidly removed from the body. By 48 hr, 90 to 100% of an administered dose can be recovered from the urine.

Paraquat poisoning must be vigorously antidoted if injury to the lung is to be avoided. Treatment should be started even in the absence of immediate symptoms. Gastric lavage and catharsis are employed to remove it from the gastrointestinal tract.

Fuller's earth and bentonite are adsorbents that bind with paraquat to form a biologically inert, nonabsorbable complex. Twenty percent mannitol accelerates movement of these adsorbents through the gastrointestinal tract (22). Both have shown special promise for selective adsorption of paraquat. They are used in preference to activated charcoal, but if neither is available, activated charcoal should be used.

Forced catharsis, even to the point of diarrhea, with sodium or magnesium sulfate is indicated. Forced diuresis with furosemide and intravenous fluids should be instituted, and is usually more effective than peritoneal dialysis. The role of hemodialysis or hemoperfusion is established, and these procedures are instituted to help remove absorbed poison. Glucocorticosteroids, antiinflammatory agents, and immunosuppressants may be recommended, but use of these agents has not met with universal success. Other symptoms are treated as appropriate. The patient should be closely monitored for

TABLE 8. *Toxicity characteristics of acute paraquat and diquat poisoning*

Stage	Toxicity characteristics
Early stage (1–5 days)	Irritation of mucosal lining of the mouth and gastrointestinal tract
Late stage (2–8 days)	Jaundice, fever, cyanosis, corrosive lung damage, focal atelectasis, respiratory distress

the next 3 to 4 weeks for development of complications of late onset.

The human LD_{50} is reported at 40 mg/kg (7). Antidoting must begin within 10 hr of ingestion, if treatment is to be effective (36).

RODENTICIDES

Rodenticides are substances that kill rodents, especially mice, rats, and squirrels. A large variety of chemicals have been used over the years, including strychnine, red squill, norbormide, several inorganic metals, and hydrogen cyanide. We will confine our study of rodenticides to the most commonly used one, warfarin, and say a few words about phosphorus, sodium fluoride, and thallium. Strychnine and cyanide, two additional chemicals used as rodenticides, are discussed elsewhere in this book.

Warfarin

Warfarin is almost universally accepted as the most effective means to control rodents. It is lethal to rodents, but safe for humans if used properly. Warfarin tablets (e.g., Coumadin®) are taken to help control blood coagulation disorders. It has also been the prototype for development of other oral anticoagulant medications. It is used in baits or added to drinking water placed where rodents congregate, and does not have to be added to the environment as such. Unfortunately, it may cause serious toxicity problems if it is repeatedly ingested by man.

Warfarin is a metabolite of vitamin K. Thus, it inhibits synthesis of the four vitamin K-dependent clotting factors in the plasma and liver, factors II (prothrombin), VII, IX, and X (Fig. 4). Consequently, prothrombin synthesis is reduced. This, in turn, promotes hemorrhage throughout the body which is the cause of death. Warfarin is reported to have a direct pathologic action on capillary walls (36), but this response is secondary to its action on prothrombin synthesis. The reason for this is that the half-lives of the four clotting factors (VII, IX, X, and II; 6, 24, 40, and 60 hr, respectively) is long. Warfarin does not affect clotting factors already formed, just those which have not yet formed. Therefore, 1 to 3 days of warfarin administration are required before a hypoprothrombinemic effect will be seen.

It is estimated that a single dose of 15 g of warfarin, or about 30 pounds of warfarin bait, would be required to cause death. However, ingestion of as little as 1 to 2 mg/kg for 6 days caused severe illness in a patient attempting suicide. A family of 14 persons accidentally consumed cornmeal containing warfarin for 15 days. Their intake of poison was estimated at 102 mg/kg/day (18). All but two of the family survived, although all persons experienced severe hemorrhaging.

Severe toxicity or death is rare following a single or few repeated doses. Major characteristics of poisoning by warfarin are all related to hemorrhage. These include bleeding of the nose (epistaxis) and gums, easy bruising of the skin, and ultimately hemorrhagic shock and death. Pain in the joints, abdomen, and back probably reflects hemorrhage into those areas. Weakness results from anemia.

Warfarin ingestion should be treated by emesis if a dose known to induce symptoms was ingested within the preceding 2 to 3 hr. This may be followed by activated charcoal. In smaller ingestions, emesis or adsorbents are not necessary. The victim should be monitored for development of symptoms.

Specific treatment of large doses, or of undetermined doses when symptoms are present, includes immediate withdrawal of the offending bait or substance and administration of vitamin K (phytonadione). Prothrombin should return to normal within 24 hr. Vitamin K_3 (menadione) and K_4 (menadiol) are not effective. Fresh blood or plasma transfusions or plasma concentrates of the vitamin K-dependent clotting factors are indicated, if hemorrhage is severe. Ascorbic acid is occasionally recommended, since it is believed to limit capillary permeability induced by warfarin.

Prognosis is good when vitamin K is given. However, death may occur 1 to 2 weeks after poisoning, so the victim must be carefully ob-

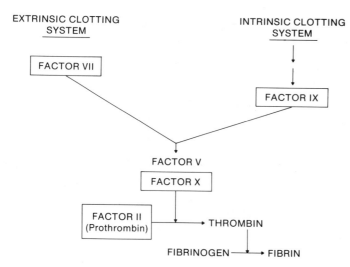

FIG. 4. Sites of action of warfarin on the blood clotting system. Factors II, VII, IX, and X are inhibited.

served and regular prothrombin times determined during this time.

Red Squill

Red squill bulbs contain at least two glycosides, scillaren-A and scillaren-B which possess potent cardiotoxic actions similar to digitalis. Signs and symptoms of toxicity are treated similarly to digitalis poisoning; those that indicate red squill poisoning has probably occurred include: blurred vision, cardiac arrhythmias, and convulsions.

Red squill has been used as a rodenticide for many years. It is considered to be of low toxic hazard to man since it possesses a powerful emetic action and most of it is therefore eliminated from the stomach before it can be absorbed. Rodents do not have a vomiting reflex and, consequently, cannot vomit. Interestingly, rodents die of chronic convulsions with respiratory failure, rather than from the cardiac effects (18).

Phosphorus

Elemental yellow (or white) phosphorus is an extremely lethal protoplasmic poison that causes disturbances to carbohydrate, fat, and protein metabolism. It impairs blood circulation and, in chronic exposure, interferes with bone growth, leading to necrosis, especially in the mandible. This is the source of the so-called "phossy jaw."

It is accidentally encountered in a number of industrial settings, although most cases of human toxicity involve its use as a rodenticide. It is incorporated into a paste which then is spread on bread, cheese, or other foods and placed where rodents (or roaches) can get to it. Unfortunately, this same food with the dark paste may be retrieved and ingested by children.

Red phosphorus is not absorbed, and consequently is not toxic. Match heads contain about 50% red phosphorus.

Phosphorus intoxication classically occurs in three stages. Initially (Stage I), intense gastrointestinal irritation with nausea, vomiting, diarrhea, abdominal pains, and mucosal burning are present. A characteristic garlic odor on the breath is detected. The vomitus and stool may be phosphorescent, and thus phorphorus poisoning has been described as the "smoking stool syndrome." Stage II may last several hours to a few days and is characterized by apparent recovery. Stage III (systemic toxicity) follows with convulsions, jaundice and hepatomegaly, coma, and death due to shock or cardiovascular failure.

A major concern in phosphorus poisoning is that the first symptoms noted, or those first taken seriously, may be those of Stage III. Many patients quickly pass through Stage I or do not interpret the period as a toxic reaction because of its lack of severity. Not all patients will have a garlic odor on their breaths or phosphorescent vomitus or feces. Too frequently, the severity of intoxication may be underrated by emergency care personnel because the victim does not have the classical symptoms (33).

Chronic exposure of low concentrations frequently causes toothache or sore jaws as the earliest perceivable symptom. This, associated with loss of appetite, weight loss, easy fracturing of bones, and anemia should alert the physician to possible phosphorus exposure.

The mortality rate is approximately 25% for victims who had early symptoms of nausea and vomiting, nearly 50% when both gastrointestinal and CNS symptoms were present, and almost 75% when the first manifestation of poisoning was restlessness, irritability, drowsiness, stupor, or coma (33). This difference in survival rates most likely reflects the time interval between time of ingestion with time of antidoting. Fifteen milligrams is the toxic dose and 50 mg may be lethal (18).

Treatment is directed at removing unabsorbed phosphorus from the gastrointestinal tract, and providing supportive care. Spontaneous vomiting after ingestion should never be interpreted as the patient being out of danger.

Gastric lavage is recommended with potassium permanganate solution to oxidize phosphorus to harmless phosphates. Hydrogen peroxide has been suggested as an alternate oxidizing agent.

Use of copper sulfate lavage is sometimes recommended. Copper salts form an insoluble coating of Cu_3P_2 over phosphorus particles to render them nonabsorbable. Copper poisoning has occurred from copper doses as little as 15 g, so the possible benefits of this procedure are questionable. Mineral oil is given to help reduce absorption and is preferred over other oils such as cottonseed or castor. Milk or other digestible fats and oils should not be used since they enhance phosphorus absorption.

Sodium Fluoride

Sodium fluoride is often described as a rodenticide (and sometimes as an insecticide) that is "no longer used for its pesticidal purposes." This statement is not true, because reports of acute toxicity encounters continue to appear in the literature. Sodium fluoride is easily obtained and inexpensive, therefore it will continue to be an important rodenticide for many years, although its popularity will never match that of warfarin. In addition, other sources of fluoride (e.g., as hydrofluoric acid, etc.) (see Chapter 8) continue to be used in industry.

Sodium fluoride is a soluble salt that readily releases its toxic fluoride ion in the gastrointestinal tract for rapid absorption. Once absorbed, fluoride is also rapidly excreted through the kidney.

Acute Fluoride Toxicity

All fluorides are protoplasmic poisons, cause hypocalcemia by removing blood and tissue calcium by precipitation, and all inhibit numerous enzyme reactions. Toxic symptoms may result after ingestion of as little as 200 mg, although the lethal dose may be closer to 4 g (6).

Death usually results from cardiac or respiratory failure, preceded by intense gastrointestinal symptoms (Table 9), hypotension, and convulsions. The responses on the nervous system and respiration are related to the calcium-binding effect of fluoride. Cardiovascular effects are due to central vasomotor depression, as well as to a direct toxic (hypocalcemic) ac-

TABLE 9. *Characteristics of fluoride poisoning*

Location	Signs and symptoms
Gastrointestinal	Abdominal pain, nausea, vomiting, diarrhea, salivation
Neurological	Paresthesias, hyperactive reflexes, clonic/tonic convulsions, positive Chvastek's sign, muscular pain and weakness
Blood	Hypocalcemia, hypoglycemia
Cardiovascular/ respiratory	Hypotension, respiratory stimulation followed by depression

Additional symptoms of fluoride intoxication are reviewed in the case study, Chapter 8.

tion on the myocardium. If death does not immediately occur, jaundice and oliguria may be seen.

Treatment of Fluoride Poisoning

Quick treatment is necessary if the fluoride-intoxicated patient is to survive. If ingestion recently occurred, a source of soluble calcium (e.g., milk, calcium chloride, lime water, etc.) should be given by lavage and/or by drinking. This calcium will react with fluoride within the gastrointestinal tract forming calcium fluoride, a relatively insoluble, nonabsorbable complex.

Calcium salts are injected intravenously to prevent rapid depletion of plasma calcium, or to replace it. Fluids are forced to increase renal clearance of the ion. Whitford et al. (44) have demonstrated in rats that administration of bicarbonate or bicarbonate with acetazolamide to induce metabolic alkalosis reduces fluoride toxicity. Although this procedure is not a part of most antidotal protocols, it merits consideration in severe toxic ingestions.

Thallium

Thallium has been used as a rodenticide and insecticide for many years. At the turn of the century it was employed therapeutically for syphilis, tuberculosis, dysentery, and ringworm. It was used topically until the early 1950s as a depilatory agent. At the present time, its use in the United States is restricted to application by qualified persons to areas where it can be shown to be needed. The incidence of poisoning by thallium has therefore declined in recent years. However, it is still the cause of an occasional report and the number of cases may increase as its use in certain industrial applications is increasing (14).

Thallium is extremely toxic with doses of approximately 1 g being lethal. It is odorless and tasteless, and this adds to its potential to cause accidental toxic ingestion. Toxicity occurs from a variety of potential mechanisms. Thallium inhibits a variety of enzyme systems in a manner similar to arsenic (Chapter 10). Sulfhydryl-containing enzymes are especially

vulnerable (20). Thallium also behaves much like potassium in the body, distributing to all tissues along with potassium. Because it substitutes for potassium in many physiological reactions, this may be part of the reason it induces severe toxic symptoms.

Signs and symptoms of poisoning (Table 10) include gastrointestinal disturbances including possible hemorrhaging. Gastric manifestations begin within hours and persist for several days.

Painful paresthesias follows within days of ingestion, followed by motor neuropathy, generalized weakness, and the Guillain-Barré syndrome. Mental capacity decreases and convulsions occur. Severe cases terminate in coma with death from respiratory depression, pneumonia, or cardiac failure. Prior to death, and about a week or more after exposure, symptoms of renal and hepatic disease, as well as necrosis to both smooth and cardiac muscle, are noted.

TABLE 10. *Characteristics of thallium poisoning*

Location	Signs and symptoms
Gastrointestinal	Nausea, vomiting, diarrhea
Neurological	Agitation, confusion, paresthesias, intense pain, neuropathy, motor weakness, Guillain-Barré syndrome, convulsions, memory loss (short-term), poor concentration, vision changes (blurred, distorted, "spots," loss)
Cardiovascular/ respiratory	Respiratory depression, pneumonia, orthostatic hypotension, cardiac failure
Other	Alopecia[a], renal and hepatic damage, smooth and cardiac muscle necrosis

[a]Diagnosis is often difficult because signs and symptoms are nonspecific. However, the appearance of alopecia, along with the other manifestations, asserts a positive diagnosis for thallium poisoning.

The most characteristic effect denoting thallium intoxication is alopecia. This begins within 1 to 3 weeks, and while other agents may also cause it, hair loss is highly suggestive of thallium intoxication. Alopecia occurs because thallium prevents incorporation of cysteine into protein, and thus prevents keratinization. While some other metals do deposit in hair and this can be used as a diagnostic means to detect their presence, thallium does not incorporate into the hair matrix.

Various chelators (see Chapter 10) have been used in an attempt to reduce thallium blood levels. Although thallium forms chelates with calcium ethyldiaminetetraacetate (Ca-EDTA), dimercaprol, and other substances, renal and pancreatic toxicity is reported. Thus, no clear-cut benefit can be derived from their use.

Since thallium and potassium have similar ionic radii and share many chemical reactions, potassium chloride is usually recommended to hasten thallium excretion. It apparently competes with thallium for reabsorption in the renal tubules. The half-life of thallium with potassium chloride therapy is lowered from 30 days normal to 3 to 10 days (14). But potassium therapy is hazardous for two reasons. First, it causes a temporary increase in plasma thallium levels. Second, potassium itself may be toxic, especially if renal function is impaired.

The latest treatment of greatest promise involves use of Prussian Blue (potassium ferri-cyano-ferrate II) to adsorb thallium from the gastrointestinal tract (36). In the alkaline pH of the intestine, thallium is substituted for potassium and prevented from being reabsorbed.

SUMMARY

Pesticides, unlike some other substances found in the home, are usually considered by most people to be extremely toxic. But instead of handling them with all the respect they deserve, pesticidal products are used carelessly and often, in great excess of amounts actually required to control the pests for which they are intended. This then leads to human poisoning and needless suffering.

Case Studies

CASE STUDY: MYSTERIOUS POISONING IN A CHILD

History

Eleven hours prior to admission to an emergency room, a 3½-year-old male began to vomit. His mother gave him children's aspirin and lemon juice. Two hours later he began to experience tremors and complained of abdominal pain and headache. He gradually became tremulous and limp. These symptoms continually worsened to the point where he was brought to the hospital.

At the hospital, the boy was awake, but lethargic. Eventually, he became flaccid and slipped into a coma. His pupils were pinpoint (1 mm). At no time were seizures noted. He did have prominent fasciculations on one thigh.

There was no evidence suggesting the ingestion of any toxic substance or prior trauma. The remaining family members remained well.

Physical examination of the young boy revealed a blood pressure of 130/60 mm Hg, pulse of 130 beats/min, and respirations of 30/min.

Laboratory findings included the following:

NA^+	= 133 mEq/L
CO_2	= 18 mEq/L
BUN	= 18 mg%
Serum creatinine	= 0.7 mg%
Hematocrit	= 35
pH	= 7.27
P_{CO_2}	= 43 mm Hg
P_{O_2}	= 150 mm Hg

A toxicology screen was negative for sedative-hypnotic drugs, alcohol, heavy metals, salicylates, phenothiazines, and opiates.

Several different diagnostic avenues were pursued in trying to delineate the reason for these symptoms. First, a 0.2-mg dose of naloxone i.v. was given. Neither respirations nor pupil size changed (thus narcotic poisoning was ruled out). Other treatment consisted of 20% mannitol, dexamethasone, ampicillin, and 40% oxygen.

Eight hours after admission, he was given 0.15 mg atropine i.v., but no response was seen until 500 mg pralidoxime (2-PAM) was given. An increase in EEG activity was noted within 2 min, and eventually consciousness was restored.

Following a visitation to the child's home, a ketchup bottle was found containing a white, milky liquid identified as a 20% solution of parathion. The mother had brought the liquid back from El Salvador for treatment of lice. The substance had been placed on the child's head for 20 min the evening before admission. (See ref. 29.)

Discussion

1. Given the information in this case study and the information about various pesticides in this chapter, can you predict what class this particular pesticide poison belongs in?

2. Is the delayed onset of symptoms consistent for this group of pesticides?

3. Explain the origin of fasciculations noted in this child.

4. Is 2-PAM expected to relieve CNS manifestations of insecticide poisonings?

CASE STUDY: LINDANE (GAMMA-BENZENE HEXACHLORIDE)

History

An 18-month-old infant male had been treated with lindane prophylactically since his older sister was diagnosed as having scabies. He was healthy, without any other apparent medical problems. The instructions were to apply a lindane lotion product for two consecutive nights, from the neck to the toes following a hot bath, and to wash it off the following morning.

The morning following the second treatment, the infant's mother forgot to wash off the lindane. Approximately 12 hr after the second treatment, the infant experienced a generalized convulsive seizure that lasted about 30 min. Shortly thereafter, he had another seizure. He was then taken to the hospital.

When he arrived, he was having some tonic-clonic movement. He was restless, lethargic, and disoriented. He was given diazepam intravenously to control seizure activity, and improved. There were no signs of head trauma or systemic illness to account for the clinical findings.

A toxicological screening of blood and urine for drugs was negative, but a qualitative test for lindane was positive. He received a thorough washing. Later, blood samples were obtained and the lindane blood levels were 0.450 ppm at 12 hr, 0.080 ppm at 24 hr, and 0.029 ppm at 96 hr after the second application.

EEGs obtained within the first 48 hr, and liver function tests were both normal. The infant was dis-

charged. Complete recovery was evident during a checkup 3 weeks later. (See ref. 41.)

Discussion

1. Would the toxic effects of lindane be more or less prominent if the solution was ingested, as opposed to percutaneous absorption? Why or why not?

2. Why was the onset of seizures delayed for at least 12 hr?

3. Lindane lotion was applied after a hot bath. Would this have possibly made a difference in the amount of poison absorbed versus if it had been applied to cold skin?

4. Is lindane effectively removed by (a) hemodialysis, (b) charcoal hemoperfusion, or (c) peritoneal dialysis?

5. To what general class of insecticide poisons does lindane belong?

CASE STUDY: PARAQUAT POISONING

History

A 17-year-old male accidentally ingested a mouthful of paraquat. An unprovoked vomiting episode occurred about 10 min later. He was brought to a local hospital 5 days following ingestion, complaining of nausea, vomiting, and burning pain in the mouth and throat. He remained at this hospital for 4 days during which time he developed a low-grade fever, was lethargic and confused. He had elevated SGOT levels and increased serum creatinine.

The patient was then transferred to a large medical center. His admitting physical examination revealed a lethargic individual with respirations of 32/min, blood pressure of 112/82 mm Hg, a temperature of 99.5°F, and pulse rate of 84/min.

The following laboratory values were obtained:

Hematocrit	= 45%
WBC	= 21,000/mm^3
BUN	= 100 mg%
Serum creatinine	= 9 mg%
pH	= 7.42
Po$_2$	= 58 mm Hg
Pco$_2$	= 33 mm Hg
CPK	6,996 mU/ml
LDH	493 mU/ml
SGOT	128 mU/ml
Alkaline phosphatase	122 mU/ml

Treatment. Initial treatment consisted of 7 g methyl prednisolone i.v. per day, along with hemodialysis. The patient remained on dialysis for 7 days, at which time his renal function recovered and an adequate urine output was maintained.

Despite this apparent recovery, the patient had a steady decline in respiratory function and increased oxygen requirement, as a result of irreversible lung damage. He died approximately 3 weeks after ingestion. (See ref. 12.)

Discussion

1. Do the symptoms and laboratory values presented in this case study correlate with the expected toxic effects of paraquat?

2. Would lavaging the patient with Fuller's earth have been of any benefit when he was admitted? How about activated charcoal?

3. Is it a consistent finding in paraquat intoxication that lung damage is delayed?

CASE STUDIES: ACUTE SODIUM FLUORIDE TOXICITY

History: Case 1

A 25-year-old male who intentionally ingested a commercially available rat poison was admitted to the emergency room 2½ hr later. An unmarked box containing a finely textured blue powder was also brought into the emergency room. It was thought, at that time, to contain arsenic. Later, it was shown to be sodium fluoride.

The physical examination was unremarkable except for tachycardia (160 beats/min) and gallop rhythm. The stool was positive for occult blood. Cyanosis was not apparent.

The following laboratory values were obtained:

Na^+	=	148 mEq/L
K^+	=	4.3 mEq/L
Cl^-	=	105 mEq/L
CO_2	=	47 mEq/L
Hct	=	48%
Hb	=	16.4 gm%

ECG demonstrated tachycardia with the QT interval of 0.45 sec. Blood and urine toxicological analyses were negative for drugs and arsenic.

Treatment. Treatment consisted of 300 mg dimercaprol i.m., since the initial diagnosis was arsenic poisoning. A nasogastric large-bore tube was inserted. Gastric lavage was performed using 3 L milk. After a while, there was profuse drainage of bright red blood from the nasogastric tube. Fluid replacement consisted of saline and dextrose.

The patient developed ventricular fibrillation about 1 hr after admission. The arrhythmia continued despite defibrillation procedures and treatment with lidocaine. He died after 30 min of unsuccessful resuscitation.

Postmortem findings showed severe congestion of the lungs and liver, along with some enlargement of the left ventricular muscle. The stomach and esophagus showed marked hyperemia, and the lumen of the stomach contained about 50 ml of a purplish-brown fluid which tested positive for fluoride. (See ref. 4.)

History: Case 2

A 2½-year-old girl ingested an undetermined amount of commercial grade laundry powder which was intended for use as a "whitener." The major ingredient was sodium silicofluoride, although this information was not made available to emergency room personnel for some time after admission. She was brought to the emergency facility because of progressive vomiting and lethargy which had been evident for about 6 hr. She experienced respiratory distress and periods of ventricular tachycardia and fibrillation for the next 2 days.

She presented in a coma with respirations of 6 to 8/min. Other vital signs were normal. She responded only to deep pain. Generalized twitching and nystagmus were also present. Chvostek and Trousseau signs were not present. Gastric lavage was performed giving a yellowish viscous material.

Laboratory findings were unremarkable for hematology, blood glucose, and supine fluid analysis. Other values included:

Na^+	=	138 mEq/L
K^+	=	6.7 mEq/L
HCO_3^-	=	13 mEq/L
Cl^-	=	107 mEq/L
+2 protein in urine		
BUN	=	31 mg%
Ca^{2+}	=	3.4 mg%

The electrocardiogram showed a normal sinus rhythm and a QT interval of 0.52 sec.

Treatment. Nine hours after admission, peritoneal dialysis was initiated with calcium chloride being added to the dialysate. The patient received a continuous infusion of calcium, and was also given 0.1% calcium hydroxide (lime water) orally. Ventricular tachycardia was controlled with lidocaine and eight separate courses of electrical cardioversion.

Nine hours after peritoneal dialysis was initiated, she became responsive and was fully conscious 2 days later. No other major problems were noted, aside from a bout of viral pneumonitis. (See ref. 46.)

Discussion

1. How does fluoride manifest its toxic actions?
2. In both cases, there was a prolonged QT interval. Why did this occur?
3. Relate fluoride poisoning to symptoms of cardiovascular and respiratory failure. How do these symptoms come about?
4. Are there any specific antidotes for fluoride toxicity? If so, what are they?
5. Patient 1 had a stool that tested positive for occult blood. Discuss what this is, and describe its potentially fatal consequences.

CASE STUDY: HERBICIDE POISONING

History

A 26-year-old male mental patient intentionally ingested 75 ml of a herbicide product containing 2,4-dichlorophenoxyacetic acid (2,4-D), and 4-chloro-2-methylphenoxypropionic acid. He was brought to an emergency facility 10 hr after the ingestion.

On admission, he was in grade 4 coma, but did not require mechanical respiratory assistance. Gastric lavage was performed. Physical examination revealed dilated pupils, but reflexes were normal and there was no indication of muscle damage. The chest and abdomen were normal. There were no corrosive burns in the mouth, but a phenolic smell was detected on his breath.

Laboratory findings revealed slight hypoxia, metabolic acidosis, and slight liver damage. Even though urinary output and adequate hydration were maintained, his BUN increased to 159 mmoles/L and serum creatinine to 165 μmoles/L. On admission, serum 2,4-D concentration was 79.6 mg/L.

Forty-eight hours following admission, the patient responded to sounds and apparently did well from that point forward. (See ref. 45.)

Discussion

1. Would herbicides, such as 2,4-D bind to activated charcoal?
2. Would forced alkaline diuresis help promote the excretion of 2,4-D? If so, why was it not employed?

CASE STUDY: PHOSPHORUS INTOXICATION

History

A 24-year-old female ingested 45 ml of Stearn's Electric Brand Paste (containing approximately 2.5% phosphorus in a 42-g tube) along with some ethyl alcohol. Forty-five minutes later, she began to vomit and experience abdominal cramping. This continued off and on for about 4 days. Afterwards, she sought medical attention at a hospital.

On admission, she was alert, cooperative, but still complained of abdominal pain, jaundice, and decreased urine output. Physical examination revealed a blood pressure of 80/68 mm Hg, pulse of 108/min, respirations of 28/min, and a temperature of 98.2°F. Her sclera were yellowed, she had shallow burns on the lips and diffuse abdominal tenderness. Arterial blood gases showed a pH of 7.51, P_{O_2} of 94 mm Hg, and P_{CO_2} of 27 mm Hg.

Other laboratory findings included:

BUN	= 113 mg%	SGOT	2,574 U
Na$^+$	= 129 mEq/L	SGPT	371 U
K$^+$	= 6.3 mEq/L	Amylase	1,826 U
Cl$^-$	= 74 mEq/L	PT	= 40% of normal
HCO$_3^-$	= 22 mEq/L	PTT	= 86.1 sec (275 second control)
Ca^{2+}	= 6.4 mg%	Creatinine	7.6 mg%
		Total bilirubin	4.4 mg%

She was stable throughout her 16-day hospital stay.

Treatment. The patient was treated with calcium chloride, vitamin K, and fluids. Urine output was severely depressed and her BUN increased to 108 mg/dl, creatinine to 9.5 mg/dl, and amylase to 2,083 U/L.

At this point, she received 50 passes of peritoneal dialysis. It was not until the eighth day postadmission that her liver function tests improved, and 10 days after admission that diuresis began. She left the hospital against medical advice on the 16th day and appeared well. She was reexamined in the medical clinic for the next 2 months and continued to make steady improvement. (See ref. 33.)

Discussion

1. Why did the phosphorus product cause burning of the oral cavity?
2. Was the patient's serum calcium level normal? If not, with what symptoms does it correlate?
3. Are the liver function tests normal or elevated? What does this suggest?

4. Can you give an explanation for the hypotension observed?

5. What is the significance of the patient's PT and PTT values?

6. What does the elevation of BUN, serum creatinine, and total bilirubin suggest?

CASE STUDIES: POISONING BY THALLIUM

History: Case 1

A 32-year-old female ingested approximately 100 mg of thallium sulfate. She was brought to the emergency room complaining of nausea, vomiting, and a burning retrosternal pain. There were no neurological or dermatological symptoms noted.

Gastric lavage was performed followed by administration of 250 mg/kg Prussian Blue given in divided doses. Due to the quantity of thallium ingested, 7 hr later she was placed on hemoperfusion (HP) and hemodialysis (HD). The initial thallium blood level was 41.50 μg%. The clearance rate for hemoperfusion was 139 ml/min, and for hemodialysis, 47 ml/min. The patient improved after 4 hr of HP-HD and was discharged 10 days later. (See ref. 10.)

History: Case 2

About 3 weeks prior to admission to a hospital, a 35-year-old female schoolteacher began to notice numbness in her extremities. She was always tired, often vomited, and no longer had an appetite. She also noticed some hair loss. Eventually, her vision deteriorated and became "fuzzy," and she experienced episodes of visual hallucinations. She had trouble judging distances, and it became progressively more difficult for her to concentrate.

Two weeks prior to her hospital admission mentioned above, she was observed at a local hospital. Physical examination revealed a blood pressure of 150/100 mm Hg with marked orthostatic changes, and pulse of 100 to 120 beats/min. Neurologic examination showed decreased sensation in the hands and feet with a decrease in muscle strength, especially in the legs. Stretch reflexes were normal. Serum potassium levels were 3.5 mEq/L. She was discharged pending urinary heavy metal analysis.

She was later admitted to a medical center hospital where she presented with severe pain in the lower extremities and marked alopecia. Her supine blood pressure was 160/110 mm Hg and while sitting erect,

140/100 mm Hg. A neurological examination was conducted and did not show any major pathological disturbances. There were some problems with attention span and difficulty with calculations.

Serum electrolytes were decreased, but hematological values were within normal limits. Suspected thallium intoxication was confirmed when urinary thallium levels were shown to be 3,100 μg%.

Treatment. The patient was treated with 15 mg of 10% KC1 every 8 hr. No other indication of additional therapy was stated, and the source of her intoxication was not determined. (See ref. 14.)

History: Case 3

A 52-year-old male deliberately ingested 20 g thallium iodide (12 g thallium) which he calculated from a chemical reference book to be 20 times the lethal dose. He was brought to the emergency facility while complaining of intense abdominal cramping and nausea.

Treatment. Treatment consisted of administering 1 g of activated charcoal 4 times a day for 5 days, a cathartic, 40 mEq of potassium chloride, 4 times a day for 6 days, and peritoneal dialysis.

The progression of signs and symptoms is given below:

Week 1: Abdominal colic, constipation, severe pain. Motor weakness of the lower extremities.
Week 2: Severe postural hypotension. Agitation, confusion, short-term memory loss.
Week 3: Alopecia.

Improvement of motor weakness and postural hypotension were noted within 1 month. He was discharged to a nursing home to regain muscle strength, and returned home a year later with some persistent neurological problems, particularly muscular weakness and trouble walking. (See ref. 25.)

Discussion

1. In Cases 2 and 3, marked orthostatic hypotension was noted. Why did this occur?

2. How does thallium manifest its toxicity?

3. What was the purpose of giving 1 g activated charcoal every 4 hr for 5 days in Case 3? Was it of any theoretical value?

4. In all three cases, potassium therapy was given. Why?

5. In Case 1, was hemoperfusion or hemodialysis more efficient in removing the poison from the blood?

6. Alopecia was present in Patients 2 and 3. What caused it?

Review Questions

1. Following ingestion of an organophosphate in-secticide, which of the following effects occur?
   A. Massive nicotinic response
   B. Massive muscarinic response
   C. Both of the above
   D. Neither of the above

2. Which of the following is a symptom character-istic of thallium intoxication?
   A. Arrhythmia
   B. Hypercalcemia
   C. Hemorrhage
   D. Alopecia

3. What does the concept of "enzyme aging" mean to the toxicity potential of an organophosphate insecticide?

4. Which of the following is a true statement?
   A. Carbamate insecticides are generally more toxic than organophosphates.
   B. Following phosphorylation of plasma cholin-esterase, several days are needed for activity to return to normal.
   C. Organophosphate insecticides cause miosis and tachycardia.
   D. Erythrocytic acetylcholinesterase levels cor-relate to levels of enzyme in the brain.

5. Appearance of a SLUD syndrome characterizes poisoning by which of the following?
   A. Phosphorus
   B. Organophosphates
   C. Warfarin
   D. Paraquat

6. Explain the probable cause of the "delayed neu-rotoxic effects" sometimes seen with organo-phosphate insecticides.

7. Organophosphate insecticides, physostigmine, and neostigmine all have a common mechanism of biologic activity. Outline this effect.

8. In treating severe organophosphate toxicity, why is it essential that both atropine and 2-PAM be given to assure maximum patient benefit?

9. Discuss why 2-PAM is contraindicated in treat-ing carbaryl intoxication.

10. Polychlorinated biphenyls are chlorinated hy-drocarbon insecticides.

A. True
B. False

11. Which of the following is true about chlorinated hydrocarbon insecticides?
    A. They are water-soluble and, hence, biode-gradable.
    B. Their use as ectoparasiticides is contraindi-cated.
    C. They are less toxic, on a milligram-to-mil-ligram basis, than organophosphates.
    D. Percutaneous absorption in man is rapid and complete.

12. Why is potassium chloride sometimes recom-mended to treat patients intoxicated with thal-lium?

13. Why is diazepam preferred over phenobarbital to antidote lindane-induced convulsions?

14. The major site of toxicity of DDT is the:
    A. Liver
    B. Brain
    C. Kidney
    D. Heart

15. Excretion of 2,4,-D can be hastened by altera-tion of the urine pH. Should the pH be raised or lowered?

16. Describe the major toxic reactions of paraquat, including site and mechanisms of toxicity. What substance will best adsorb paraquat from the gastrointestinal tract?

17. Symptoms of diquat poisoning are identical to those caused by paraquat.
    A. True
    B. False

18. A major toxic outcome of sodium fluoride inges-tion is:
    A. Hypocalcemia
    B. Hyperkalemia
    C. Hypokalemia
    D. None of the above

19. What is the specific rationale for performing gastric lavage with solutions of copper sulfate in victims of phosphorus ingestion?

20. Discuss the major symptoms associated with each stage of phosphorus poisoning.

21. "Phossy jaw" is a symptom of phosphorus intoxication. What are the events that lead to this problem?

22. Describe the mechanism of toxic action of warfarin. Why are single acute ingestions of even large doses not especially toxic?

23. Labels of products containing pyrethrins warn persons with hayfever or severe allergies to avoid inhaling the products. What is the specific reason for this precaution?

24. A victim of "derris" intoxication should receive antidotal treatment for poisoning by:
    A. 2,4-D
    B. diquat
    C. rotenone
    D. pyrethrins

25. An acute poisoning with nicotine causes initial muscle stimulation followed by muscular weakness. How does nicotine act to cause this cyclic effect?

26. Discuss the toxic potential of dioxin. What is its source(s) and how can accidental exposure to it best be avoided?

27. Describe the probable mechanism of toxicity of chlorinated hydrocarbon insecticides.

28. Discuss the relationship between chlorinated hydrocarbons and catecholamines, as these relate to myocardial response.

29. Which of the following produces symptoms of poisoning largely identical to DDT: lindane (I), methoxychlor (II), or TEPP (III)?
    A. I only
    B. II only
    C. I and II only
    D. II and III only

30. A victim of insecticide ingestion was admitted to the hospital for observation. The symptoms that developed did not correlate to those expected from the specific insecticide contained in the bottle. List all the various factors that could cause appearance of these unexpected symptoms.

References

1. Anon. (1979): Organophosphate insecticide poisoning. *Clin. Toxicol.*, 15:189–191.
2. Anon. (1979): EPA halts most use of herbicide 2,4,5-T. *Science*, 203:1090–1091.
3. Arena, J. M. (1979): *Poisoning: Toxicology, Symptoms, Treatment*, 4th ed. Charles C Thomas, Springfield, Illinois.
4. Baltazar, R. F., Mowers, M. M., Reider, R., Funk, M., and Soloman, J. (1980): Acute fluoride poisoning leading to fatal hyperkalemia. *Chest*, 78:660–663.
5. Casida, J. E. (1970): Mixed-function oxidase involvement in the biochemistry of insecticide synergists. *J. Agric. Food. Chem.*, 18:753.
6. Chernick, W. S. (1971): The ions: Potassium, calcium, magnesium, fluoride, iodide, and others. In: *Pharmacology in Medicine*, 4th ed., edited by J. R. DiPalma, pp. 940–957. McGraw-Hill, New York.
7. Conning, D. M., Fletcher, K., and Swan, A. A. (1969): Paraquat and related bipyridyls. *Br. Med. Bull.*, 25:245–249.
8. Cremlyn, R. (1978): *Pesticides—Preparation and Mode of Action*. John Wiley, New York.
9. Dale, W. E., Gaines, T. B., Hayes, W. J., and Pearce, G. W. (1963): Poisoning by DDT: Relation between clinical signs and concentration in rat brain. *Science*, 142:1474–1476.
10. DeBacker, W., Zachee, P., Verpooten, G. A., Majelyne, W., Vanhuele, A., and DeBroe, M. E. (1982): Thallium intoxication treated with combined hemoperfusion-hemodialysis. *J. Toxicol. Clin. Toxicol.*, 19:259–264.
11. Dreisbach, R. H. (1980): *Handbook of Poisoning*, 10th ed. Lange Medical Publications, Los Altos.
12. Fairshter, R. D., Rosen, S. M., Smith, W. R., Glauser, F. L., McRae, D. M., and Wilson, A. (1976): Paraquat poisoning: New aspects of therapy. *Quart. J. Med.*, 180:551–565.
13. Gage, J. C. (1968): The action of paraquat and diquat on the respiration of liver cell fractions. *Biochem. J.*, 109:757–761.
14. Gastel, B. (1978): Thallium poisoning. *Johns Hopkins Med. J.*, 142:27–31.
15. Gehring, P. J., Krames, C. G., Schultz, B. A., Rose, J. Q., and Rowe, V. K. (1973): The fate of 2,4,5-trichlorophenoxyacetic acid (2,4,5-T) following oral administration to man. *Toxicol. Appl. Pharmacol.*, 26:352–361.
16. Hayes, W. J. (1963): *Clinical Handbook on Economic Poisons*. Public Health Service Publication No. 476. U.S. Government Printing Office, Washington, D.C.
17. Hayes, W. J. (1969): Pesticides and human toxicity. *Ann. NY Acad. Sci.*, 160:40–54.
18. Hayes, W. J. (1971): Insecticides, rodenticides, and other economic poisons. In: *Pharmacology in Medicine*, 4th ed., edited by J. R. DiPalma, pp. 1256–1276. McGraw-Hill, New York.
19. Hayes, W. J. (1975): *Toxicology of Pesticides*. Williams & Wilkins, Baltimore.
20. Herman, M. M., and Bensch, K. G. (1967): Light and electron microscopic studies of acute and chronic

thallium intoxication in rats. *Toxicol. Appl. Pharmacol.*, 10:199–222.

21. Hill, E. C., and Carlisle, H. (1947): Toxicity of 2,4-dichlorophenoxyacetic acid for experimental animals. *J. Ind. Hyg. Toxicol.*, 29:85–89.

22. Hoffman, S., Jedeikin, R., Korzets, Z., Shapiro, A. L., Kaplan, R., and Bernheim, J. (1983): Successful management of severe paraquat poisoning. *Chest*, 84:107–109.

23. Howard, J. K. (1983): The myth of paraquat inhalation as a route for human poisoning. *J. Toxicol.-Clin. Toxicol.*, 20:191–193.

24. Klaassen, C. D. (1980): Nonmetallic environmental toxicants: Air pollutants, solvents and vapors, and pesticides. In: *The Pharmacological Basis of Therapeutics*, 6th ed., edited by A. G. Gilman, L. S. Goodman, and A. Gilman, pp. 1638–1659. Macmillan, New York.

25. Koshy, K. M., and Lovejoy, F. H. (1981): Thallium ingestion with survival: Ineffectiveness of peritoneal dialysis and potassium chloride diuresis. *Clin. Toxicol.*, 18:521–525.

26. Kutz, F. W., Strassman, S. C., Sperling, J. F., Cook, B. T., Sunshine, I., and Tessari, J. (1983): A fatal chlordane poisoning. *J. Toxicol.-Clin. Toxicol.*, 20:167–174.

27. Lange, E. P., Nelson, A. A., Fitzhugh, O. G., and Kunze, F. M. (1950): Liver cell alteration and DDT storage in the fat of the rat induced by dietary levels of 1 to 50 p.p.m. DDT. *J. Pharmacol. Exp. Ther.*, 98:268–273.

28. Lee, B., and Grath, P. (1977): Scabies: transcutaneous poisoning during treatment. *Pediatrics*, 59:643–645.

29. Lotti, M., and Becker, C. E. (1982): Treatment of acute organophosphate poisoning: Evidence of a direct effect on central nervous system by 2-PAM (Pyridine-2-aldoxime methyl chloride). *J. Toxicol. Clin. Toxicol.*, 19:121–127.

30. Mahieu, P., Hassoun, A., Van Binst, R., Lauwerys, R., and Deheneffe, Y. (1982): Severe and prolonged poisoning by fenthion. Significance of the determination of the anticholinesterase capacity of plasma. *J. Toxicol.-Clin. Toxicol.*, 19:425–432.

31. Matthew, H., Logan, A., Woodruff, M. F. A., and Heard, B. (1968): Paraquat poisoning: Lung transplantation. *Br. Med. J.*, 3:759–763.

32. Mayer, S. E. (1980): Neurohumoral transmission and the autonomic nervous system. In: *The Pharmaco-logical Basis of Therapeutics*, 6th ed., edited by A. G. Gilman, L. S. Goodman, and A. Gilman, pp. 56–90. Macmillan, New York.

33. McCarron, M. M., Gaddis, G. P., and Trotter, A. T. (1981): Acute yellow phosphorus poisoning from pesticide pastes. *Clin. Toxicol.*, 18:693–711.

34. Mellanby, K. (1970): *Pesticides and Pollution.* Collins, London.

35. Moore, J. A., and Courtney, K. D. (1971): Teratology studies with the trichlorophenoxyacid herbicides, 2,4,5-T and Silvex. *Teratology*, 4:236–240.

36. Murphy, S. D. (1980): Pesticides. In: *Toxicology—The Basic Science of Poisons*, 2nd ed., edited by J. Doull, C. D. Klaassen, and M. O. Amdur, pp. 357–408. Macmillan, New York.

37. Nogue, S., Mas, A., Pares, A., Nadal, P., Bertran, A., Milla, J., Carrera, M., To, J., Pazos, M. R., and Corbella, J. (1982–83): Acute thallium poisoning: An evaluation of different forms of treatment. *J. Toxicol.-Clin. Toxicol.*, 19:1015–1021.

38. O'Leary, J. F., Kunkel, A. M., and Jones, A. H. (1961): Efficacy and limitations of oxime-atropine treatment of organophosphorous anticholinesterase poisoning. *J. Pharmacol. Exp. Ther.*, 132:50–55.

39. Rose, M. S., and Smith, L. L. (1977): Tissue uptake of paraquat and diquat. *Gen. Pharmacol.*, 8:173–176.

40. Taylor, P. (1980): Anticholinesterase agents. In: *The Pharmacological Basis of Therapeutics*, 6th ed., edited by A. G. Gilman, L. S. Goodman, and A. Gilman, pp. 100–119. Macmillan, New York.

41. Telch, J., and Jarvis, D. A. (1982): Acute intoxication with lindane (gamma benzene hexachloride). *CMA Journal*, 126:662–663.

42. Wachs, H. (1947): Synergistic insecticides. *Science*, 105:530.

43. Wells, W. D. E., Wright, N., and Yeoman, W. B. (1981): Clinical features and management of poisoning with 2,4-D and mecoprop. *Clin. Toxicol.*, 18:273–276.

44. Whitford, G. M., Reynolds, K. E., and Pashley, D. H. (1979): Acute fluoride toxicity: Influence of metabolic alkalosis. *Toxicol. Appl. Pharmacol.*, 50:31–39.

45. Wolfe, H. R., Durham, W. F., and Armstrong, J. F. (1967): Exposure of workers to pesticides. *Arch. Environ. Health*, 14:622–633.

46. Yolken, R., Konecny, P., and McCarthy, P. (1976): Acute fluoride poisoning. *Pediatrics*, 58:90–93.

Metals

10

Over forty substances are classified as metals. Most are not significant causes of human poisoning. Others possess great potential for toxicity, but the circumstances of poisoning are that the event occurs only in limited industrial exposure. But a few metals are still considered to be significant causes of acute or chronic poisoning in a fairly large number of persons.

This chapter will focus on five such poisons: arsenic, cadmium, iron, lead, and mercury. Three additional metals are also discussed, but to a lesser extent. These are either less commonly reported as causes of toxicity than the other five (e.g., copper), or are in the news as being contemporary sources for potential poisonings because of their use as part of fad diets or "nutritional" programs (e.g., selenium, zinc).

It is no surprise to anyone that metals are everywhere. They have been carelessly used in the past or have been casually discarded into the air, water, or food supplies. They have been used as medicinals (e.g., sugar of lead, calomel, etc.) for centuries, or as legitimate insecticides or pesticides; and fossil fuels rich in metal content have been freely burned. The end result is that we have not had much to say in the past about our own destiny when it came to avoiding toxic exposure to metals.

It is tempting to state that the incidence of heavy metal poisonings will decrease in the future, as we learn more about the sources and properties of the toxic agents. This indeed has already occurred with some metals. Lead, for example, causes fewer poisonings today than in past years. By removing it from paint used on surfaces that children frequently place in their mouths, we have significantly reduced the incidence of lead poisoning.

At the same time, increasing our knowledge of metals and their potential uses may actually prove to be a disadvantage. As new technologies are developed, new uses will undoubtedly be designed for metals. We have seen this happen with the space program, and it will probably occur with other endeavors. As a result, lead, mercury, and arsenic poisonings may continue to decrease, but they will probably be replaced with nickel, cadmium, selenium, or other metals.

Toxicity from metals may occur by any route of exposure—inhalation, oral ingestion, or percutaneous absorption. In industry, inhalation of metallic fumes is the most significant route for exposure. At home, oral ingestion is more frequently encountered. On occasion, a metallic salt will be absorbed across inflamed or abraded skin to cause systemic effects. Even more rarely, someone will inject a metal substance, usually with suicidal intentions.

TREATMENT OF METAL POISONING

Chelation

The art of using chemicals to specifically antidote metal toxicity is only four decades old (33). Dimercaprol (British antilewisite:BAL) was the first antidote specifically designed to antagonize metal poisoning. Lewisite was a vesicant arsenical war gas. BAL is one of several substances (Fig. 1) called *chelators* (G: *chela* = claw) that bind directly with metal ions to form stable complexes which remove the metal from competition with the body's cells (79). Because a chelated metal is water soluble, it is readily excreted through the kidney. By definition, then, a *chelate* is a cyclic complex formed between a metal and a compound that contains two or more ligands (binding sites). The most stable chelates are those with a five- or six-membered ring. They tend to be less stable at lower pH values, and may partially dissociate in an acidic urine releasing free metal atoms to be reabsorbed back into the body.

Although chelators are generally perceived as having specific affinity for a particular metal, this is actually not the case. There is a great amount of nonspecific affinity for metals. For example, ethylenediaminetetraacetic acid (EDTA), which is generally used to antidote lead ingestion, will also form tight complexes with several other metals including calcium. Thus, the possibility exists of producing hypocalcemic tetany. For this reason, when EDTA antidotal action is desired, the substance is ad-

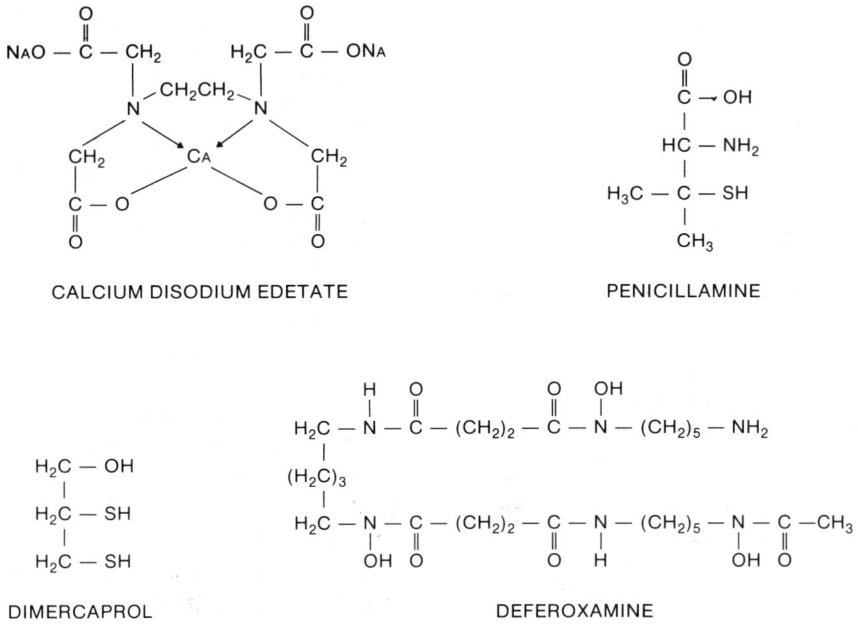

FIG. 1. Chelators used to antidote metal poisoning.

ministered as the calcium disodium salt (CaNa$_2$-EDTA).

The properties of an ideal chelator are listed in Table 1. Unfortunately, there is no such item.

ANTIDOTE TOXICITY

The old pharmacological adage that "no drug has a single effect" ("drugs are two-edged swords") carries over to the chemical chelating substances. Each has its own array of side-effects and special precautions must be closely

TABLE 1. *Properties of an ideal chelating agent*

Have a greater affinity for the metal than the ligands of tissue
Possess high water solubility
Be able to penetrate into tissue areas of metal storage
Be resistant to metabolism or degradation
Form tight bonds with metal that are stable and nontoxic at physiologic pH values
Be readily excreted as chelate with little or no dissociation
Have a low affinity for calcium
Possess minimal inherent toxicity
Be absorbed via oral administration

adhered to when they are used. The physician is always confronted with the difficult decision of whether to start or withhold chelation therapy.

It could well be that the metal is stored in one of the body's tissues, such as fat or bone and, therefore, is away from the tissues where it would normally exert its toxic action. This way it would slowly leach out of its storage depot into the blood, and as long as blood concentrations never exceeded the critical level, no significant toxicological effect would result. So administering a chelator to this person might be subjecting him to unnecessary problems.

Dimercaprol

Dimercaprol (BAL) was designed specifically to bind with arsenicals (Fig. 2) (69). Subsequent work showed that it would also chelate other metals (Table 2) reducing their concentration in the tissues. For maximum effect, it should be given soon after exposure to the poison, since it acts better as a sulfhydryl group protector than a reactivator. This will be discussed later.

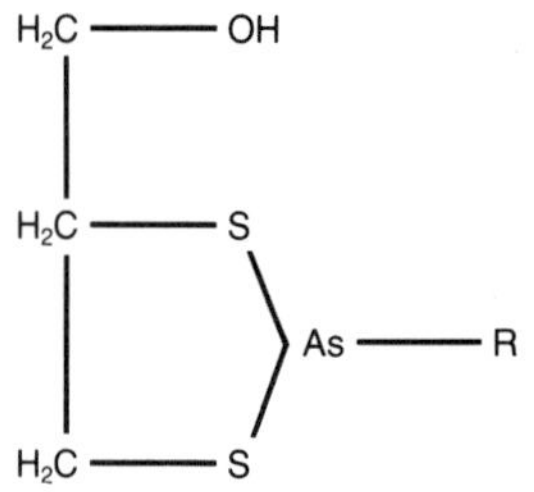

FIG. 2. Chelate formed when dimercaprol binds with arsenic.

TABLE 2. *Clinical usefulness of chelating agents*

Chelating agent	Metals reported to be chelated
Calcium disodium EDTA	Beryllium
	Cadmium
	Cobalt
	Copper
	Iron
	Lead
	Manganese
	Mercury
	Nickel
	Zinc
Deferoxamine	Iron
Dimercaprol (BAL)	Arsenic
	Cadmium
	Lead
	Mercury
Penicillamine	Copper
	Lead
	Mercury
	Zinc

TABLE 3. *Toxicity reported for dimercaprol*

Increased systolic and diastolic pressures
Tachycardia
Nausea and vomiting; abdominal cramps
Headache; sweating forehead
Painful or burning sensation in mouth, lips, throat, and penis
Conjunctivitis, rhinorrhea, lacrimation, salivation
Constriction in throat and chest
Paresthesias
Painful (sterile) abscesses at injection site
Anxiety and unrest
Fever in children

Dosage of BAL is designed to assure formation of a 2:1 complex (i.e., 2 molecules of dimercaprol and 1 molecule of metal). These complexes are both more stable and soluble in water than a 1:1 complex. This assures that the substance will chelate strongly with the metal but, at the same time, be readily excreted from the body. BAL blood levels are achieved and maintained by giving repeated and frequent doses. It must be given parenterally. Excessive single doses should be avoided because of possible side-effects.

The antidote causes a variety of toxicities of its own (Table 3), which are reported to occur in up to 50% of those who receive it. For rea-

sons stated earlier, the physician may thus elect to simply observe the patient for development of metal poisoning symptoms and treat the patient symptomatically, rather than subject him to these adverse effects.

BAL is clinically useful in treating acute and chronic poisoning by either organic or inorganic arsenicals, and protecting against mercury-induced renal damage. It is generally not effective in treating neurological conditions or symptoms of brain damage (21,29). Although theoretically active as a chelator for cadmium, the chelate may partially dissociate within the kidney and actually enhance renal damage from free cadmium (18,20).

Calcium Disodium Edetate

Calcium disodium edetate will chelate with any metal that has a higher binding affinity for it than Ca^{2+}, but the substance also chelates calcium, and in some cases causes hypocalcemic tetany. Providing the antidote as the calcium disodium salt, $CaNa_2$-EDTA, largely prevents this occurrence.

The chelator does not enter host cells, but relies on excretion of lead into the blood from bone (its major storage site) (24,25). Lead chelates with $CaNa_2$-EDTA to form a complex that is 10^7 times greater than that of the calcium complex (22). Lead that remains in blood and soft tissues redistributes into bone, where it later can also be removed through chelation.

Other metals have a greater affinity for the chelator and, in theory, will displace calcium and become part of the chelator complex. However, they simply do not form strong enough complexes to significantly alter their blood levels. The antidote is generally reserved only for lead poisoning. Future studies may broaden its clinical applications.

Toxicity to CaNa$_2$-EDTA partly restricts its usage. Following intravenous administration, severe proximal nephron degeneration may occur. This is believed to be due to the massive quantity of chelated complex which probably partially dissociates to release free lead causing the renal damage. Alternatively, the chelator may remove other essential metals from the nephron. Other symptoms of chelator toxicity are occasionally seen (e.g., fever, nasal congestion, dermatitis), but are secondary to the renal effects.

Penicillamine

The chelator, penicillamine, is formed from hydrolysis of penicillin. Penicillamine forms tight chelates with copper, lead, mercury, and zinc, and lowers the blood level of each. It is not recognized by all physicians as the first-choice antidote for lead or mercury. An advantage of this chelator is that it is well absorbed from the gastrointestinal tract following oral administration. Consequently, it is often given for long-term treatment of chronic metal poisoning after the patient has been removed from immediate danger using a parenterally administered chelator (i.e., CaNa$_2$-EDTA for lead; BAL for mercury). An added advantage is that penicillamine, unlike BAL, facilitates removal of methylmercury (3) and enhances urinary mercury excretion following inhalation of mercury vapor (66).

Penicillamine should be recognized by most of us as the treatment for Wilson's disease (hepatolenticular degeneration). This is a genetically determined disorder associated with a deficiency of ceruloplasmin, the protein that normally transports copper through the blood. As a result, free copper deposits in the liver and brain causing a wide variety of hepatic and neurological symptoms.

It has also found favor in treating severe forms of rheumatoid arthritis when more conventional therapy has failed. It is not used routinely for this purpose because of its toxicity.

Penicillamine may cause acute allergy-like reactions that are thought to be due to histamine release. In large doses, symptoms appear identical to pyridoxine (vitamin B$_6$) deficiency. In both animal and human studies, these symptoms have been reversed when the vitamin was given.

Allergy to penicillin must be carefully considered before penicillamine is given. Patients allergic to the antibiotic may also be allergic to the chelator agent.

Deferoxamine

Deferoxamine has a high affinity for both ferrous and ferric iron. It readily binds with iron of hemosiderin and ferritin, sparing that of the cytochromes and hemoglobin which bind iron more tightly. It is given parenterally, since less than 15% is absorbed from the gastrointestinal tract.

Its toxicity includes those related to histamine release (e.g., urticaria, gastrointestinal irritation, and hypotension).

SITE OF TOXIC METAL ACTION

Metals are toxic because they bind with ligands of biologic structures. Major sites include the various enzyme systems of the body. This binding, with subsequent inactivation of the enzyme system, is the primary reason metals are toxic.

It is difficult to pinpoint a single target tissue site or enzyme system for each metal. Their affinities for enzymes are great. However, for each metal there is a "most sensitive" area, and most signs and symptoms caused by the metal can be traced to it. But keep in mind that other sites may also be affected. The specified site is based on the tissue most sensitive at the lowest dose that will cause toxicity. When larger doses are encountered, additional sites (enzymes) may also be affected. Thus, the dose of the metal is an important factor in determining what therapeutic approaches need to be followed, as well as in predicting a probable prognosis.

ARSENIC

Arsenic is one of the legends of folklore history. It has been used as a therapeutic agent prior to the birth of Christ, and as a poison for probably as many years. Actually, when we think of arsenic, one of our first associations is "poison." It has gained notoriety throughout the ages as a very effective means for homicide.

Metallic arsenic is a gray, brittle metal, and is considered nontoxic. The most common commercial form is arsenic trioxide (As_2O_3) which is a white solid that looks like sugar. Arsenic trioxide is an inorganic salt of the trivalent form of arsenic acid (H_3AsO_4). Arsenic also exists in the pentavalent oxidation state (As_2O_5). The arsenates (e.g., lead arsenate:$PbHAsO_4$), which are salts of arsenic acid, are the most abundant forms present in nature and are less toxic than trivalent arsenic. Organic arsenicals also exist and, in this form, arsenic is covalently bonded to an aliphatic carbon chain or a ring structure, with arsenic existing in either the trivalent or pentavalent form. This form of arsenic is also considered to be less toxic than the trivalent inorganic salts.

The most toxic form of arsenic is arsine gas (AsH_3) which can be generated when acids are combined with arsenic-containing metals. Poisoning by arsine is relatively rare. When it does occur, it is generally via an industrial accident.

Acute arsenic poisonings are most commonly the result of suicidal or accidental ingestions, although some authors still list homicide as the most common cause of arsenic poisoning (23). Arsenic trioxide is odorless and tasteless, thus it could be easily added to most liquids without notice. Chronic arsenic poisonings are usually from environmental or industrial exposures.

Table 4 lists the various sources of arsenic. It is a common industrial nuisance around factories where ores, such as gold and copper, are being smelted. It is also used in the manufacturing of certain kinds of glass, pigment production, and the hardening of copper and lead alloys. Because of many years of carelessness with by-products of metal smelting, much arsenic has been released into the environment (50). It has been found as a contaminant of some water supplies and soil samples. It is also an excellent insecticide and herbicide and has been widely used as such for many years. No

TABLE 4. *Sources of arsenic exposure*

Environmental
Water, soil, air
Fish, shellfish
Industrial
Metallurgy
Manufacturing of glass
Pigment production
Manufacturing of arsenical chemicals
Household
Weed killers
Ant and roach control
Arsenic-containing pharmaceuticals

doubt this has also contributed to the environmental burden. Its use in medicinals is now limited to treatment of a few tropical diseases. Rarely does an arsenical drug cause poisoning in the United States.

Daily arsenic exposure by man reaches 900 μg (42). The source is primarily food and water and, to a lesser extent, air. About four-fifths of absorbed arsenic is stored in the body, especially the liver, kidney, walls of the gastrointestinal tract, the spleen, and lung. The arsenicals are deposited in fine hair and nail beds, and can be detected in these tissues several years after chronic exposure. The body burden for arsenic is approximately 21 mg, and normal, unexposed blood levels are in the range of 0.2 μg%. Toxic exposures have been correlated with blood levels greater than 10 μg%, and lethal blood levels in the range of 60 to 90 μg% (5).

Mechanism of Arsenic Toxicity

Arsenic is a general protoplasmic poison. It produces its toxic effects by combining with sulfhydryl (−SH) groups, particularly those contained within enzymes. One such enzyme system is the pyruvate dehydrogenase complex which is necessary for the oxidative decarboxylation of pyruvate to acetyl CoA and CO_2 before it enters into the TCA cycle. This enzyme system is comprised of several enzymes and co-factors as shown in Fig. 3. One reaction involves a transacetylase which combines with coenzyme A (CoA-SH) to form acetyl CoA and a dihydrolipoyl-enzyme complex that contains

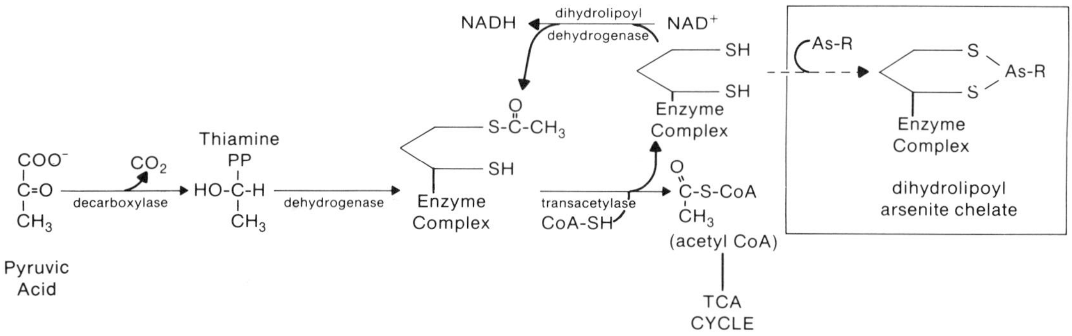

NADH ← dihydrolipoyl dehydrogenase ← NAD⁺

Thiamine PP

COO⁻
|
C=O   CO₂
| ↘   decarboxylase
CH₃

Pyruvic
Acid

HO-C-H
|
CH₃   dehydrogenase   → Enzyme Complex

$$\text{S-C-CH}_3 \quad (O)$$

SH

transacetylase
CoA-SH

$$\text{C-S-CoA} \quad (O)$$
CH₃
(acetyl CoA)

TCA
CYCLE

SH
SH
Enzyme Complex

As-R

S
S   As-R
Enzyme Complex

dihydrolipoyl arsenite chelate

FIG. 3.   The effect of arsenic on sulfhydryl related enzyme systems.

two sulfhydryl groups. These sulfhydryl groups are extremely vulnerable to the trivalent form of arsenic, thus forming a chelate. This dihydrolipoyl-arsenite chelate then prevents the reoxidation of the dihydrolipoyl group necessary for continued enzymatic activity. As a result of arsenic binding to this enzyme system, there is an accumulation of pyruvic acid in the blood (see *far left side* of Fig. 3).

Arsenate also uncouples oxidative phosphorylation in the second stage of glycolysis by competing with phosphate in the glyceraldehyde dehydrogenase reaction. As shown in Fig. 4, the binding of arsenate to glyceraldehyde-3-phosphate and its subsequent nonenzymatic hydrolysis to 3-phosphoglycerate does not produce ATP, in contrast to the normal glycolytic pathway. Since arsenic has an affinity for −SH groups and there are several SH-containing enzymes, it is likely then to expect high concentrations of arsenic in the liver binding to metabolic enzymes. There are structural proteins which also contain sulfhydryl groups, and that is the reason arsenic has an affinity for hair, nails, and, to a lesser extent, bone. Because of its tight binding with −SH groups, arsenic can still be detected in hair and bones years after the poisoning event.

Clinical Manifestations of Arsenic Poisoning

Acute

Due to restrictions imposed by FDA, EPA, and OSHA on arsenic, there has been a de-

crease in the allowable amount of arsenic content in food and in the atmosphere. In addition, the homicidal and suicidal modes of arsenic poisoning have also decreased.

If the amount ingested is small, the signs and symptoms discussed below may not be seen, so a positive diagnosis of arsenic as the cause of toxicity may be missed. On the other hand, if a large quantity was involved, death ensues rapidly and usually without any significant effects to label the ingestion as an arsenic poisoning. A garlic-like odor on the breath or in perspiration should always suggest arsenic poisoning. Death is due to circulatory collapse.

At first, the capillary beds are dilated then arteriolar and myocardial damage occur. If the patient survives an acute arsenic poisoning, ECG abnormalities may still be seen months later. In general, acute arsenic ingestions usually have a delayed onset of toxic action. Symptoms can be delayed for 30 min to hours.

The initial effects of acute arsenic poisoning are listed in Table 5 and are associated with extreme gastroenteritis beginning with burning esophageal pain, difficulty in swallowing, and unbearable stomach pain. These are accompanied by nausea, projectile vomiting, and explosive diarrhea. The diarrhea consists of watery feces containing shreds of mucus, similar to the rice-water stools seen with cholera, which soon progresses to a bloody diarrhea. This is due to intense irritation and swelling of the gastric mucosa. The metal causes capillary transuda-

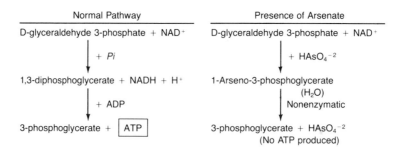

FIG. 4. Binding of arsenic to glyceraldehyde-3-phosphate resulting in inhibition of ATP production.

tion of plasma under the gastrointestinal mucosa, with vesicle formation. As these rupture into the gastrointestinal tract, the tissue sloughs off, and the plasma leaks into the intestine where it coagulates. This increased volume of fluid within the intestine causes a "bulk laxative" effect and, also, because of the epithelial irritation, intense vomiting and catharsis occur. If the local irritation is sufficiently strong, epithelial cell proliferation is halted, which further potentiates the damage. Bleeding soon occurs and is the source of blood in the stool and vomitus. This also adds further insult to the circulatory system and the blood pressure progressively decreases.

Of course, these symptoms by themselves would not automatically indicate an arsenic poisoning. Sudden, unexplained violent gastroenteritis is followed by inflammation of the respiratory tract and conjunctival membranes, and erythematous and vesicular skin eruptions. Renal dysfunction, blood dyscrasias, cardiomyopathies, and liver damage may also be present.

Kidney damage is seen within the renal capillaries, tubules, and glomeruli. Initially, the glomeruli are destroyed and filled with plasma protein as the renal capillaries dilate. The tubules become necrotic. Urine outflow is decreased or halted.

Blood cells exhibit morphological changes as well as a significant decrease in red blood cell and white cell counts.

Eventually the liver shows signs of fatty infiltration with central necrosis and cirrhosis.

Delayed actions of an acute arsenic poisoning include alopecia, and peripheral neuropathy characterized by paresthesias of the lower extremities, foot drop, wrist drop, abnormal gait, and slow reflexes.

Chronic

At one time, arsenic (e.g., as Fowler's solution) was a popular medication for treating certain skin diseases. Taken in low doses, it caused a "milk and roses" appearance by its vasodilation action on facial capillaries. Prolonged usage also produced hyperkeratosis, keratosis of the palms and soles, and dermatitis, especially in areas where there was a high concentration of sweat glands, such as the groin area and armpits. The dermatitis was due to the primary irritation and sensitization action of arsenic.

Chronic arsenic poisoning may begin insidiously with the victim complaining of weakness, tiredness, lack of appetite, weight loss, and irritability. It is obvious that these are rather nonspecific indicators and could be the result of a number of different toxic exposures, as well as other generalized causes. More specific characteristics of chronic arsenic poisoning are noted by the effects of arsenic on the integumentary system. This results in the appearance of dark brown pigmentation and a thickening of the skin's horny layer. The nails thicken and characteristic white bands (referred to as Mee's lines) develop above the lunulae.

Peripheral neuropathies sometimes develop in the latter stages. The legs are affected more than the arms, causing paralysis of both the

TABLE 5. *Characteristics of arsenic poisoning*

Acute arsenic toxicity
  Severe nausea
  Profuse diarrhea; rice-water stools
  Projectile vomiting
  Abdominal pain
  Skin eruptions
  Severe irritation of the nose, throat, conjunctiva
  Loss of fluid
  Uremia
  ECG abnormalities
  ST-segment and T-wave abnormalities
  Hypoxic convulsions
Chronic arsenic toxicity
  Weight loss
  Anorexia
  General malaise
  Garlic odor on breath
  Hyperpigmentation—mottled brown spots
  Hyperkeratosis—palmar and plantar surfaces
  Mee's lines—white lines on the lunulae of the
    nails
  Peripheral neuritis
  Tremors
  Ulceration of gastrointestinal tract
  Chronic hepatitis
  Liver cirrhosis
  Pancytopenia
  Anemia

motor and sensory pathways. There is also a tendency for ulcerations to develop in the gastrointestinal tract, with hepatitis and cirrhosis also appearing with occupational exposure to arsenic.

Laboratory examination of peripheral blood shows pancytopenia, especially neutropenia. Prominent features of chronic arsenic poisoning include a decrease in red blood cell production and basophilic stippling. Occasionally, hypochromatic normoblasts and megaloblastic anemia associated with folic acid deficiency has been observed.

Epidemiological studies have shown a correlation between long-term exposure to both the trivalent and pentavalent arsenic compounds and the incidence of lung cancer, lymphatic cancer, and skin cancer (6,12).

Treatment of Arsenic Poisoning

For acute arsenic poisoning, all possible measures should be undertaken to initiate suppor-

tive and symptomatic treatment. To prevent neuropathy, chelation therapy should be started as soon as possible. The specific chelator most often used is BAL.

The standard regimen used for BAL is 3 to 5 mg/kg given every 4 hr for 2 days, followed by 2.5 mg/kg every 6 hr for 2 days, then 2.5 mg/kg every 12 hr for 1 week. During this time, 24-hr urine samples should be obtained, and chelation therapy should be discontinued when the 24-hr urine arsenic concentration is less than 50 mg. BAL treatment is often followed by treatment with oral penicillamine given every 6 hr for 5 days.

Treatment for chronic arsenic poisoning should begin with removal of the source. Chelation therapy is not usually indicated, since the half-life of arsenic is 3 to 4 days.

CADMIUM

Although sporadic cases of toxicity to cadmium have been reported since the mid-1850s, it was not until nearly a century later that its toxic potential generally became understood. It is not even mentioned in many books that discuss heavy metal poisoning except in the most recent editions. However, cadmium now ranks as one of the heavy metals of greatest toxicologic concern (17).

Cadmium and its salts are widely employed in numerous industrial processes and it is a component of many commercial products. Electroplating is the major use of the pure metal. It is also used in process engraving and storage batteries. Its salts find use in photography, glass and silver-alloy manufacture, in production of photoelectric cells, photoconductors, and phosphorus. Cadmium acetate is used in production of an iridescent glaze used in pottery and procelain. Cadmium is also used in production of paper, textiles, soaps, rubber, inks, fireworks, and in hundreds of other items.

Cadmium is found in nature in close association with lead and zinc (79). Thus, when one or the other metal is mined and extracted, the others, if not specifically processed, are released into the environment. Of course, today all three would be extracted, since each has widespread technological uses. Unfortunately, this has not always been the case for cadmium, and, as a result, the environment has been freely contaminated with cadmium.

We can assume that one of the reasons cadmium poisoning has not always been of great concern is that toxicities previously reported as due to lead may actually have been due to cadmium. It is a repeat of the same old adage, "if you are not looking for something, you are not likely to find it."

There is no known biological use for cadmium. Still, the average 50-year-old American has about 30 mg of cadmium stored in his body (19). In fact, cadmium is the heavy metal most prone to accumulate in the body. Its level increases throughout life as its biological half-life is 10 to 30 years (38). Thirty days after rats were exposed to inhaled cadmium, more than 40% of the inhaled quantity was still present in the blood. Greater than 90% remained 30 days after an intravenous or intraperitoneal dose (49). Most of this burden accumulates from contaminated foodstuff, water, and inhalation of airborne cadmium, including cigarette smoking. Coal and other fossil fuels release cadmium into the air, and areas around metal-processing plants are especially high in cadmium. Actually, cadmium is only poorly absorbed from the gastrointestinal tract with as little as 5% entering the blood (58). This is contrasted to inhalation, whereby cigarette smokers may absorb up to 40% cadmium (19). Thus, intoxication via the oral route is relatively unimportant, contrasted to inhalation.

Mechanism of Cadmium Toxicity

Cadmium inhibits enzymes that contain sulfhydryl groups. It also binds to other ligands including the carboxyl, cysteinyl, histidyl, hydroxyl, and phosphatyl groups of protein and purines. Its major toxic effects probably result from such interactions. However, it has also been reported to compete with various other metals in the body. For example, cellular uptake of copper and zinc may be depressed. The clinical significance of most of these effects is still unknown.

One plasma enzyme that cadmium inhibits is α_1-antitrypsin (9). A deficiency of this enzyme has been linked to emphysema, and this may be the mechanism that is at least partially responsible for the pulmonary symptoms.

Clinical Manifestations of Cadmium Poisoning

As we learned earlier, cadmium is more toxic if inhaled than if swallowed, and most cases of acute toxicity to cadmium follow from inhalation of cadmium dusts and fumes (especially cadmium oxides).

Within several hours, the victim complains of intense irritation to the respiratory passages, nausea and vomiting, dizziness, and chest pains. Death is usually attributed to severe pulmonary edema. If the patient survives, life-long bouts of emphysema and other respiratory disorders will be encountered. Important clinical manifestations of toxicity are summarized in Table 6.

Cadmium is probably stored in all tissues, but seems to have special affinity for liver and kidney with about half of all cadmium located in these two tissues. The reason for this high affinity may be due to the presence of a low molecular weight protein called metallothionein (35). Metallothionein is rich in sulfhydryl groups

TABLE 6. *Characteristics of cadmium toxicity*

Oral
Severe nausea, vomiting, diarrhea
Muscular cramps
Salivation
Dizziness
Proteinuria
Glycosuria
Osteomalasia
Inhalation
Rhinorrhea
Dyspnea
Chest pain
Pulmonary edema
Progressive emphysema
Azotemia
Proteinuria

and has a high binding affinity for cadmium, as well as zinc, and perhaps silver, mercury, and even other metals. However, this binding is reversible, and since cadmium does accumulate in the body, it is doubtful if this protein offers the only mechanism for binding.

Following chronic exposure by inhalation, symptoms are not unlike those from acute exposure of high levels.

Cadmium also causes nephrotoxicity. Proteinuria, glycosuria, and aminoaciduria are noted, and glomerular filtration rate is decreased.

Of major research interest in recent years have been the effects of chronic cadmium exposure on the cardiovascular system. Several studies have suggested that cadmium was a cause of hypertension (63,71,74). This observation has been extended to rat studies where animals receiving cadmium in drinking water developed hypertension. The suggestion is especially appealing because of the high renal tissue affinity for cadmium. However, hypertension is not a consistent finding of chronic industrial poisonings.

Cadmium is reported to cause osteomalacia, perhaps by interfering with calcium and phosphate balance in the kidney. Residents of Toyama, Japan were shown several years ago to have severe cadmium poisoning, with symptoms largely referable to bone and muscle pain. The disease was termed I'tai-I'tai Byo (the "ouch-ouch" disease) and resulted from contamination of rice fields by cadmium released from a metal processing plant upstream (73). Osteomalacia was a prominent feature of these victims.

A major direction in animal research has been toward studying cadmium accumulation in the testis. The interstitial cells and the testicular vascular endothelium seem to be mainly involved (52,77). The extent of damage seems to be species-dependent. Testicular damage has not been proven in man, although it has been suggested. For example, in men exposed to chronic cadmium inhalation, impotence is not an uncommon event. However, whether this impotence was caused by cadmium or by other toxic substances in the industrial environment cannot be stated for certain (41).

Acute and chronic exposure of animals have also demonstrated that cadmium causes growth retardation and is carcinogenic. The clinical significance of these effects is not known.

Treatment of Cadmium Poisoning

Treatment methods for cadmium are not as clear-cut as for some of the other metals. It is largely supportive. Vitamin D has been recommended for relieving bone pain.

While chelators will increase renal excretion, they may also increase renal toxicity (18,20). This occurs because the chelated complexes readily dissociate in the kidney, releasing free cadmium.

IRON

Accidental ingestion of iron-containing preparations is relatively common among children, whereas intentional overdoses with iron are occasionally seen in adults (4). Even though these exposures are rarely fatal, they can result in mental retardation and possibly death. The reason for the high incidence of accidental iron poisoning among children is easily understood if we examine the types of dosage forms that are available for iron-containing preparations. Comparing iron tablets with pieces of candy (refer back to Chapter 1, Fig. 4) reminds us of their similarity in appearance, shape, and color.

Iron is the fourth most abundant element in the earth's crust and was probably the first metal used by ancient peoples. Iron is essential to all organisms, animals, and plants. Metallic iron is chemically unstable and is slowly converted to the ferrous or ferric state. The iron content in animals varies according to the state of health, nutrition, age, sex, and species.

The major source of atmospheric contamination of iron is the iron and steel industry. Inhalation of iron oxide fumes or dust, especially in mining communities, causes a benign pneumoconiosis referred to as "siderosis." Iron poisoning is not a common environmental event.

Practically every tissue of the body contains iron. The human body burden is near 4 g. Most of the iron normally exists bound to proteins. Some of these iron-containing proteins are porphyrins and heme compounds such as hemoglobin and myoglobin. Other proteins involved with binding of iron include ferritin, transferrin, and hemosiderin.

The daily diet of an average man contains about 10 to 15 mg of elemental iron, only a small portion of which is actually absorbed. The minimum lethal dose (MLD) for iron is about 200 to 250 mg/kg body weight.

Iron is commonly available in many preparations, including iron supplement tablets as the sulfate, gluconate, and fumarate salts, in multiple vitamin-mineral preparations, and in prenatal vitamin-mineral preparations. An important consideration to remember is that all discussion about iron toxicity is related to the actual amount of elemental iron that is actually absorbed. Therefore, for the salt that forms, the actual amount of iron content must be calculated. It is reported that prior to the introduction of deferoxamine, the death rate in children from iron poisoning exceeded the rate for aspirin (65).

Mechanism of Iron Toxicity

The primary site for control of body iron content is the small intestine. It acts both as an absorptive and excretory organ. Iron is absorbed in its divalent (ferrous) form into the gastrointestinal mucosa and converted there to the trivalent (ferric) form. It then combines with apoferritin to form ferritin. Ferrous iron is absorbed more easily than the ferric form. Ferritin passes into the bloodstream and then is converted to transferritin. In the bloodstream, the iron remains in the trivalent state or is transported to the liver or spleen where it is either stored as ferritin or hemosiderin. Toxicity occurs whenever its binding sites become saturated.

Serious acute iron poisoning in children can occur following ingestion of as little as 1 g, although most ingestions involve larger quantities (16). The normal iron intake for children is about 10 to 20 mg/kg. Acute toxicity from iron is primarily manifested toward irritation to the gastrointestinal tract.

Most deaths occur in children between ages 12 and 24 months (15). The frequency of iron poisoning is usually related to the presence of an overabundant supply of prenatal vitamins or postnatal iron supplement vitamins that remain in the house. The shiny sugar coating of these tablets are often too great a temptation to a small infant.

The exact mechanism of action of iron poisoning is not understood. It is thought that death is due to shock secondary to a local gastrointestinal irritation. On autopsy, the pathology usually involves hemorrhage and necrosis of the stomach and intestinal mucosa.

In iron poisoning, capillary permeability increases and plasma is lost. This decreased blood volume then leads to a lowered cardiac output and shock. Since tissues are receiving less nutrition, cellular hypoxia and resultant acidosis ensue.

Animal studies have shown acute iron poisoning produces prolongation of coagulation time and prothrombin time, as well as an increase in thrombocytes. In addition, serum enzyme assays such as glutamic acid oxalacetic transaminase (SGOT) and glutamic pyruvate transaminase (SGPT) have also been shown to increase (61). These results indicate that some sort of hepatic degenerative process occurs following acute oral administration of massive doses of iron. Iron does accumulate in the mitochondria of hepatic cells (32,40). There it causes mitochondria to swell, which is probably the cause of their dysfunction. Fatty degeneration of the myocardium and the kidney have also been reported.

Clinical Manifestations of Iron Poisoning

There are five critical stages associated with iron poisoning (11), although some writers combine phases three and four. These stages are listed in Table 7.

The first phase lasts from 30 min to 2 hr after ingestion and may be characterized by abdom-

TABLE 7. *Characteristics of acute iron poisoning*

Phase	Time	Signs and symptoms
Phase 1	30 min–2 hr	Irritability Seizures Restlessness Abdominal pain Vomiting Bloody diarrhea Tachypnea, tachycardia
Phase 2	Immediately follows Phase 1	"Period of apparent recovery"
Phase 3	8–16 hr after Phase 1	Shock Refractive acidosis Cyanosis Fever
Phase 4	2–4 days postingestion	Hepatic necrosis Elevated SGOT, SGPT
Phase 5	2–4 weeks postingestion	Gastrointestinal obstruction

inal pain, explosive diarrhea, or vomiting brown or bloody vomitus, and possibly CNS irritation. Tachypnea, tachycardia, and hypotension may be seen. The person may be lethargic, restless, and experience severe abdominal pain. Iron produces a direct corrosive effect, and, consequently, the gastrointestinal mucosa will show signs of hemorrhage and possibly shock. Victims seldom die from problems encountered in Phase 1, but it is still possible. Presence of shock or coma during this early phase is indicative of a grave prognosis.

Assessment of iron poisoning may be difficult during this early phase. As could be expected, especially from a single dose, iron is rapidly cleared from the plasma and deposited in the liver (61). Thus, when the patient is observed for workup, the blood level may be normal or near normal. However, it must always be remembered that, even in the absence of elevated blood levels of iron, toxicity is progressing.

The second phase is a lapse phase of quiescence in which an apparent recovery is suspected, but the patient usually progresses into the third phase which occurs 8 to 16 hr after the initial phase. During the third phase there is an abrupt onset of shock, and acidosis causing hyperventilation, hypoglycemia, cyanosis, and fever.

The fourth phase occurs 2 to 4 days postingestion and is characterized primarily by liver injury. It is thought that hepatic necrosis is due to a direct action of iron on the mitochondria in the hepatocyte.

The final phase of iron toxicity occurs 2 to 4 weeks after ingestion and is generally characterized by gastrointestinal obstruction, including pyloric stenosis and gastric fibrosis.

Treatment of Iron Poisoning

The most meaningful laboratory test to determine acute iron poisoning is a serum iron level. If the concentration of iron in the serum exceeds 300 μg%, chelation therapy is indicated. However, therapy should not be delayed until a serum iron level can be obtained if the history and clinical evidence strongly suggest iron ingestion.

The most important consideration in treating acute iron poisoning is to prevent continued absorption. This can be achieved by several means. First, emesis is indicated in the absence of vomiting when large amounts of iron have been ingested. Lavage may be performed with a 5% solution of sodium bicarbonate which produces nonabsorbable ferrous carbonate. A Fleet's® enema or Fleet's Phospho-Soda® diluted 1:4 with water can be given to form a nonabsorbable iron phosphate complex. Bicarbonate forms a more insoluble iron product than phosphate, but both solutions actually complex less than one-eighth of available iron (8).

The use of the Fleet's® enema serves two purposes: (a) to convert soluble ferrous salt to the less soluble carbonate and phosphate, and (b) to evacuate the stomach. Administration of a saline cathartic, such as magnesium sulfate, is also indicated for removal of large quantities of iron tablets.

Chelation therapy with deferoxamine is recommended when serum iron levels exceed 300 μg%, even if clinical signs of poisoning are not evident. Deferoxamine complexes preferentially, but not exclusively, with ferric iron. One hundred milligrams of deferoxamine will bind with approximately 9 mg elemental iron (43). It can be given orally to bind with iron in the gut and reduce its absorption. At this point, an oral dosage form is available only for experimental use. Deferoxamine is typically administered intravenously at 15 mg/kg/hr. Also it should be administered cautiously because of drug-induced hypotension. If it is a milder poisoning, then intramuscular administration of deferoxamine at 90 mg/kg can be given. The urine should be monitored for the characteristic reddish-orange (vin rosé) color, which indicates excretion of the chelated complex. Chelation therapy should be continued until the urine returns to a normal color, indicating termination of iron complexation.

Deferoxamine should be given quickly after toxic iron ingestion, since its efficacy decreases with time (55).

LEAD

Lead is another metal whose toxicity has plagued man since early civilization. Lead was found in almost all of the early utensils, storage containers, and vessels used for cooking. Today, it is produced in larger quantities than any of the other toxic heavy metals. It is estimated that the world production exceeds 3.5 million tons per year (79). More is known about lead toxicity than about any other metal.

Besides the metallic form, lead may exist in both an inorganic and organic form. For all practical purposes, the inorganic forms of lead have the same action in the body. Organic lead compounds, primarily the tetraethyl- and tetramethyl-forms (TEL, TML), act similarly to each other, but differently from inorganic salts.

Sources of exposure to lead are listed in Table 8. Lead is a cumulative poison that causes both chronic and acute intoxication. Although acute poisoning from lead is rare, chronic poisoning is a serious problem.

Lead toxicity is of special concern to workers such as miners and smelters, automobile finish-

TABLE 8. *Sources of lead exposure*

Environmental
Water
Air
Soil
Food
Household
Crayons and toys
Paper and clothes
Dirt and sand
Paint flakes
Furniture
Wallpaper
Lead-glazed dishes, cups, glasses, etc.
Persons at high industrial risk
Miners
Smelters
Automobile finishers
Storage battery workers
Sheet metal workers
Spray painters

ers, foundry and storage battery workers, typesetters, sheet metal workers, and spray painters. Lead (as well as potentially toxic levels of copper and zinc) may also be a contaminant in illegally produced or "moonshine" whiskey (28,53). Sometimes old automobile radiators are used as condensers, and the beverage becomes contaminated with lead from solder used in the original construction of the radiator. Prior to World War II, paints containing lead concentrations of up to 40% dry weight were commonly used as house paints for both exterior and interior surfaces. The Lead Poisoning Prevention Act was passed by Congress in 1971 which limited the acceptable lead concentration in residential paint to 1%. In 1977, this legislation was amended to reduce the acceptable level to 0.06%. Even though the use of paint with a high concentration of lead has been largely discontinued, there still exists a major potential hazard for children obsessed with pulling paint chips from walls and woodwork of older homes and buildings. A tiny flake or paint chip from one of these old houses may contain as much as 100 mg lead. If a child ingested a few of these chips, this would exceed the daily permissible intake by a factor of 30. In 1970, 3,500 cases of lead poisoning from such causes were reported in Chicago alone (59).

Some small children seem to possess an abnormal craving for placing unnatural, nonnutritional substances in their mouths. Such substances include paint chips, plaster, and paper. Also, it includes chewing on the painted surface of lead pencils, etc. This unusual habit is referred to as *pica*. While the term is often described as the child's having this craving for paint or plaster chips, pica is, in reality, a generic term that describes the craving for anything abnormal for the mouth. Most lead poisoning in children occurs between the ages of 1 and 5 years. Also, there is a higher incidence of child-related lead poisoning during the warmer months.

Standards currently in effect for paints used on furniture, pencils, and toys, or on internal house surfaces, limit the amount of lead used to 1% of total dried solids (51,56).

Lead is ubiquitous. In other words, it is present in soil, water, food, air, and in numerous industrial products. The lead content of soil varies depending upon the surroundings. Areas near a lead smelter, or where lead-based spray paints were once used, show a high lead content. Since most plumbers today use copper, galvanized, or even plastic piping, lead water pipes are no longer a major source of water lead content. A theory often stated is that one of the factors that led to the eventual fall of the Roman Empire was the lead pipes this early civilization used to transport its water supply. These people, it is said, eventually consumed enough lead from this water to cause toxic, and often fatal, poisonings. If true, this theory might also account for the decline of numerous other civilizations who used lead-lined containers to store or transport their drinking water. Soft and acid waters dissolve more lead from pipes on plumbing fixtures than hard water.

The major source of environmental lead intake today by humans is in food. Plants may take up lead through the leaf respiratory mechanism. Plants can absorb soluble lead through their roots and transport it above ground. Vegetable farms and fruit orchards located near heavily travelled highways have been shown to produce fruit and vegetables with a high lead content. Also, lead used in the canning process of some foods adds to the total lead intake in humans.

Therefore, there are several sources of lead exposure to man. It has been estimated that the average body burden of lead among children and adults in the United States is 100 times greater than the so-called "natural" burden. Also, the amount of lead in the body is directly proportional to the amount of lead in the air. The good news, however, is that the average blood level of lead in Americans has dropped approximately 37% from 1976 to 1980 (1).

Organic lead intoxication is even more rare than inorganic lead poisoning and will probably decrease in the future. Organic lead compounds have been used in gasoline as "anti-knock" additives. With the nation rapidly converting its automotive fuel needs to "nonleaded" gasoline, the risk of organic lead poisoning is declining.

Mechanism of Lead Toxicity

Lead manifests its toxicity primarily by binding to sulfhydryl groups of protein molecules. This causes inactivation or inhibition of several vital enzyme systems. Lead interferes with heme synthesis by preventing the conversion of delta-aminolevulinic acid (δ-ALA) to porphobilinogen and incorporation of iron into protoporphyrin IX to form heme, by inhibiting the enzymes δ-aminolevulinic acid dehydrotase and ferrochelatase, respectively (Fig. 5). This causes an increase in urinary coproporphyrin and δ-ALA excretion, and a decrease in heme synthesis.

To compensate for the decreased heme synthesis produced by lead, the bone marrow increases production of red blood cells. These cells are then released as immature reticulocytes and stippled cells. Basophilic stippling occurs as part of the metabolic disturbances of heme synthesis which occurs with lead poisoning. The red blood cells fail to completely mature, and they retain some of the cellular organelles which usually disappear during cell maturation. When peripheral blood smears are stained, the irregular polyribosomes and associated RNA aggregate and produce the characteristic stippled cell.

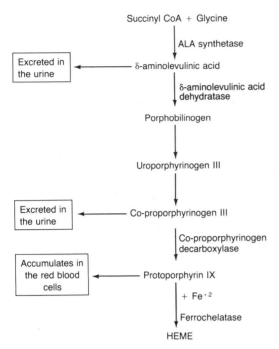

Succinyl CoA + Glycine

| ALA synthetase

δ-aminolevulinic acid ──→ Excreted in the urine

| δ-aminolevulinic acid dehydratase

Porphobilinogen

Uroporphyrinogen III

Co-proporphyrinogen III ──→ Excreted in the urine

| Co-proporphyrinogen decarboxylase

Protoporphyrin IX ──→ Accumulates in the red blood cells

| + Fe⁺²
| Ferrochelatase

HEME

FIG. 5. The inhibition of heme production by lead.

Basophilic stippling is not pathognomonic of lead poisoning. The ultimate effect of lead on the hematopoietic system is a resultant microcytic hypochromic anemia which is usually not severe, even in children. The anemia is a result of a decrease in the lifespan of the red blood cell, as well as interference with hemoglobin synthesis.

In vitro experiments have suggested that the accumulation of δ-ALA and protoporphyrins may produce a toxic effect on some tissues. For example, animal studies have shown that quantities of δ-ALA have been found in the hypothalamus, and that protoporphyrin accumulates in the dorsal root ganglion. There is a good chance these may be responsible for the lead encephalopathy. The peripheral neuropathies associated with lead poisoning appear to be related to demyelination and degeneration of the peripheral nerves.

Lead circulates through the blood, following absorption, mostly in association with erythrocytes. It is initially distributed to the soft tissues such as the renal tubules and liver, but

it eventually incorporates into bone, hair, and teeth for storage (38), with up to 90% storing in bones (26). A small quantity stores in the brain.

In bone, lead is found as the tertiary lead phosphate. In theory, as long as lead remains bound to bone, it is unavailable to vulnerable tissues of the body.

There is a special problem with lead poisoning that must be considered. Any factor that affects calcium absorption or desorption can affect the stability of this stored lead. For example, a diet low in phosphate favors release of lead into the blood, whereas a high phosphate intake promotes storage. Vitamin D promotes lead deposition, if the phosphate concentration is sufficient, and parathyroid hormone causes its removal.

Clinical Manifestations of Lead Poisoning

Acute lead poisoning is occasionally observed, but this rare. Most cases of acute poisoning result from accidental ingestion of large quantities of one of the acid soluble salts of lead. Characteristics of lead poisoning are listed in Table 9. Presenting signs and symptoms of acute lead poisoning are rather nonspecific and include severe abdominal pain, vomiting, constipation or diarrhea, thirst, malaise, and anorexia. The stool will be black from lead sulfide. Acute CNS effects include muscle weakness and pain, and paresthesias. Intense anemia and hemoglobinuria may be seen following severe poisoning. Urinary output decreases due to renal damage, and if the dose is large enough, the patient is likely to die as a result of cardiovascular collapse. If the patient survives an acute poisoning, symptoms of chronic toxicity are commonly seen.

Chronic lead poisoning (plumbism) results in a wide variety of symptoms that primarily involve the hematopoietic system, the gastrointestinal tract, and, in the more advanced stages of plumbism, the nervous, renal, and neuromuscular systems. These symptoms may occur singly or in combination. In general, chronic lead intoxication usually is manifested by CNS

TABLE 9. *Characteristics of lead poisoning*

Acute lead poisoning (rare)
   Sweet metallic taste
   Salivation
   Vomiting
   Intestinal colic

Chronic lead poisoning (plumbism)
   Hematological
      Basophilic stippling
      Hypochronic normocytic anemia
   Neurological (lead encephalopathy)
      Ataxia, nausea, vomiting
      Restlessness
      Irritability
      Convulsions
      Coma
   Gastrointestinal (lead colic)
      Anorexia
      Constipation
      Metallic taste
   Neuromuscular (lead palsy)
      Wrist drop, foot drop
      Fatigue
      Muscular weakness
   Renal
      Fanconi-like syndrome (reversible)
      Chronic nephritis (irreversible)

toxicity. In adults the symptoms are primarily gastrointestinal (38).

In the early stages of plumbism, the victim is anemic and, therefore, feels tired and weak. These hematological changes result from a decreased life-span of the red blood cells and an interference in the synthesis of the heme portion of hemoglobin. As a result, a hypochromic, microcytic anemia and reticulocytosis are evident. The cells are hypochromic because of the reduction in heme synthesis as discussed earlier, and the increase in reticulocytes is a compensatory process responding to the decreased number of red blood cells. The effects of lead on the hematopoietic system are seldom life-threatening.

Lead stimulates the smooth muscle of the gastrointestinal tract, and abdominal pain is a striking feature of plumbism in both children and adults. In fact, it may become so severe as to suggest possible bowel obstruction on preliminary diagnosis. Early symptoms are mild and nondescript, however, as lead intoxication progresses, anorexia and constipation (adults) or diarrhea (children) appears, and intestinal spasms

increase in frequency and intensity to produce even more severe abdominal pain commonly referred to as lead colic. A persistent metallic taste appears in the mouth. As the term "colic" implies, the gastrointestinal attacks are paroxysmal. That is, they occur sporadically and without warning. The victim's abdominal muscles become rigid and the pain can be excruciating.

Lead also produces a toxic effect on the kidney by causing damage to the proximal tubules, producing a Fanconi-like syndrome. This results in impaired tubular reabsorption of glucose, phosphate, amino acids, bicarbonate, and uric acid. Lead also causes irreversible nephritis characterized by progressive interstitial fibrosis, sclerosis of the renal blood vessels, and glomerular atrophy. This irreversible damage is usually observed in individuals who have been exposed to high concentrations of lead for prolonged periods of time.

Lead palsy is another characteristic of chronic lead poisoning and results in an action of lead on the neuromuscular system. Lead causes demyelination of the median nerve which innervates the extensor muscles of the hand, to produce a "wrist drop" phenomenon. A similar effect is seen in the foot, but with less frequency and severity.

The most serious manifestation of lead poisoning is the encephalopathy which occurs more often in children than adults. Local edema, hemorrhage, and necrosis of brain tissue are seen. The first indications of encephalopathy include clumsiness, lethargy, insomnia, restlessness, and irritability. It may eventually progress to delirium, convulsions, and even coma. Projectile vomiting and visual disturbances are also commonly associated with encephalopathy. One-fourth of all victims with encephalopathy will not survive. Of those who do, up to 40% will experience intense neurological dysfunctions (62,67).

Lead sulfide may deposit as a thin line along the gingival margin. This line, which appears blue-to-black, is called a "Burtonian" line and is characteristic of chronic lead poisoning. However, a similar discoloration of the gums along a line just above the teeth may be caused by chronic accumulation of other metals such as silver, iron, or mercury.

Treatment of Lead Poisoning

The Center for Disease Control has established guidelines for the standardization of lead intoxication (7). Diagnostic laboratory tests for lead poisoning include: blood lead greater than or equal to 80 μg%, or red blood cell protoporphyrin greater than or equal to 190 μg% with or without symptoms of toxicity, or blood lead between 50 to 79 μg% with symptoms, or a sharp elevation in erythrocyte protoporphyrin, urinary δ-ALA, or urinary coproporphyrins (Table 10).

A patient with a blood lead of 80 μg% or greater and an erythrocyte protoporphyrin of 190 μg%, even without symptoms, should be hospitalized and chelation therapy started immediately in order to prevent lead encephalopathy.

When indicated by the above criteria, the chelators of choice are BAL, CaNa$_2$-EDTA, and penicillamine. BAL aids in lead poisoning by chelating lead in serum and cerebral spinal fluid. The stable complex formed is rapidly excreted in the urine. Some of the common side-effects include transient hypertension, increased heart rate, nausea, vomiting, fever, and since it is given intramuscularly, pain at the injection site.

CaNa$_2$-EDTA will chelate lead from bone and soft tissue. It also forms a stable complex which

TABLE 10. *Diagnostic tests for lead poisoning*

Test	Toxicity	Normal
Blood		
Lead	≥ 80 μg%	< 40 μg%
Erythrocyte protoporphyrin concentration	≥ 190 μg%	40–100 μg%
Urine (24 hr)		
Lead	≥ 0.15 mg/L	< 0.08 mg/L children
		< 0.15 mg/L adults
δ-ALA	> 19 mg/L	1.3–8.5 mg/L
Coproporphyrin III	> 150 μg/L	0–60 μg/L
		50–160 μg/24 hr

is rapidly excreted in the urine. Some of the side-effects of CaNa$_2$-EDTA therapy include fever, headache, nausea, vomiting, anorexia, myalgias, decreased blood pressure, and histamine-like reactions.

Penicillamine has also been successfully used to chelate lead.

MERCURY

Mercury compounds are divided into three chemical classes: elemental mercury (quicksilver, mercury vapor), inorganic, and organic mercury salts. Quicksilver is a silver-white, heavy, liquid metal. The inorganic mercury salts exist either in the mercurous (Hg^{1+}) or mercuric (Hg^{2+}) state. Mercuric salts are more toxic than the mercurous salts. Aryl, alkyl, and alkoxyalkyl mercury compounds represent the organic mercury compounds that are of greatest toxicologic significance.

Poisonings due to mercury have been recognized since ancient times. Among the writers of ancient Greek history, Hippocrates, Theophrastus, Pliny, and Dioscorides, to name a few, discussed mercury poisoning. Most of those poisonings were due to mining and cleaning of elemental mercury.

Throughout the years mercury has been used in medicine, agriculture, and industry. Medicinal uses of mercury originated as early as 1500 A.D., when mercury was used in treatment of syphilis. Calomel (mercurous chloride) was used as a cathartic until just a few decades ago when physicians became firmly convinced of its toxicity potential. Organic mercury compounds, used for a number of years as diuretics, have also been carefully scrutinized because of toxicity. Most have now been removed from therapy in the United States. Mercury alloy is the amalgam used in dentistry.

Mercury has been popular in agricultural use because of its ability to counteract fungi and mold, and therefore it has been widely used to prevent grain spoilage. A serious outbreak of poisoning occurred in the early 1970s when grain treated with methylmercury was inadvertently ground into flour and consumed. Over

500 people who consumed it died (2). Organic mercury compounds are commonly used on apple trees, tomato and potato plants, and rice fields.

The two principal industrial users of mercury compounds are the paint and paper manufacturing industries. Again, the organic materials are used because of their ability to decrease mold growth. In the paper industry, mercury protects wood pulp stored for processing so that mold growth does not occur. Other industrial applications of mercury include use as catalysts, particularly in the vinyl chloride industry, which is important in the synthesis of many plastics. Many of the sources of airborne mercury are due to its industrial uses.

In recent years there has been a decrease in toxic episodes from medicinal products, but an increase in toxic effects due to environmental pollution. In some areas, mercury pollution has expanded to epidemic proportions.

As previously stated, mercury exists in three different chemical forms. Elemental mercury vapor is the most volatile of all mercury compounds. Intoxication is mainly an occupational problem, usually a chronic poisoning. Elemental mercury has a high vapor pressure. At a saturated atmosphere of 20°C, approximately 15 mg/m^3 mercury vapor is present; at 24°C, 18 mg/m^3; and at 40°C, 80 mg/m^3. Exposure to an atmosphere of 0.7 mg/m^3 for 5 hr/day is associated with symptoms of mercury poisoning (26,48).

Solid elemental mercury may be accidentally spilled onto carpeting or into crevices of the floor from where it is slowly released over a period of months to years. Along the same lines, mercury that is swallowed because of a thermometer accidentally breaking in one's mouth will not generally pose any particular problem, as far as the mercury itself is concerned. The more significant problem is the glass particles that may have been inadvertently swallowed.

Suicide attempts by injecting elemental mercury have been documented (1,27). Whereas elemental mercury is considered nontoxic when ingested, it can be toxic when introduced subcutaneously (70). Toxic mercury salts may form

and enter the blood to cause dangerously high levels.

The inorganic mercury salts exist in two oxidation states. Mercurous salts include calomel (Hg_2Cl_2), which was used in the past as a cathartic, and mercuric chloride ($HgCl_2$, corrosive sublimate), formerly used as an antiseptic. Mercuric chloride is still widely employed in industry. Mercuric nitrate was commonly used in the felt hat industry and has been associated with neurological changes in individuals working in that industry. In fact, the phrase "mad as a hatter" is derived from mercuric nitrate exposure and one wonders if Lewis Carroll knew a real-life hatter after whom he patterned the *Alice's Adventures in Wonderland* character.

Differences in toxicity among the organic mercurials are due their ease of dissociation between the organic moiety and the anion attached. The alkyl mercury salts are of greatest toxicological importance because they are incorporated into the food chain. The most toxic of all the alkyl mercurials is methylmercury. Characteristic and usually irreversible CNS damage has been associated with methylmercury exposures (48,57).

Mechanism of Mercury Toxicity

Mercury ions produce their toxic effect by protein precipitation, enzyme inhibition, and by a generalized corrosive action. Mercury binds to sulfhydryl groups, as well as to phosphoryl, carboxyl, amide and amine functional groups. Mercury is known to react with several enzymes and other proteins which contain these functional groups and, thus, mercury interferes with cellular enzymatic reactions.

The toxic effects produced by the various compounds of mercury are functions of their chemical form, route of administration of the compound, and duration of exposure. For example, it was mentioned previously that mercuric salts are more toxic than mercurous salts. This is partly because the divalent inorganic mercury compounds (e.g., $HgCl_2$) are much more soluble than the monovalent mercury compounds (e.g., Hg_2Cl_2) and, therefore, when ingested, $HgCl_2$ will be more rapidly absorbed and produce a greater toxic effect.

On the other hand, at least 90% of a methyl-mercury dose is absorbed from the gastrointestinal tract, compared to about 10% with the soluble inorganic salts. Consequently, organic mercurials are less corrosive to the intestinal mucosa than the inorganic compounds, such as mercuric chloride. They also cross the blood-brain barrier and placenta, and cause teratogenic and neurological disorders more readily than do the inorganic salts (46). They also show less specificity for various tissues than the inorganic salts (37).

Unlike for lead, there are no specific biochemical tests which can be used to determine if mercury exposure has occurred. The only indicator available is the concentration of mercury itself in blood and/or urine. Also, since concentrations in hair may be several hundred times that in the blood, hair samples may be checked.

Elemental mercury vapor presents some unique toxicological problems. There are two important properties of elemental mercury that make it a potential hazard to man. First, it crosses cell membranes with little difficulty. This is due to its high lipid solubility and lack of charge. Consequently, it readily crosses the blood-brain barrier and accumulates in the brain.

The second, and more critical, property of elemental mercury is its ability to easily oxidize to the mercuric form. Even though elemental mercury is rapidly oxidized to the mercuric ion (10), chronic exposure to these two forms of mercury produces significant toxic effects to two separate organ systems.

To illustrate, in mercurialism due to chronic inhalation of mercury vapor, mercury preferentially attacks the CNS (31). Chronic exposure to inorganic mercury compounds leads to renal complications. Again, this can be explained on the basis of the high lipid solubility of mercury vapor. After elemental mercury has rapidly accumulated in the brain, it oxidizes to the mercuric form and the expected reactions occur.

Independent of the chemical form of mercury, two major target organs have been iden-

tified: the CNS and the kidney. CNS specificity is characteristic of elemental mercury vapor and short-chain alkyl mercury compounds. When these mercury compounds enter the CNS, degenerative changes occur from the action of mercury on the structural proteins and enzyme systems. Synaptic and neuromuscular transmission is blocked.

Mercury compounds are nonspecific enzyme inhibitors. Therefore, it is difficult to pinpoint specific enzymes which may be inactivated. The cell membrane is the most obvious point of attack, since sulfhydryl groups are throughout the membrane structure. The Na^+, K^+-ATPase system is inevitably involved, causing shifts in intracellular and extracellular ions.

Although the kidney is the principal target organ for the inorganic mercurials, all mercury compounds concentrate in the kidney to some degree. Inorganic compounds, though, produce the majority of the toxic effects. Mercurial diuretics have been shown to selectively inhibit the proximal tubular resorption of sodium, even at nontoxic doses.

Clinical Manifestations of Mercury Poisoning

Mercury poisoning is characterized by a variety of clinical manifestations. Symptoms will be qualitatively and quantitatively dependent on the chemical structure of the compound, the amount and duration of exposure, and individual sensitivity to the particular mercury compound. Table 11 lists the clinical manifestations according to the chemical form of mercury encountered.

Elemental mercury does not produce significant toxicity when ingested. When inhaled at high concentrations, however, the volatile, lipid-soluble vapor can easily be absorbed across the alveolar membrane. As a result of its high lipid solubility and lack of charge (Hg^0), the dissolved mercury vapor easily crosses the blood-brain barrier and accumulates in the CNS. Likewise, placental transfer can occur leading to an accumulation of mercury in the fetus.

Acute exposure to high concentrations of elemental mercury can cause bronchial irritation

TABLE 11. *Characteristics of mercury poisoning*

Chemical form	Elemental	Inorganic	Organomercurial
Primary route of exposure	Inhalation	Oral	Oral, food chain
Target organ	CNS, kidney	Kidney	CNS, liver
Clinical manifestations Local			
Lungs	Bronchial irritation	—	—
	Pneumonitis	—	—
GI tract	Metallic taste	Metallic taste	—
	Stomatitis	Stomatitis	—
	Gingivitis	Gastroenteritis	—
	Excessive salivation	—	—
Skin	—	Urticaria	—
	—	Vesication	—
Systemic			
CNS	Erethism	—	Ataxia, chorea, athetosis, tremor
	Tremors	—	Convulsions, paresthesias, erethism
Kidney	Tubular necrosis (limited)	Tubular necrosis	—
Treatment	BAL	BAL	Chelators are *not* effective
	$CaNa_2$-EDTA		
	N-acetylpenicillamine		
Biological half-life	10–15 days	65–70 days	70–90 days

associated with shortness of breath, coughing, chest pains, and tremor. Postmortem examinations usually reveal diffuse pneumonitis with marked interstitial edema and alveolar exudation. In mild cases, the symptoms persist for about 2 weeks, followed by complete recovery.

Classical mercurialism may result from continued exposure to moderately high concentrations of mercury vapor. Prolonged exposure to mercury vapor at concentrations greater than 100 mg/m³ will result in an insidious onset of mercurialism. Anorexia, weight loss, fatigue, and muscular weakness are some of the nonspecific clinical manifestations of chronic exposure. Due to accumulation of mercury in the cerebral and cerebellar cortex, chronic mercury toxicity is evidenced by a variety of neurological and behavioral problems.

Fine muscle tremors are among the early signs of mercurialism. Tremor usually begins in the fingers, eyes, or tongue. Sometimes it progresses to affect an entire limb. Handwriting suffers severely and can be used as a qualitative measurement of the success of treatment. The magnitude of these tremors may also affect the facial muscles resulting in slurred speech. In extreme cases, there might be generalized tremor involving the entire body.

The emotional state of the individual who has been repeatedly exposed to mercury is also altered. Sudden attacks of anger, increasing irritability, loss of memory, and drowsiness occur. The person loses interest in his life and becomes withdrawn from society. The syndrome is referred to as *erethism*. The origin of the word is based on the blushing and sweating that also occurs.

Elemental mercury also causes a brownish or yellowish discoloration of the lens, but this is of little clinical significance to visual acuity.

Acute inorganic mercury poisonings result from accidental or intentional ingestions. Although mercuric chloride taken orally is an unpleasant approach to death, it once ranked sixth in frequency of use as a suicidal agent. At one time, mercuric chloride was available as a blue coffin-shaped tablet with the skull and crossbones depicted on one side and the inscription, <u>POISON</u>, on the other side (Fig. 6). Despite these obvious warnings, the tablets were often ingested (usually accidentally). A 0.5-g tablet dissolved in water and swallowed will quickly produce immediate injury to the mucosa of the mouth, throat, esophagus, and stomach. The reason for these gastrointestinal effects is because mercuric chloride is a corrosive and causes protein precipitation. As a result the mouth, pharynx, and gastric mucosa will appear ashen, and these areas are intensely painful. If a large quantity of an inorganic salt is ingested, intense epigastric pain, profuse vomiting of mucoid material, bloody diarrhea, circulatory collapse, shock, and sudden death may occur. A metallic taste is also usually present.

After mercuric chloride produces its local corrosive effect, it is absorbed into the bloodstream where its major target organ is the kidney. Localization of the mercuric ion in the kidney leads to proximal tubular necrosis. Within an hour or so after ingestion, the concentration of mercury in the kidney increases. Renal dysfunction is noted as a transient diuresis followed by oliguria or anuria. As urine output decreases, azotemia, electrolyte imbalances, and acid-base disturbances become evident. The victim may die as a result of uremia. If the victim survives, renal insufficiency will usually last for 1 to 4 weeks. After there is sufficient time for regeneration of the tubular epithelium

to occur, renal function slowly returns to normal.

Hypersensitivity reactions to mercury preparations have been known to occur, especially in children. In the past, calomel was used by children as a teething powder. This practice results in acrodynia or pink gum disease. A severe erythematous rash developed followed by desquamation, loss of hair, and ulceration. Neurological symptoms included tremor, decreased tendon reflexes, and muscle weakness.

Other hypersensitivity reactions include those due to mercury fulminate, an explosive used in detonators which can produce contact dermatitis, and mercuric sulfide, a red pigment used in tattooing, which may also cause an allergic dermatitis.

The organomercuric compounds are classed into two separate groups, based on chemical structure and relative toxicity. These two classes are the long-chained aryl mercury compounds and the short-chained alkyl mercury compounds. The group which poses the greater hazard to man is the short-chained alkyl compounds such as methylmercury. These compounds are the more hazardous because they possess the greater inherent toxicity, and because they are a major threat to the environment (14).

As evidence of the environmental threat of mercury, Minamata's disease is often cited (14,47,68). Effluent from plastic manufacturing

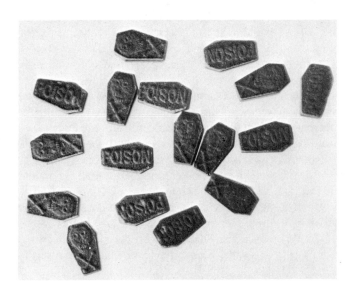

FIG. 6. Mercuric chloride (coffin-shaped) tablets.

factories was released into the Minamata Bay in Japan. This effluent contained high concentrations of methylmercury. Methylmercury is absorbed by the flora and also by fish, and eventually proceeds through the food chain until the contaminated fish and shellfish are consumed by man. Minamata's disease is the name given to a puzzling neurological disorder which appeared in epidemic proportions from 1953 to 1960, affecting over 1,000 people, killing more than 40. Eventually, the neurological signs and symptoms were attributed to the high mercury content in the fish and shellfish from Minamata Bay.

The alkylmercury compounds are almost completely absorbed from the gastrointestinal tract; distributed to the brain, liver, and kidney; and excreted primarily in the feces. The arylmercury compounds are excreted as the mercuric ion.

Differences between acute and chronic toxicity are minimal. A characteristic feature is that symptoms may occur weeks to months after an acute exposure. The severity and clinical manifestations of organic mercury poisoning are dependent on daily intake, duration of exposure, age of the patient, and individual sensitivity. The neurological manifestations of organic mercury poisoning are due to toxic effects on the cerebellum and can lead to ataxia, tremors, unsteady gait, and difficulty in maintaining equilibrium. Simple tasks such as buttoning a shirt become difficult to perform. Illegible handwriting and slurred speech are also noted. Sensory involvement includes paresthesias of the lips, hands, and feet, as well as visual and hearing impairment. Emotional disturbances and erethism are also manifestations of organic mercury poisoning. If the poisoning is severe, the symptoms may not be reversible.

It has been previously noted that alkylmercury compounds can easily penetrate the blood-brain barrier. Similarly, the placental membrane is no obstacle for methylmercury. Congenital intoxications have been noted especially from pregnant women who ate fish from Minamata Bay contaminated with methylmercury. The infants suffered from palsy, convulsions, and mental retardation.

Aryl organic mercury poisonings are rare. When they do occur, poisonings show signs of gastrointestinal and renal toxicity. This is because these compounds are metabolized to mercuric ions.

The biological half-life of methylmercury is approximately 70 to 90 days. Elimination is slow and irregular and accumulation of mercury can easily produce toxicity. Mercury concentrations in the blood at about 10 to 20 μg% are usually not associated with toxic symptoms, but blood levels around 50 to 100 μg% are associated with toxic manifestations.

Treatment of Mercury Poisoning

The choice of treatment of mercury poisoning depends on the form of mercury involved. For example, mild exposure to mercury vapor may only require that the victim be removed from the source of the vapor. In the case of acute oral inorganic mercury poisoning, the initial concern is the neutralization of mercury in the gastrointestinal tract with egg whites or milk.

A considerable amount of mercuric chloride can be removed from the body by spontaneous or ipecac-induced vomiting and gastric lavage. This can then be followed with a generous slurry of activated charcoal.

The most effective means to eliminate inorganic mercury for both chronic and acute poisoning is by using chelators. The choices include BAL, penicillamine, and its *N*-acetyl derivative, *N*-acetylpenicillamine. CaNa$_2$-EDTA is contraindicated in mercury poisoning because it poorly binds to mercury and is potentially nephrotoxic in its own right.

BAL is usually reserved for those patients who cannot take penicillamine orally. The BAL-Hg complex is excreted through the liver as well as the kidney; hence, it is the chelator of choice for cases of poisoning complicated by severe oliguria or anuria. Daily measurement of urinary mercury levels is necessary to assess the efficiency of chelator therapy. Also, it is important to monitor the patient's fluid and electrolyte balance throughout the treatment period.

At present, no effective drug therapy is available for treatment of alkyl mercury intoxication. None of the chelators will remove appreciable quantities of the toxic substance from the CNS. Prognosis for patients with poisoning due to methyl or ethyl mercury is poor. Poisoning is often fatal.

OTHER METALS

In addition to the metals already discussed, several others are occasionally the cause of toxic reactions. They are discussed at this time. An additional metal, thallium, was discussed in Chapter 9.

Copper

Copper occurs throughout nature in a variety of salt forms, as well as in the pure metallic form. It is widely used in industry and in the home as metallic copper in electrical wiring and components. Copper sulfate is added to farm ponds and swimming pools as an algicide. It is also occasionally recommended for use as an emetic, although this use, as was discussed in Chapter 3, is outmoded and potentially dangerous. Death has resulted from ingestion of 10 g. Trace quantities are required for proper functioning of the body.

Poisoning usually always results from acute oral ingestion of a copper salt such as copper sulfate. It has also resulted from repeated washing of burned skin with copper sulfate (30). It is generally felt that chronic exposure to excessive copper does not result in poisoning.

Although not a form of poisoning in the true sense, victims of Wilson's disease have abnormally high blood levels of copper. An inborn error of metabolism, Wilson's disease is a hereditary disorder in which levels of ceruloplasmin are decreased. Ceruloplasmin is one of the plasma α-globulins that normally transports copper through the body. Wilson's disease is an uncommon disorder resulting in the accumulation of copper in the CNS which destroys nerve cells in the putamen, caudate nucleus, and cerebral cortex. The neurologic syndrome which results from copper accumulation in the brain consists of tremors of the extremities, muscle rigidity, choreoathetoid movements, and personality changes progressing to dementia. Centrilobular hepatic necrosis develops producing cirrhosis with ascites, edema, and progressive hepatic failure. Also, a golden-brown ring is deposited on the cornea due to copper deposits. These are known as Kayser-Fleischer rings, and are present in 50% of the patients with Wilson's disease. While incurable, therapy with chelating agents can control copper levels so that the patient can lead a nearly normal life.

Characteristics of Copper Poisoning

Following ingestion of an excessive dose of copper, victims experience severe nausea with vomiting, bloody vomitus and stool, diarrhea, hypotension, and jaundice (Table 12). Repeated exposures have been associated with hemolytic anemia (45). Death usually occurs within 24 hr, preceded by coma. In hepatic or renal complications, it may be hastened.

Treatment of Copper Poisoning

The most effective medical means to manage copper poisoning is with penicillamine. This chelator is also widely used in treating patients with Wilson's disease and certain other diseases such as rheumatoid arthritis.

TABLE 12. *Characteristics of copper toxicity*

Acute exposure
  Nausea, vomiting
  Bloody diarrhea
  Hypotension
  Hemolytic anemia
  Uremia
  Cardiovascular collapse

Chronic exposure
  Sporadic fever
  Vomiting
  Epigastric pain
  Diarrhea
  Jaundice

Inhalation
  Ulceration and perforation of nasal septum
  Necrotic hepatitis

Selenium

Selenium is produced mainly as a by-product of copper refining. While technically not a metal from a chemist's standpoint, it does have metallic characteristics. It has a variety of industrial applications including use in electronics, glass, and paint industries. It is a vulcanizing agent for rubber. Selenious acid is a gun blueing agent. Selenium is used as a drench for sheep and cattle. Selenium sulfide is employed as a shampoo for dandruff control, and aside from causing irritation to the eyes or mucous membranes, this form of selenium is nontoxic. More recently, selenium has been widely promoted as a nutritional element and food additive. It is because of this latter use that contemporary interest in potential selenium toxicity has emerged.

Most experts agree that trace levels of selenium are required by man for proper functioning of the body. Its precise purpose is unknown. Animals receiving a diet deficient in selenium develop liver, kidney, heart or skeletal muscle necrosis, depending on the species. Advocates of supplementing the diet with selenium claim that cancer is caused by deficiencies of this metal. Their claims are largely based on inferential evidence that links selenium levels in the soil to cancer occurrence (64). Selenium is concentrated in plants and enters the body through the diet. (In fact, selenium is often cited as the only element that is absorbed by plants in sufficient concentration to kill animals that eat the plants.) In some geographic areas where soil selenium concentration is lowest, the cancer rate seems higher, and vice versa. It should be pointed out, however, that these same areas that are generally deficient in soil selenium are highly industrialized, and this information is not usually part of the advocate's argument. On the other hand, selenium will protect some animals against tumor formation by a variety of known carcinogens (76).

Selenium plays an essential role in biosynthesis of ubiquinone (coenzyme Q) and aids in vitamin E utilization.

Mechanism of Selenium Toxicity

The precise mechanism of toxicity of selenium is not understood. It has a high affinity for thiol groups (13). Selenium may thus inhibit certain sulfhydryl-containing enzymes.

Characteristics of Selenium Poisoning

Acute poisoning causes a variety of gastrointestinal and CNS effects (Table 13). Nervousness, drowsiness, and convulsions are common occurrences. The bizarre behavior expected from horses that grazed on "loco" weed in western movies of the 1930s and 1940s may well have been due to selenium intoxication. Loco weed accumulates selenium to 15,000 or more ppm (78). A fatal case of poisoning from ingestion of gun blueing produced widespread focal hemorrhages and edema, with death probably resulting from cardiovascular collapse. Death is usually due to depression of the respiratory or cardiovascular centers.

Chronic poisoning may induce pallor, a "garlic" breath, metallic taste, liver and spleen damage, and anemia, in addition to gastrointestinal and CNS effects. Fatty necrosis of the liver is a frequent finding. Selenium is believed to be teratogenic in humans (60), and may be carcinogenic.

TABLE 13. *Characteristics of selenium toxicity (selenosis)*

Acute exposure
  Nervousness
  Drowsiness
  Fever
  Vomiting
  Decreased blood pressure
  Convulsions
  Death due to respiratory or
    cardiovascular failure

Chronic exposure
  Depression
  Garlic-like odor on breath
  Pallor
  Loss of nails and hair
  Hemolytic anemia
  Liver and spleen damage
  May be teratogenic and carcinogenic

Inhalation
  Chemical pneumonitis

Treatment of Selenium Poisoning

Treatment of selenium poisoning by ingestion or inhalation includes controlling symptoms. The influenza-like symptoms may be controlled with salicylates. The individual must be immediately removed from inhalation exposure. Contaminated skin and eyes should be thoroughly rinsed.

Zinc

Zinc is widely used industrially in galvanizing processes, in paints, and as $ZnCl_2$ for preserving wood. Zinc is another essential trace element, necessary for numerous enzyme reactions, protein synthesis, and carbohydrate metabolism. It is a component of numerous enzymes including alcohol dehydrogenase, carbonic anhydrase, carboxypeptidase, and lactic dehydrogenase.

Over the years, various zinc salts have been employed in numerous medicinal preparations as a topical astringent, antiseptic, and antifungal agent. Zinc sulfate, like copper sulfate, has been recommended as an emetic.

Characteristics of Zinc Poisoning

Poisoning by zinc occurs most commonly by inhalation of zinc oxide fumes, or ingestion of one of the salts. A syndrome known as metal fume fever results from inhalation of freshly formed fumes of zinc oxide. This occurs as zinc fumes are produced when zinc is heated to high temperatures such as in welding, metal cutting, or smelting zinc alloys. Victims complain of nausea and vomiting, chills and fever, muscular aches and pains, and weakness (Table 14). No fatalities have been recorded to date, with recovery occurring in 24 to 48 hr. Zinc chloride fume has caused fatalities, with death occurring due to pulmonary edema. While metal fume fever may occur from heating other metals, it is most common with zinc.

Treatment of Zinc Poisoning

Treatment of zinc poisoning includes immediate removal of the victim from the source of poisoning. The victim is treated symptomati-

TABLE 14. *Characteristics of zinc toxicity*

Oral
Lassitude
Enteritis
Diarrhea (bloody, watery)
Intense abdominal pain
CNS depression
Tremors
Inhalation
"Fume fever"—sudden onset of thirst, fever, chills, myalgias, and headaches

cally. Aspirin helps control the influenza-like symptoms. Glucocorticoids are useful in treating pulmonary edema.

SUMMARY

Symptoms of metal poisoning are classic and usually predictable. Their antidoting involves specific chelating chemicals but, more importantly, symptomatic treatment is just as valid. Many of the chelators form complexes that are toxic in their own right. Thus, the best treatment may be to remove the poison from the victim's environment and control his symptoms.

Case Studies

CASE STUDY: ACUTE ARSENIC EXPOSURE

History

When found in the backyard of her home, a 16-month-old 10-kg female was holding a wafer from a package of Grant's Ant Control. Her face had traces of a gel-like substance around the mouth, so her parents washed her hands and face. However, approximately 30 min later, the child began to vomit and she had a watery bowel movement.

She was rushed to a local emergency facility and there was given 15 ml of syrup of ipecac which provoked further vomiting. Following a bout of copious emesis, she was then given 20 g of activated charcoal and 2.5 g of sodium sulfate. A short while later, the child became lethargic and had three rice-watery stools. At this point she was transported to a larger medical facility for further care.

It was later estimated that she ingested about 2 to 3 g of ant killer resulting in the consumption of 9 to 14 mg of arsenic trioxide. Because of the severity of her symptoms, it was assumed she had swallowed a toxic dose.

Treatment. While she was being transported, she was given 25 mg BAL intramuscularly. She presented with a heart rate that varied between 130 to 156 beats/min, blood pressure of 110/55 mm Hg, respiratory rate was 36, and rectal temperature was 36.7°C. Arterial blood gases, electrolytes, renal and liver function tests were all within the normal limits. A total of 185 mg of BAL was administered over an 18-hr period. This was then followed by 250 mg of penicillamine every 6 hr for 5 days.

A charcoal stool was passed about 22 hr postingestion. During her hospital stay, there were no seizures, arrhythmias, vomiting, watery diarrhea, or changes in laboratory values.

The patient was released from the hospital on her third day of confinement. Penicillamine treatment was continued by her private physician for 5 days. Her arsenic blood level on admission was in excess of 7 μg%, and on the second day had decreased to approximately 2 μg%. (See ref. 75.)

Discussion

1. With the exception of some early gastrointestinal symptoms, this young patient did not experience many of the symptoms listed in Table 5. What are some possible reasons for this omission?

2. Why was D-penicillamine initiated and BAL discontinued?

3. Was the initial blood arsenic level suggestive of toxic exposure?

4. Compare poisoning by arsenic trioxide with what would be expected had the ingested substance been arsenic pentaoxide.

5. What is the significance of knowing that a charcoal stool was passed?

CASE STUDY: CADMIUM FUME POISONING

History

A 25-year-old male Hull Technician First Class military person was cleaning the sanitary tank (approximately 428 ft³) of a submarine. The job required heating a pipe joint that had previously been brazed with a cadmium-containing grade of silver braze alloy. After heating the joint he began coughing, dis-

continued work, and left the area. He had worked about eight minutes in the confined area.

The coughing ceased after exposure to fresh air, but he experienced a mild sore throat and some dyspnea which rapidly improved. The dyspnea reappeared four hours later and his cough worsened, forcing him to report to the sick bay the following morning.

The patient presented with moderate respiratory distress. Auscultation of the chest revealed bilateral rales over the posterior aspect of the thorax. Vital signs were: blood pressure 130/80 mm Hg, pulse 120/minute, respiratory rate 40/minute, and very shallow. A chest X-ray revealed a diffused, bilateral infiltrate in the lungs, indicating pulmonary edema.

Treatment. Treatment consisted of furosemide and dexamethasone. The patient recovered completely within two days. No arrhythmias were noted. He was discharged two days later and returned to full duty. (See ref. 72.)

Discussion

1. In this case study, there was an asymptomatic period following some initial pulmonary irritation. Is this typical of cadmium intoxication?

2. Which organ is most sensitive to the toxic effects of cadmium? Did this patient experience problems to this system? If so, what were they?

3. Is chelation therapy indicated for most acute cadmium exposures?

4. How would the symptoms this victim experienced have differed if poisoning would have been by ingestion?

5. Discuss what a fume is. How are they produced?

CASE STUDY: IRON POISONING

History

In what was believed to be a suicide attempt, a 17-year-old pregnant female ingested 90 325 mg ferrous sulfate capsules. On admission to the emergency department one-half hour later, her physical examination revealed no strikingly abnormal values, and her vital signs were all within the normal limits.

Vomiting was induced with 30 ml of syrup of ipecac. The vomited material contained many partially digested iron capsules.

An unprovoked emesis resulted about 4 hr later. This was followed by diarrhea. Both were positive for the presence of blood. But physical examination was still unremarkable, except for hypoactive bowel sounds. About 12 hr after admission, she vomited bloody material.

Laboratory results revealed hypoglycemia, metabolic acidosis, bleeding tendencies, and renal dysfunction. She had tachycardia, and eventually developed renal impairment.

Treatment. Treatment consisted of fluids, dextrose, sodium bicarbonate, and diuretics. Deferoxamine was not given for two reasons: (a) her pregnant state, and (b) because of renal failure. Instead, she underwent an exchange transfusion 30 min after admission, after which she spontaneously aborted a 16-week fetus.

Her condition became progressively worse. In addition to the hypotension, hypoglycemia, and clotting deficiency, she became febrile (105°F), tachypneic, cyanotic, continued vomiting dark-brown material, and experienced a seizure 74 hr after admission. She was intubated and given a pressor agent because of progressively decreasing blood pressure but, unfortunately, died 80 hr after admission.

It was later reported that the victim did not mean to commit suicide, but intended only to get attention. (See ref. 44.)

Discussion

1. Based on your knowledge of the toxic action of compounds like ferrous sulfate, what would you expect the autopsy findings to reveal?

2. Comment on the production of hypoglycemia with iron poisoning. Why did it occur?

3. What was the mechanism of death of the victim? What caused the fetus to abort?

4. Did this case study exhibit all five clinical phases of toxicity?

5. At what serum iron concentration is chelation therapy usually started? What indicator is used to stop chelation therapy?

CASE STUDIES: INTOXICATION WITH LEAD

History: Case 1

A 3-year-old female was brought to the emergency room by her parents after trying unsuccessfully to awaken her. Her father had noticed over the past 2 days that she had become lethargic, always being fatigued and sleepy. Her personality had also changed and she complained of abdominal pains and headaches.

She was given acetaminophen, 0.8 ml, three times daily for her aches and pains. The previous day she had vomited three times. Her dietary intake was restricted to orange juice which was one of her favorite beverages. The family suspected that the little girl had picked up some kind of a virus while vacationing, and that was the reason for the flu-like symptoms.

When responding to a physician's questioning in order to obtain a complete history, the father remembered that his daughter had taken a special interest in a pink, "funny-faced" Indian mug, and whenever she drank liquids she used this particular mug. She drank at least 5 to 6 glassfuls of orange juice per day. This admission provided the clue for the young girl's problem. It was assumed that the acid in orange juice had mobilized lead from the noncommercially glazed mug, and it was the cause of her poisoning.

The girl was admitted with a pulse of 80 beats/min, temperature 101°F, blood pressure 130/90 mm Hg. She was in the lighter stages of a coma and able to awaken on verbal commands. Her physical examination also revealed questionable blurring of the optic disc and hyperactive reflexes.

The laboratory values showed a hemoglobin content of 12 g% hematocrit of 38%, and a mean corpuscular volume of 78. The WBC was 8,000 cells/mm^3. The differential count showed 60% leukocytes, 35% polys, 3% eosinophils, and 2% mononucleocytes. The free erythrocytic protoporphyrin (FEP) level was 300 µg/dl.

Treatment. The patient received treatment with CaNa$_2$-EDTA, improving with time. She was discharged without apparent sequelae. (See ref. 8.)

History: Case 2

A 59-year-old female was admitted to the hospital with diffuse pains and anemia. About one year previously, she injured her back. She was treated with acupuncture by an herbalist-chiropractor on two separate occasions. She was given two herbal products to be ingested daily.

A few months after initiating therapy, she began to complain of pain in her knees, hips, and abdomen. Also, she became unusually irritable and could not sleep well. It was difficult for her to hold objects in her hands and she often felt constipated.

On admission, the following laboratory results were obtained:

		Normal
Hematocrit	= 27%	(36–42%)
Reticulocyte count	= 5.6%	(0.5–2.0%)

Blood iron	= 98 μg%	(80–160%)
Total iron-binding capacity	= 260 μg%	(250–350 μg%)
RBC protoporphryn	= 403 μg%	(40–100 μg%)
Urine ALA (24 hr)	= 51.9 mg	(1.5–7.5 mg)
Urine lead (24 hr)	= 0.281 mg	(less than 0.100 mg)
Blood lead	= 90 μg%	(less than 60 μg%)

Peripheral blood smears showed marked basophilic stippling

Her symptoms and laboratory values were suggestive of lead poisoning. Her husband's blood and urine showed lead levels within the normal limits. The herbal pills were therefore suspected to be a possible source. They were analyzed, and found to contain 0.5 mg of lead. She had been ingesting 30 pills per day for 2 to 3 months. Therefore, she had a daily lead intake of 15 mg.

Treatment. The patient was started with chelation therapy, CaNa$_2$-EDTA given at the rate of 2 g/24 hr intravenously, with intravenous fluids. Marked reduction in symptoms occurred within 24 hr. She was also given antibiotics, chlordiazepoxide for anxiety, and vitamins. Her improvement was remarkable and quick. After the first day of treatment, the blood level of lead decreased to 70 μg%. She was released after 10 days. (See ref. 36.)

History: Case 3

A 23-year-old male amateur painter was admitted to the hospital after experiencing violent abdominal cramps. The only physical findings were facial pallor and mild icterus.

The following laboratory findings were obtained:

Hematocrit	= 25.5%
Hemoglobin	= 8.9 g%
RBC count	= 288×10^4 cells/mm^3
Total bilirubin	= 4.3 mg%
Indirect bilirubin	= 2.7 mg%
Serum iron	= 201 μg%
Total iron-binding capacity	= 86%
Urine δ-ALA	= 144 mg/day
Urine coproporphyrin	= 1,800 μg/day
Serum lead	= 112 μg%

Treatment. At the time of admission, the source of this apparent lead intoxication was not established, and the patient denied exposure to lead. But treatment with CaNa$_2$-EDTA was initiated. Although treatment was continued over the next 50 days, the chelator caused the reversal of the abdominal colic and hyperbilirubinemia within 2 weeks.

Thirty days after the final CaNa$_2$-EDTA treatment, the following laboratory values were obtained:

Urine δ-ALA	= 1.9–3.9 mg/day
Urine coproporphyrin	= 60–140 μg/day
Serum lead	= 47 μg%
Serum iron	= 67 μg%

The patient finally identified the source of lead exposure. He had been ingesting lead white (basic lead carbonate), about 15 g a month. His intent was to produce hallucinations so that he could be more artistically creative in his work. (See ref. 54.)

Discussion

1. The preceding case studies have dealt with a variety of sources of lead exposure. What are some of the common clinical findings in all three cases?

2. In Case 3, which laboratory tests were indicative of jaundice? What is the cause of the jaundice? How do the toxic actions of lead account for these changes?

3. Is CaNa$_2$-EDTA the only chelator used for lead toxicity? If not, what others might be used, and when?

4. Patient 2 received intravenous fluid therapy and it can be assumed that the others did likewise. Comment on why this was given.

CASE STUDY: MERCURY POISONING

History

A 49-year-old somnolent female ingested 125 g of a fungicide, containing 3.5% methoxyethylmercury chloride, in a suicide attempt. She vomited a blue liquid. She presented with no outstanding physical symptoms relating to the caustic nature of mercury poisoning. Two hours after ingestion she was admitted to an emergency facility where she was intubated and gastric lavage was performed, and forced diuresis was initiated. Two hours after ingestion, charcoal hemoperfusion was utilized for 4 hr. This was repeated 15 hr after ingestion. Chelators used included penicillamine and dimercaprol.

All laboratory results were within normal limits, except for a slight increase in SGOT. The patient continued under examination for the next 3 months without experiencing further problems. Blood levels of mercury remained high throughout the period. (See ref. 39.)

Discussion

1. Why was there no kidney damage with this intoxication?

2. Three months after ingestion, the patient had no toxic symptoms but had high blood levels of mercury. How could this be?

3. Could a better choice of chelator antidotes have been made to treat this patient?

CASE STUDIES: METALLIC MERCURY POISONING

History: Case 1

A 53-year-old man had been working on an amateur ore distillation experiment. He had heated mercury on his kitchen stove on two separate occasions within a 2-week period.

After the first exposure he presented to the emergency room, cyanotic, with chills, fever, dyspnea, and severe abdominal cramping. He often saw red spots in front of his eyes, and became partially blinded. The symptoms gradually disappeared over 2 days from the first exposure to mercury vapor.

On the second occasion, he noted the room becoming dark, and the red spots reappeared. He was again admitted to the hospital with acute respiratory distress and with severe abdominal cramping. He was given a tracheostomy and mechanical assistance for breathing. Urinary mercury level, at this time, was 5 mg% (0–2.0 μg% normal). He was transferred to another facility so that charcoal hemoperfusion could be initiated.

Physical examination showed the blood pressure to be 130/100 mm Hg, respirations 18/min, and pulse 76 beats/min. A chest X-ray depicted extensive bilateral pulmonary infiltrates, but no signs of cardiomegaly.

Laboratory findings included:

Na^+	= 131 mEq/L
Cl^-	= 94 mEq/L
Glucose	= 172 mg%
BUN	= 45 mg%
Uric acid	= 9.6 mg%
LDH	= 2,400 U
Urinary Hg	= 0.37 mg%
Serum creatinine	= 1.5 mg%

Treatment. The patient was given 500 ml 5% dextrose over 4 hr. He also received a course of BAL. Urine mercury levels were 0.06 mg% by the seventh day and renal function improved. He temporarily recovered, but later developed a nosocomial pneumonia, which proved to be fatal. He died during his third week of hospitalization. (See ref. 34.)

History: Case 2

The patient was a 17-year-old male storekeeper who ingested the metallic mercury content of a clock pendulum, i.e., approximately 204 g or 15 ml. (For comparison, a clinical fever thermometer contains approximately 1 g mercury.) He arrived asymptomatic at the hospital 2 hr following the ingestion. Blood urea, electrolytes, and hematology were normal.

Treatment. Treatment consisted of a mild laxative and bed rest. X-rays of the abdomen were used to follow the passage of the mercury through the gastrointestinal tract, and by 3 weeks all the mercury was excreted in the feces. Daily urine mercury excretions were all less than 15 μg. There were no gastrointestinal symptoms, and apparently a significant portion was not absorbed. He was discharged without further problems. (See ref. 80.)

Discussion

1. Is the delayed onset of respiratory distress with mercury vapor exposure typical? What other signs and symptoms of this type of exposure were consistent with the text information from the chapter?

2. In Case 2, why was chelator therapy and other aggressive therapy *not* given following this massive ingestion?

3. If anuria or renal shutdown had occurred with either of these patients, describe the procedure which could be used to decrease the concentration of mercury.

4. Patient 2 ingested a much greater amount of mercury than Patient 1. However, Patient 1 was more seriously intoxicated. Discuss the reasons why this occurred.

Review Questions

1. Chronic exposure to which of the following heavy metals is the cause of "ouch-ouch" disease?
   A. Cadmium
   B. Lead
   C. Mercury
   D. Selenium

2. Throughout the chapter, we refer to the "body burden" of metals. What does this term mean?

3. Following iron ingestion, lavage with a bicarbonate or phosphate solution may be undertaken.

What is the specific reason these substances are employed?

4. Contamination of "moonshine" whiskey with lead is a continual problem. What is the source of this metal?

5. Which of the following is a reported symptom of toxicity of BAL: bradycardia (I), sedation (II), or paresthesias (III)?
   A. I only
   B. III only
   C. I and II only
   D. II and III only

6. A characteristic odor on the breath may be detected following selenium ingestion. Describe it.

7. Which of the following is the antidote of first choice for treating an overdose of iron?
   A. CaNa$_2$-EDTA
   B. Deferoxamine
   C. Dimercaprol
   D. Penicillamine

8. One of the following salts is extremely toxic and the other has limited toxic potential. Which is which? Cite their common names.
   A. HgCl$_2$
   B. Hg$_2$Cl$_2$

9. A young girl has been brought to the emergency room, a victim of having a fever thermometer broken within the rectum. Discuss the problems.

10. Which of the following is the principal site of toxic action of inorganic mercurials?
    A. Kidney
    B. Brain
    C. Heart
    D. Bone

11. A physician treating a patient for chronic mercurialism will monitor the victim's handwriting. Why?

12. Discuss the cause and symptoms of erethism.

13. Which of the following forms of organomercuric compounds is more toxic?
    A. Long-chain aryl compounds
    B. Short-chain alkyl compounds

14. What specific property of dimercaprol makes it a chelator of choice for cases of mercury poisoning complicated by severe oliguria or anuria?

15. Copper poisoning has resulted from topical application of copper sulfate.
    A. True
    B. False

16. A rule of thumb is that chronic lead poisoning will manifest mainly as CNS toxicity.
    A. True
    B. False

17. The toxic action of lead on erythrocytes is usually life-threatening.
    A. True
    B. False

18. What is lead colic? What are its major symptoms?

19. Discuss the "wrist drop" phenomenon associated with lead poisoning. Why does it occur?

20. Which of the following is a true statement?
    A. Pica refers solely to ingestion of lead-based items.
    B. Each of the inorganic forms of lead produces symptoms of poisoning that are specific for that form.
    C. Acute poisoning from lead is rare; chronic intoxication is a serious problem.
    D. Inorganic lead poisoning is more rare than organic lead poisoning.

21. What is "basophilic stippling," and why does it occur with lead poisoning?

22. Following ingestion of a lead salt, the stool may appear unusually black. What is the source of this abnormal color?

23. A request to supply BAL should be acknowledged by providing which of the following?
    A. CaNa$_2$-EDTA
    B. Deferoxamine
    C. BAL
    D. Penicillamine

24. The text discusses the approximate lethal dose of iron in children. Translate this into an average number of tablets/capsules of popular proprietary products that would need to be ingested to be fatal.

25. Describe the major symptoms associated with the various stages of iron poisoning. What are the inherent dangers of Stage 2?

26. Heavy metals cause corrosive action on the gastrointestinal tract. Following ingestion, is emesis indicated or contraindicated?

27. Which of the following is a true statement about deferoxamine?
    A. It imparts a greenish-blue color to the urine.
    B. It complexes more tightly with ferric iron.
    C. Rapid injection is associated with hypertensive crises.
    D. Therapy is indicated when the serum iron concentration exceeds 100 mg%.

28. Discuss the mechanisms of toxicity for each of the heavy metals. How are they similar in many instances, and different in others?

29. A delayed symptom of arsenic poisoning is the presence of Mee's lines. What are these?

30. In the latter stages of arsenic poisoning, peripheral neuropathies may develop. Discuss the physiological problems that these disorders may cause.

31. It has been stated that many older reported instances of toxicity to lead and zinc may actually have been due to cadmium. What are the factors that can lead to this conclusion?

32. What are the toxic effects of selenium on the CNS?

33. Based on their average biological half-lives, which heavy metal has the greatest potential to accumulate in the body to high levels?

34. Which of the following forms of mercury is the most potentially toxic to the CNS?
    A. Hg^0
    B. Hg^{1+}
    C. Hg^{2+}

35. Discuss the physical characteristics of arsenic trioxide that may be partially responsible for its activity as a highly toxic material.

36. Arsine gas is produced when acid reacts with arsenic-containing metals.
    A. True
    B. False

37. Cadmium has been shown to inhibit α_1-antitrypsin activity. What is the physiological significance of this inhibition?

38. Which of the following tissues has the highest binding affinity for cadmium?
    A. Bone
    B. Brain
    C. Kidney
    D. Heart

39. Discuss why vitamin D is sometimes given to treat chronic cadmium toxicity.

40. The term "siderosis" refers to toxic symptoms produced by inhalation of which of the following metals?
    A. Zinc
    B. Lead
    C. Iron
    D. Arsenic

41. Which of the following is the antidote of first choice for treating a toxic ingestion of arsenic?
    A. $CaNa_2$-EDTA
    B. Deferoxamine
    C. BAL
    D. Penicillamine

42. Discuss the pros and cons of using a chemical chelator to antidote heavy metal intoxication. Why might a physician decide against using a chelator, even if the victim has seriously high blood levels of metal?

43. The dosage of BAL is calculated to provide a particular drug-metal ratio complex. What is this ratio, and why is it ideal?

44. BAL is not recommended to antidote cadmium poisoning. State the reason why this is so.

45. Which of the following chelator substances is commonly given by the oral route?
    A. BAL
    B. Deferoxamine
    C. Penicillamine

46. Lead is stored by the body primarily in what tissue?

47. A victim of heavy metal poisoning has an odor of garlic on his breath. What is the most probable cause of poisoning?
    A. Mercury

B. Lead

C. Zinc

D. Arsenic

48. Describe a "Burtonian" line. What is its significance?

49. Which of the following is the antidote of first choice for treating a toxic ingestion of copper?
A. CaNa$_2$-EDTA
B. Deferoxamine
C. BAL
D. Penicillamine

50. Discuss the cause, symptoms, and treatment of zinc fume fever.

References

1. Annest, J. S., Pirkle, J. L., Makug, D., Neese, J. W., Bayse, D. D., and Kovar, M. G. (1983): Chronological trend in blood levels between 1976 and 1980. *N. Engl. J. Med.*, 308:1373–1377.

2. Bakir, F., Damluji, S. F., Amin-Zaki, L., Mortadha, M., Khalidi, A., Al-Rawi, N. Y., Tikriti, S., Dhahir, H. I., Clarkson, T. W., Smith, J. C., and Doherty, R. A. (1973): Methylmercury poisoning in Iraq. An interuniversity report. *Science*, 181:230–241.

3. Bakir, F., Al-Khalidi, A., Clarkson, T. W., and Greenwood, R. (1976): Clinical observations on treatment of alkylmercury poisoning in hospital patients. *Bull. WHO*, 53:87–92.

4. Banner, W., and Czajka, P. A. (1981): Iron poisoning. *Am. J. Dis. Child.*, 135:484–485.

5. Baselt, R. C., and Crarey, R. H. (1977): A compendium of therapeutic and toxic concentrations of toxicologically significant drugs in human biofluids. *J. Anal. Toxicol.*, 1:81–103.

6. Blat, W. J., and Fraumeni, J. F. (1975): Arsenical air pollution and lung cancer. *Lancet*, 2:142.

7. Centers for Disease Control (1975): Increased lead absorption and lead poisoning in young children. *J. Pediatr.*, 87:824–830.

8. Chiba, M., Toyoda, T., Inaba, Y., Ogihara, K., and Kikuchi, M. (1980): Acute lead poisoning in an adult from ingestion of paint. *N. Engl. J. Med.*, 303:459.

9. Chowdhury, P., and Louria, D. B. (1976): Influence of cadmium and other trace metals on human α_1-antitrypsin; an *in vitro* study. *Science*, 191:480–481.

10. Clarkson, T. W. (1972): The pharmacology of mercury compounds. *Ann. Rev. Pharmacol.*, 12:375–406.

11. Covey, T. J. (1964): Ferrous sulfate poisoning: A review, case summaries, and therapeutic regimen. *J. Pediatr.*, 64:218–226.

12. Department of Labor (1975): Standard for exposure to inorganic arsenic. *Fed. Reg.*, 40:3392.

13. Diplock, A. T. (1976): Metabolic aspects of selenium action and toxicity. *Crit. Rev. Toxicol.*, 4:271–329.

14. Elhassani, S. B. (1982–83): The many faces of methylmercury poisoning. *J. Toxicol.: Clin. Toxicol.*, 19:875–906.

15. Fairbanks, V. F., Fahey, J. L., and Beutler, E. (1971): *Clinical Disorders of Iron Metabolism*, 2nd ed. Grune & Stratton, New York.

16. Finch, C. A. (1980): Drugs effective in iron-deficiency and other hypochromic anemias. In: *The Pharmacological Basis of Therapeutics*, 6th ed., edited by A. G. Gilman, L. S. Goodman, and A. Gilman, pp. 1315–1330. Macmillan, New York.

17. Flick, D. F., Kraybill, H. F., and Dimetroff, J. M. (1975): Toxic effects of cadmium: A review. *Environ. Res.*, 4:71–85.

18. Friberg, L. (1956): Edathamil calcium-disodium in cadmium poisoning. *Arch. Ind. Health*, 13:13–23.

19. Friberg, L., Piscator, M., Norberg, G., and Kjellstrom, T. (1974): *Cadmium in the Environment*, 2nd ed. CRC Press, Cleveland.

20. Gilman, A., Philips, F. S., Allen, R. P., and Koelle, E. (1946): The treatment of acute cadmium intoxication in rabbits with 2,3-dimercaptopropanol (BAL) and other mercaptans. *J. Pharmacol. Exp. Ther.*, 87:85–101.

21. Glomme, J., and Gustavson, K. H. (1959): Treatment of experimental acute mercury poisoning by chelating agents BAL and EDTA. *Acta Med. Scand.*, 164:175–182.

22. Goldstein, A., Aronow, L., and Kalman, S. M. (1974): *Principles of Drug Action: The Basis of Pharmacology*, 2nd ed. John Wiley, New York.

23. Goldstein, N., McCall, J. I., and Dyck, P. J. (1962): Metal neuropathy. In: *Peripheral Neuropathy*, edited by P. J. Dyck, P. K. Thomas, and F. Lambert, pp. 1227–1262. Saunders, Philadelphia.

24. Hammond, P. B., Aronson, A. L., and Olson, W. C. (1967): The mechanism of mobilization of lead by ethylenediaminetetraacetate. *J. Pharmacol. Exp. Ther.*, 157:196–206.

25. Hammond, P. B. (1971): The effect of chelating agents on the tissue distribution and excretion of lead. *Toxicol. Appl. Pharmacol.*, 18:296–310.

26. Hammond, P. B., and Beliles, R. P. (1980): Metals. In: *Toxicology—The Basic Science of Poisons*, 2nd ed., edited by J. Doull, C. D. Klaassen, and M. O. Amdur, pp. 409–467. Macmillan, New York.

27. Hannigan, B. G. (1978): Self-administration of metallic mercury by intravenous injection. *Br. Med. J.*, 2:933.

28. Havelda, C. J., Sohi, G. S., and Richardson, C. E. (1980): Evaluation of lead, zinc, and copper excretion in chronic moonshine drinkers. *South. Med. J.*, 73:710–715.

29. Hay, W. J., Richards, A. G., McMenemey, W. H., and Cummings, J. N. (1963): Organic mercurial encephalopathy. *J. Neurol. Neurosurg. Psychiatry*, 26:199–202.

30. Holtzman, N. A., Elliott, D. A., and Miller, R. H. (1966): Copper intoxication. Report of a case with observations on ceruloplasmin. *N. Engl. J. Med.*, 275:347–352.

31. Hryhorczuk, D. O., Meyers, L., and Chen, G. (1982): Treatment of mercury intoxication in a dentist with

N-acetyl-D,L-penicillamine. *J. Toxicol.: Clin. Toxicol.*, 19:401–408.

32. Hunter, F. E., Gebicki, J. M., and Hoffstein, P. E. (1963): Swelling and lysis of rat liver mitochondria induced by ferrous ions. *J. Biol. Chem.*, 288:828–835.

33. Jones, M. M. (1982): Newer trends in therapeutic chelating agents. *Trends Pharmacol. Sci.*, 3:335–337.

34. Jung, R. C., and Aaronson, J. (1980): Death following inhalation of mercury vapor at home. *West. J. Med.*, 132:539–543.

35. Kagi, J., and Vallee, B. (1960): Metallothionein: A cadmium- and zinc-containing protein from equinine renal cortex. *J. Biol. Chem.*, 235:3460–3465.

36. Kalman, S. M. (1977): The pathophysiology of lead poisoning: A review and a case report. *J. Anal. Toxicol.*, 1:277–281.

37. Klaassen, C. D. (1975): Biliary excretion of mercury compounds. *Toxicol. Appl. Pharmacol.*, 33:356–365.

38. Klaassen, C. D. (1980): Heavy metals and heavy-metal antagonists. In: *The Pharmacological Basis of Therapeutics*, 6th ed., edited by A. G. Gilman, L. S. Goodman, and A. Gilman, pp. 1615–1637. Macmillan, New York.

39. Koppel, C., Baudisch, J., and Keller, F. (1982): Methoxymethylmercury chloride poisoning: Clinical findings on *in vitro* experiments. *J. Toxicol.: Clin. Toxicol.*, 19:391–400.

40. Lehninger, A. L. (1962): Water uptake and extrusion by mitochondria in relation to oxidative phosphorylation. *Physiol. Rev.*, 42:467–517.

41. Lerner, S., Hong, C. D., and Bozian, R. C. (1979): Cadmium nephropathy—A clinical evaluation. *J. Occup. Med.*, 21:409–412.

42. Lisella, F. S., Long, K. R., and Scott, H. G. (1972): Health aspects of arsenicals in the environment. *J. Environ. Health*, 34:511–518.

43. Lovejoy, F. H. (1982–83): Chelation therapy in iron poisoning. *J. Toxicol.: Clin. Toxicol.*, 19:871–874.

44. Manoguerra, A. S. (1976): Iron poisoning: Report of a fatal case in an adult. *Am. J. Hosp. Pharm.*, 33:1088–1090.

45. Manzler, A. D., and Schreiner, A. W. (1970): Copper-induced acute hemolytic anemia. A new complication of hemodialysis. *Ann. Intern. Med.*, 73:409–412.

46. Marsh, D. O., Myers, G. J., Clarkson, T. W., Amin-Zaki, L., Tikriti, S., and Majeed, M. A. (1981): Dose-response relationship for human fetal exposure to methylmercury. *Clin. Toxicol.*, 18:1311–1318.

47. McAlpine, D., and Shukuro, A. (1958): Minamata disease. An unusual neurological disorder caused by contaminated fish. *Lancet*, 2:629–631.

48. McIntyre, A. R. (1971): The toxicities of mercury and its compounds. *J. Clin. Pharmacol.*, 11:397–401.

49. Moore, W., Stara, J. F., Crocker, W. C., Malanchuk, M., and Iltis, R. (1973): Comparison of 115m cadmium retention in rats following different routes of administration. *Environ. Res.*, 6:473–478.

50. Morse, D. L., Harrington, J. M., Houseworth, J., Landrigan, P. J., and Kelter, A. (1979): Arsenic exposure in multiple environmental media in children near a smelter. *Clin. Toxicol.*, 14:389–399.

51. National Academy of Sciences (1972): *Lead: Airborne lead in perspective.* National Research Council, Washington, D.C.

52. Parizek, J. (1957): The destructive effect of cadmium-ion on testicular tissue and its prevention by zinc. *J. Endocrinol.*, 15:56–63.

53. Patterson, M., and Jernigan, W. C. T. (1969): Lead intoxication from "moonshine." *GP*, 40:126–130.

54. Pearce, J., and Burg, F. D. (1982): Lead poisoning in children. *Drug Therapy*, May, 87–102.

55. Peck, M. G., Rogers, J. F., and Rivenbark, J. F. (1982–83): Use of high doses of deferoxamine (Desferal) in an adult patient with acute iron overdosage. *J. Toxicol.: Clin. Toxicol.*, 19:865–869.

56. Pichirallo, J. (1971): Lead poisoning: Risks for pencil chewers? *Science*, 173:509–510.

57. Pierce, P. E., Thompson, J. F., Likosky, W. H., Nickey, L. N., Barthel, W. F., and Hinman, A. R. (1972): Alkyl mercury poisoning in humans—Report of an outbreak. *JAMA*, 220:1439–1442.

58. Rahola, T., Aaran, R. K., and Mietinen, J. K. (1972): Half-time studies of mercury and cadmium by whole body counting. International Atomic Energy symposium on the assessment of radioactive organ and body burdens. In: *Assessment of Radioactive Contamination in Man.* The Agency, Vienna.

59. Rennert, O. M., Weiner, P., and Madden, J. (1970): Asymptomatic lead poisoning in 85 Chicago children. *Clin. Pediatr.*, 9:9–13.

60. Robertson, D. S. E. (1970): Selenium—A possible teratogen. *Lancet*, 1:518–519.

61. Robotham, J. L., and Lietman, P. S. (1980): Acute iron poisoning. *Am. J. Dis. Child.*, 134:875–879.

62. Sanford, H. N. (1955): Lead poisoning in young children. *Postgrad. Med.*, 17:162–169.

63. Schroeder, H. A. (1965): Cadmium as a factor in hypertension. *J. Chronic. Dis.*, 18:217–228.

64. Shamberger, R., and Willis, C. (1971): Selenium distribution and human cancer mortality. *Clin. Lab. Sci.*, 2:211–221.

65. Sisson, T. R. C. (1960): Acute iron poisoning in children. *Q. Rev. Pediatr.*, 15:47–49.

66. Smith, A. D. M., and Miller, J. W. (1961): Treatment of inorganic mercury poisoning with N-acetyl-D,L-penicillamine. *Lancet*, 1:640.

67. Smith, H. D., Boehner, R. L., Carney, T., and Majors, W. J. (1963): The sequelae of pica with and without lead poisoning. *Am. J. Dis. Child.*, 105:609–616.

68. Smith, W. E., and Smith, A. M. (1975): *Minamata.* Holt, Rinehart & Winston, New York.

69. Stocken, L. A., and Thompson, R. H. S. (1949): Reactions of British antilewisite with arsenic and other metals in living systems. *Physiol. Rev.*, 29:168–194.

70. Teitelbaum, D. T., and Ott, J. E. (1969): Elemental mercury self-poisoning. *Clin. Toxicol.*, 2:243–248.

71. Thind, G. S., and Fischer, G. (1976): Plasma cadmium and zinc in human hypertension. *Clin. Sci. Mol. Med.*, 51:483–486.

72. Tibbits, P. A., and Milroy, W. C. (1980): Pulmonary edema induced by exposure to cadmium oxide fume: Case report. *Milit. Med.*, 145:435–437.

73. Tsuchiya, K. (1969): Causation of Ouch-Ouch disease, an introductory review. *Keio J. Med.*, 18:181–194.

74. Voors, A. W., and Shuman, M. S. (1977): Liver cadmium levels in North Carolina residents who died of heart disease. *Bull. Environ. Contam. Toxicol.*, 17:692–696.

75. Watson, W. A., Veltui, J. C., and Metcalf, T. S. (1981): Acute arsenic exposure treated with oral D-penicillamine. *Vet. Hum. Toxicol.*, 23:164–165.

76. Wattenberg, L. W. (1978): Inhibitors of chemical carcinogenesis. *Adv. Cancer Res.*, 26:197–226.

77. Webb, M. (1972): Biochemical effects of Cd^{2+}—injury in the rat and mouse testis. *J. Reprod. Fertil.*, 30:83–98.

78. Wilber, C. G. (1980): Toxicology of selenium: A review. *Clin. Toxicol.*, 17:171–230.

79. Williams, D. R., and Halsted, B. W. (1982–83): Chelating agents in medicine. *J. Toxicol.: Clin. Toxicol.*, 19:1081–1115.

80. Wright, N., Yeoman, W. B., and Carter, G. F. (1980): Massive oral ingestion of elemental mercury without poisoning. *Lancet*, 1:206.

Household Products

11

Every home contains a variety of products that are intended to meet most domestic needs, from cleaning the floor or bathroom bowl, to treating minor skin cuts and abrasions. The number of such products may run into the hundreds and while some are not of toxicological concern (refer back to Chapter 1, Table 3), many others are, if they should be accidentally ingested or misused.

The purpose of this chapter is to discuss those products that are commonly found in the home. While some of the products have been examined in previous chapters, others have not. Whenever necessary, we will refer to the appropriate chapter for a complete discussion of symptoms and management of the specific poisoning. For the products not considered in other chapters, those discussions will be dealt with here.

HOUSEHOLD POISONINGS

People may come into contact with household products either by accident or on purpose. Accidental poisoning includes the inadvertent ingestion of a quantity of cleaning agent or other substance intended for inanimate or noninternal use. Purposeful poisoning includes any application or ingestion of a substance that the victim uses correctly and in good faith, but for some reason reacts adversely to it. In general, children under 3½ years of age have the highest incidence of accidental poisoning, and usually consume only one swallow (5 ml) or a small bite of the toxic agent, whereas poisoning in children over the age of 6 is rarely accidental.

It is important again to realize that swallowing a product is technically an *ingestion*, rather than poisoning. Poisoning occurs only if symptoms develop. On the other hand, this distinction may be more academic than practical, because any time a substance is misused, either accidentally or intentionally, even in the absence of clinically perceivable symptoms, the event should be considered a possible medical emergency until it can be ruled otherwise. If the victim of such an ingestion is a child, the event should never be brushed off casually because it could be (and there is a good chance it will be) repeated again, the second time with a less favorable outcome.

The reasons for these poisonings, the persons most likely poisoned, and all other important general considerations of poisoning were discussed in Chapter 1. We assume that this comprehensive information is now well understood. However, a few minutes spent in review of the basic principles outlined in that chapter will aid in our understanding of the principles explained here.

Many products that are found in the home are not adequately labeled to indicate their true potential for poisoning. There is a feeling among many persons representing the household products industry that indiscriminate use of warning labels may foster a generalized disinterest in poisoning prevention measures in the public, especially if they are told that everything is dangerous. Consequently, the public is frequently left on its own to distinguish between products that are safe versus products that have a potential for causing serious problems if ingested.

The toxic agents in many household products vary widely and their product formulations are constantly changing. Unless an individual is astute and reads the label each time a new product is purchased or an old product is replaced, he may be dealing with a product having the same trade name, but entirely different constituents or concentrations. Whereas an earlier formulation may have been of little toxicological concern, the newer one may pose significant toxicological concern if ingested.

Antidoting information on labels is not always accurate and up-to-date; even the wrong information may be stated. We are reminded of products containing strong alkali which inform the individual to administer a weakly acidic "antidote" in case of ingestion. As was pointed out in Chapter 3, the results of such a suggestion may be disastrous.

Other times, a product may inform the user to induce emesis with a salt solution. As was also discussed in Chapter 3, this procedure is no longer considered safe and should never be attempted. Many products that were purchased years ago, and were not used in their entirety at that time, still remain in the home. Should the user ingest one of these and read the outdated antidoting information, a disastrous outcome could result.

Another problem relates to an individual's understanding of commonly used words. For example, the term "soap" to some individuals may refer to soap, per se, which is relatively nontoxic; to others it may imply a strong detergent product which is highly alkaline and extremely toxic. Consequently, questions must be asked of the individual to ascertain the exact nature of the product before specific recommendations can be made for antidoting the poisoning.

CLEANING AIDS

Soaps and Detergents

Soaps and detergents constitute the largest class of household products found in greatest quantity around most households. A true soap is a salt of a fatty acid that usually results from reacting a natural fat or oil with a strong alkali, such as sodium or potassium hydroxide. A detergent, on the other hand, is technically any cleaning agent. More specifically, the term refers to the cleaning products primarily used for automatic dishwashers and laundering purposes. They are usually based on nonsoap surfactants (1). Most soaps are relatively nontoxic and possess an emetic action that is possibly as effective as syrup of ipecac (Table 1). Soap-induced emesis is mediated through a direct effect on the gastrointestinal tract, rather than through systemic action (4). Ingestion of many soap products is not especially dangerous because the product is self-eliminating, and few symptoms, other than gastric upset, will be experienced.

While the same general statement about the emetic action of a detergent is true, ingestion of a strong detergent product will cause a variety of reactions, depending on the specific product. This is because detergents contain a wider variety of ingredients than soap products. Most consist of mixtures of inorganic and or-

TABLE 1. *Emetic action of household cleaning products in dogs*[a]

Products	Mean emetic dose (g/kg)	Mean time for emesis (min)
Heavy-duty granular laundry detergent	0.02–0.05	1–4
Light-duty liquid detergent	0.3–1.5	15–45
General purpose liquid household cleaner	0.1–1.0	0.5–10
Bleach, liquid (sodium hypochlorite)	0.25	1–2
Toilet soap	5.0	30–60
Syrup of ipecac	0.1	30–50

[a]From ref. 1.

ganic substances. Surfactants may be anionic, cationic, or nonionic, but most products contain anionic or nonionic surfactants.

Builders are added to detergents to improve the product, for example, by inactivating calcium and other minerals. Common builders include carbonates, silicates, aluminosilicates, and sulfates. The use of phosphates as a builder was popular in previous years. It has largely been replaced in recent years because of the concern by many of its effect on the environment. The major problem from ingestion of most detergent products is the builder. Because of their high alkalinity, they may induce intense gastrointestinal damage.

Other ingredients including whitening agents, fabric softeners, suds-controlling agents, and enzymes are frequently added. These are of no great toxicologic concern.

Bar soaps have a low order of toxicity. The most significant symptoms produced by their ingestion are usually nausea and vomiting, although diarrhea can appear and may be severe in certain people. No treatment is usually required. However, if vomiting or diarrhea is especially severe, electrolyte replacement therapy may be indicated. With mild nausea, a demulcent may bring quick relief.

Shampoos have a similar low order of toxicity, although their gastric irritation action may cause a greater incidence of nausea and vomiting. Treatment of their ingestion usually requires no more concern than indicated for ingestion of bar soap. However, the addition of "antidandruff agents" to shampoos increases the toxicity of the product. Many of the shampoos are irritating to the eyes and mucous membranes and often can be managed by washing these areas well with copious quantities of water.

Granular soaps and detergents generally have a low order of toxicity. The exception is those products intended for automatic dishwashing machines (18). These frequently are highly alkaline and may induce severe mouth and esophageal irritation as was explained in Chapter 8.

Except for dishwasher cleaning products, ingestion of any of the other substances should be antidoted as explained above for bar soaps and shampoos. However, if carbonates are present, an acidic antidote should not be administered. Large quantities of carbon dioxide gas will be formed and may distend the stomach to cause premature emptying of its contents into the intestine. Also, it may cause increased esophageal irritation and generalized gastrointestinal discomfort.

Treatment for ingestion of automatic dishwasher granules should be undertaken as was discussed in Chapter 8 for alkaline materials.

Liquid laundry and dishwashing detergents have a slightly greater order of toxicity. Their ingestion should also be treated as for bar soaps. Fabric softeners are of low toxic potential, so their ingestion is usually of little concern.

Liquid hard-surface cleaners frequently contain pine oil or petroleum distillates. While the quantity of such substances contained within these products is generally of little toxic concern, their chance for being aspirated during emesis is great. Consequently, victims who ingest one of these products should be kept as quiet as possible and not made to vomit. (Refer to Chapter 7.)

Disinfectant cleaners may contain phenolic compounds, quaternary amines, or detergents. They are more toxic than plain soaps and detergents, and require specific antidoting procedures. Generally, phenol-containing products are less toxic than those containing quaternaries

or detergents since the former is more likely to induce vomiting and, thus, be removed from the gastrointestinal tract. Both phenol and quaternary compounds are discussed later in this chapter.

Ammonia, oven cleaners, and drain cleaners are highly alkaline, and thus extremely caustic. Ammonia solution (household ammonia), per se, ranges from 5 to 10% ammonia, but an industrial strength greater than 50% is also available. Ammonia is used in a wide variety of products, and its corrosive action is seen on all cells. Ingestion of stronger solutions must be treated as for any caustic substance that was discussed in Chapter 8.

A distinction must be made between ammonia, per se, and products advertised as "having ammonia." These latter products contain small quantities of the substance and are usually of little toxic concern.

Toilet bowl cleaners may be acidic or alkaline. Acidic substances are liquid (usually hydrochloric acid) or granular (commonly sodium bisulfate). Their ingestion should be treated as for an acid (Chapter 8).

"Automatic toilet bowl cleaners," those which are added to the tank, may also be liquid or granular and are usually strongly alkaline. Generally, they are composed of calcium hypochlorite. Their ingestion is treated as for chlorine bleach which is discussed later. Some other "automatic" cleaners contain only detergents, without a chlorine source. Their ingestion should be treated as for any liquid laundry detergent.

The flow chart scheme that is presented in Fig. 1 illustrates the action that should be taken if a soap or detergent product is ingested.

Bleach

Most bleach products are solutions of 3 to 6% sodium hypochlorite in water. The pH is approximately 11, which makes them highly alkaline. Symptoms of ingestion of bleach include severe irritation and corrosion of mucous membranes with pain and vomiting. There may be a fall in blood pressure with delirium and coma. On the other hand, the amount of bleach ac-

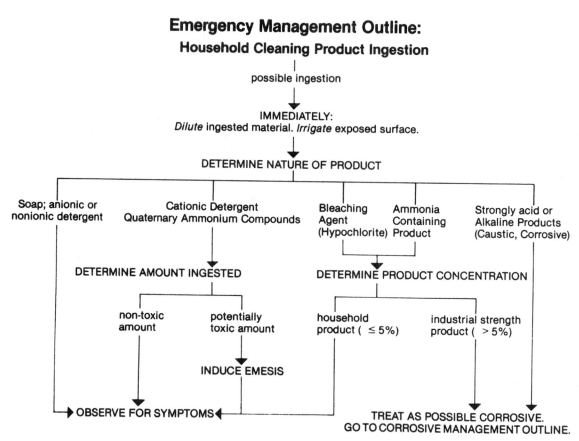

FIG. 1. Flow chart illustrating the steps involved in assessment and management of a victim of poisoning by a household product. (Reproduced with permission of The Soap and Detergent Association.)

tually ingested by most people is usually small. This is probably due to the extremely bad taste of bleach. Therefore, severe toxicity is usually avoided.

Treatment of bleach intoxication includes demulcent therapy. Although the pH of a bleach solution is alkaline, acidic antidotes should not be given. The reason for this caution is that hypochlorus acid is formed in the stomach when sodium hypochlorite reacts with hydrochloric acid. Hypochlorus acid is not toxic when absorbed in small quantities, since it is buffered by the blood. However, it is extremely irritating to both the mucous membranes of the esophagus and the gastrointestinal tract.

Bleach should never be mixed with strongly acidic or alkaline cleaning agents, although this apparently is a common procedure in many households. When bleach reacts with either acid or base, as shown in Fig. 2, chlorine gas or chloramine gas may be released. Although inhalation of small quantities of either of these gases does not produce severe toxicity, either can cause lacrimation, and irritation of the mucous membranes and respiratory passages if they are inhaled in sufficient concentrations in a confined area. In a high concentration, both could cause asphyxiation.

A particularly important concept that should also be remembered is that some bleaches, especially the powdered ones, contain other oxidizing agents such as peroxides or perborates. When these substances are present, their ingestion must be antidoted because they may be more toxic than the bleach, per se.

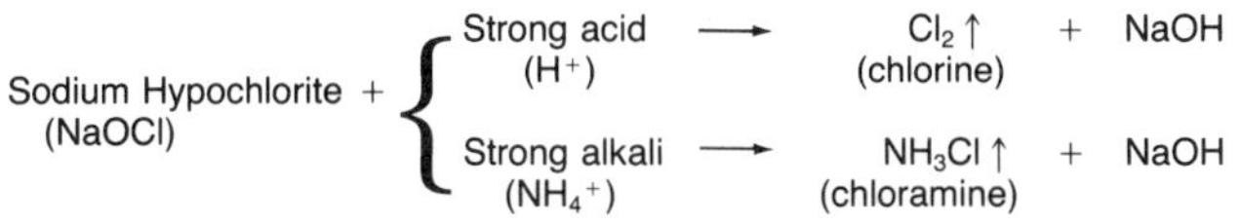

Sodium Hypochlorite + {
    Strong acid $\longrightarrow$ $Cl_2 \uparrow$ +   NaOH
(NaOCl) (H^+) (chlorine)

    Strong alkali $\longrightarrow$ $NH_3Cl \uparrow$ +   NaOH
    (NH_4^+) (chloramine)

FIG. 2. Sodium hypochlorite (bleach) mixed with strong acid or strong alkali results in formation of chlorine or chloramine gas.

Carbon Tetrachloride

Although the use of carbon tetrachloride is now largely limited to industrial applications, it is still available in many households. A pint bottle purchased years ago, from which only an ounce or two was removed, still contains enough carbon tetrachloride to inflict severe toxicity if ingested. Carbon tetrachloride has long been a favorite substance for cleaning grease from clothing and numerous other items. Thus, it will continue to be a source of poisoning for many years.

Carbon tetrachloride was at one time used as a general inhalational anesthetic with its pharmacologic action resembling chloroform. It was also used orally, until the early 1940s, for treatment of hookworm infestations. However, its medical use for both purposes was discontinued with the introduction of more potent (and less toxic) alternative drugs. Since the oral dose needed to cause death may be less than 2 ml (2,20), we must wonder about the many people who possibly suffered the consequences of receiving carbon tetrachloride to treat an intestinal worm infestation. On the other hand, the fatal dose is reported to be as high as 100 ml (19).

Carbon tetrachloride ingestion inflicts severe damage to both the liver and kidney, with the more significant changes occurring to hepatic tissue. The most characteristic change is fatty necrosis of the liver that occurs in all animal species. The fat that accumulates is primarily triglyceride which is produced by the liver. This would normally be secreted into the blood, but because the secretory mechanism is blocked by the poison, it accumulates. After some time, this blocks important hepatic processes and frank liver failure occurs.

The precise mechanism for toxic action has been studied in detail, and carbon tetrachloride is still the classic hepatotoxic chemical to which all other substances that cause liver damage are compared (6,17). However, many questions do remain regarding its exact mechanism of action. Some specific sites for injury that have been identified include the mitochondria, endoplasmic reticulum membrane, and the lysosomes. Whatever the effect is on the liver, the same action is thought to occur on the kidney.

Mechanism of Carbon Tetrachloride Toxicity

It is believed that in order to exert its toxic action, carbon tetrachloride must be converted to a toxic intermediate product (6,17). The theory of greatest interest is that it is converted to free radicals (i.e., $\cdot CCl_3$), or eventually to CCl_3CCl_3 which could occur from condensation of two molecules of the free radical. This conversion may be brought about by the microsomal mixed-function oxidase system. For example, if these enzymes are stimulated (e.g., by ethanol) prior to carbon tetrachloride ingestion, its overall toxicity is greater. (We will also observe the same effect later, when we study acetaminophen.) Furthermore, one of the means used to antidote toxicity is to administer antioxidants such as vitamin E.

Clinical Manifestations of Carbon Tetrachloride Poisoning

Characteristics of carbon tetrachloride ingestion are nonspecific, including gastrointestinal irritation, along with liver and kidney changes (Table 2). Gastric effects normally appear within hours of ingestion. Changes in the liver can also be detected within hours and usually reach a maximum in 24 to 48 hr. In nonlethal quantities, hepatic repair may start within days, but the victim's prognosis will remain guarded over the next several months to a year. Hepatic complications (e.g., cirrhosis) are common, and death

TABLE 2. *Characteristics of carbon tetrachloride poisoning*

Ingestion
    Nausea, vomiting, abdominal cramping, gastrointestinal bleeding
    Hepatic injury (e.g., elevated enzymes, ferritin, and bile acids; cholestasis; jaundice; swollen, tender liver)
    Dizziness
    Confusion
    Depressed respirations
    Renal failure (e.g., oliguria, edema, azotemia, uremia)
    Coma
Inhalation
    Fatigue, weakness
    Dizziness
    Blurred vision
    Paresthesias
    Tremors
    Nausea, abdominal discomfort

---

may not occur until months after ingestion. In the event of surviving the hepatic damage, renal failure due to tubular necrosis is the second most significant cause of death.

Symptoms from inhalation are identical to those of any other CNS depressant. These are potentiated if the victim has consumed alcohol or has taken a CNS sedative drug. The depression is caused by a generalized sedative action on the brain.

Treatment of Carbon Tetrachloride Poisoning

Carbon tetrachloride ingestion of any quantity must be considered a toxic emergency. Its early presence in the gastrointestinal tract can be confirmed radiographically (2). Emetics, activated charcoal, and cathartics will aid in its removal from the gastrointestinal tract. Treatment must begin immediately. Inducers of microsomal enzymes (e.g., phenobarbital, ethanol) must not be administered for reasons stated earlier. Hemodialysis should begin at the onset of renal failure. Total parenteral nutrition may be helpful in reducing protein catabolism (10).

An interesting report in the literature of an accidental observation may shed new light on methods to prevent serious toxicity (22). A victim of poisoning was believed to have been intoxicated by carbon monoxide, so he was given hyperbaric (2.5 atm) oxygen therapy. Later (8–16 hr after ingestion), the confusion was recognized and the actual cause of poisoning (carbon tetrachloride, approximately 250 ml) was identified and conventional treatment was started. At that time, symptoms were mild and it appeared that oxygen therapy had helped, so it was repeated. The patient survived. The authors concluded that the oxygen may have corrected regional tissue hypoxia in the liver and thus prevented hepatic damage from this otherwise lethal dose.

The report is mentioned because we are constantly impressed with the notion that sometimes the least conventional methods do the most good. In managing patients who have been poisoned by any type of substance, the nonconventional methods should not be withheld, especially if the patient is not responding to the more traditional means.

MISCELLANEOUS PRODUCTS

Mothballs, Toilet and Diaper Pail Deodorants

Most products used as mothballs, and toilet and diaper pail deodorants contain naphthalene or paradichlorobenzene. Today, naphthalene is used less often than previously because of its great potential for toxicity. It has been replaced with the less toxic substance, paradichlorobenzene, which if ingested, may induce local irritation of the gastrointestinal tract. However, it requires no antidotal therapy, except possibly for a demulcent, and treatment of nausea and vomiting, if severe.

Naphthalene, on the other hand, is a powerful toxic substance that requires immediate medical treatment if ingestion occurs. Most immediate danger from naphthalene occurs in infants who find a mothball in some out-of-the-way place and decide that it is candy. Adults are rarely poisoned. At special risk are those persons with erythrocytic glucose-6-phosphate dehydrogenase (G6PD) deficiency (8). G6PD is an enzyme that reduces NADP to NADPH as shown below:

$$\text{NADPH} \underset{\text{Reduction}}{\overset{\text{Oxidation}}{\rightleftharpoons}} \text{NADP} + \text{H}^+$$

NADPH is the active form required by erythrocytic membranes to maintain their structural integrity. In the normal individual, oxidizing chemicals convert NADPH to NADP which is then quickly converted back to NADPH. In a person with G6PD deficiency, however, reduction of NADP to NADPH proceeds much more slowly and, therefore, erythrocytic membranes begin to break down. Hemolysis, then, is the major outcome, and all significant clinical manifestations of naphthalene intoxication (Table 3) can be traced to this event (12).

Treatment is largely supportive and nonspecific.

Nail Polish Remover (Acetone)

Acetone forms the basis for most commercial fingernail polish remover products. However, many other products for this same use are also available which do not contain acetone. Some products may also contain mineral seal oil, castor or olive oil, lanolin, or glycerin. Thus, the label should be checked for the product's contents. Acetone may also be readily recognized by its sweet, pungent odor.

Intoxication by acetone is a potential health hazard in industrial settings where it is employed as a solvent for a variety of lipids. Most industrial poisonings are by inhalation, with irritation of the eye, nose, and throat produced at exposures of 500 to 1000 ppm (7). Higher concentrations cause CNS depression.

In the home, acetone poisoning is less frequent, but it does occur. Ingestion of small

TABLE 3. *Characteristics of naphthalene poisoning*

Nausea, vomiting, diarrhea
Excitement
Convulsions
Coma
Jaundice
Hemolysis, anemia
Pain on urination
Oliguria, hematuria

quantities ranging from 10 to 20 ml does not normally produce symptoms, while 200 ml has caused severe coma in an adult (21). Two to 3 ml/kg is a toxic dose in a child. Acetone is absorbed through the skin, but the quantity that may be absorbed from nail polish removers poses no medical problems. Acetone imparts an intense drying effect on the skin as it dissolves dermal lipids. Unless occurring over a large area, this is not serious.

Ingestion of toxic amounts of acetone induces a variety of signs and symptoms. Nausea with vomiting and gastric hemorrhage may occur. CNS sedation with respiratory depression, ataxia, and paresthesias is common. Coughing and bronchial irritation may be the only clues to ingestion of quantities that are too small to produce sedation. Depression may proceed to coma. Hyperglycemia and ketonemia that resemble acute diabetic coma are often reported, and renal tubular necrosis may occur.

Treatment of symptoms following oral ingestion or inhalation of quantities sufficient to produce toxicity is purely symptomatic. Unless the patient is comatose, emesis should be performed, followed by activated charcoal and saline catharsis. Diazepam will control seizures.

Disinfectants and Antiseptics

Most households contain a large number of products that are used for various disinfectant purposes. Their potential for serious toxicity varies greatly, and, consequently, they cannot be studied as a single group.

Boric Acid

At one time boric acid was recommended for more than 40 medical purposes. This weakly bacteriostatic substance has gained considerable notoriety of late, however, because of its great potential to cause toxicity. Due to this and because it does not possess strong disinfectant action, there may eventually be a curtailment of its use. On the other hand, boric acid is an excellent insecticide for roaches and other crawling insects. It is used in large quantities where these insects are present. Borates (e.g., as sodium tetraborate, etc.) are widely used as cleaning aids. So it is doubtful that, even with an eventual decrease in use of boric acid for its alleged medical purposes, the incidence of poisoning by borates will decline.

The usual circumstance for poisoning is by accidental ingestion. For example, boric acid has been taken in error for epsom salts ($MgSO_4$). A boric acid solution has been mistakenly used to prepare baby formula in several cases, resulting in numerous deaths.

Boric acid is readily absorbed through abraded tissue (15). Many cases on record attest to the problems encountered when the solution or powder is applied to a wound, especially with occlusion. Systemic effects commonly occur.

Boric acid is toxic to all cells. Its greatest danger is in areas where it concentrates highly, such as in the kidney (9). The fatal dose is estimated to be 15 to 20 g (14).

Following exposure, the signs and symptoms listed in Table 4 may be seen. A characteristic of poisoning is a severe erythematous rash ("boiled lobster rash") that is seen on the palms, soles, and buttocks. The immediate cause of death is usually CNS depression. However, if the patient survives the acute poisoning event, complications such as hepatic fatty necrosis, cerebral edema, or renal failure may be the cause of death.

Treatment of poisoning is nonspecific and symptomatic. A fatality rate of 50% of those who ingest a toxic dose is reported.

Phenol (Carbolic Acid)

Phenol was one of the oldest disinfectants/deodorizers and is still used alone, as well as an ingredient in many commercial products. Phenol is a significant cause of poisoning.

Intoxication can occur following absorption of phenolic substances through intact skin, or by ingestion. Most poisonings occur from accidental exposure. Preparations containing phenol that are intended for topical use should never contain a concentration greater than 1%. Phenol has a strongly characteristic odor and its presence can be readily detected on the breath.

Phenol is a protein precipitant which induces strong corrosive actions. It is a cellular depressant and causes a variety of signs and symptoms (Table 5). Death immediately following poisoning usually occurs from respiratory depression. Survival beyond a day or two is often met with renal damage that eventually leads to death. Although esophageal stricture is rare, it is a long-term complication that may develop.

Immediate emesis or lavage of ingested poison is important. Egg whites, milk, or gelatin solution should be given quickly. These serve as a source of protein which any phenol remaining in the stomach will precipitate, in preference to the protein of the stomach lining. Nonabsorbable oils (e.g., olive or mineral) are indicated to absorb phenol and, thus, reduce its chance for transport into the blood. Castor oil is frequently recommended as the antidote of choice because phenol has high affinity for it, and because castor oil produces a cathartic ac-

TABLE 4. *Characteristics of boric acid poisoning*

Skin: erythematous ("boiled lobster") rash, blistering, desquamation, excoriation
Lethargy, weakness
CNS depression, collapse, coma
Cardiovascular collapse
Twitching, tremors, convulsions
Hyperpyrexia
Hypotension
Cyanosis
Jaundice
Renal failure

TABLE 5. *Characteristics of phenol (carbolic acid) poisoning*

Nausea, vomiting, bloody diarrhea, abdominal cramping
Sweating (profuse)
Cyanosis
CNS stimulation, hyperactivity, convulsions, followed by CNS depression
Stupor
Hypotension
Increased respirations followed by depressed respirations
Pulmonary edema, pneumonia
Esophageal stricture
Hemolysis, methemoglobinemia
Jaundice
Renal failure
Cardiovascular collapse, shock
Skin: blanching, erythema, corrosion

tion which helps to remove the poison from the gastrointestinal tract quickly. This use for a stimulant cathartic is one of the few times in antidotal therapy where a *stimulant* cathartic is specifically indicated.

Iodine

Iodine has been used as a topical disinfectant since the early 1800s. It is also used to sterilize contaminated water by placing several drops of a 2% tincture in each quart of water.

The toxicity potential for iodine is usually overstated and overemphasized. Deaths are rare (5). It is doubtful that the quantity contained in 0.5 to 1 ounce, which is the normal quantity found in most homes, would inflict serious injury. Most of the fears of iodine or reasons for its bad image probably resulted from use, in previous years, of the 7% tincture which is no longer used except in veterinary practice.

Iodine is a direct protein precipitant which is corrosive to mucous membranes. In the intestine it is converted to the less toxic iodide, and it also is rapidly deactivated by foodstuff in the gut. Furthermore, it causes a strong vomiting reflex which removes much of the poison. All of these factors help to minimize its toxicity.

Major symptoms of ingestion are seen on the gastrointestinal tract, with nausea, vomiting, diarrhea, and gastroenteritis being paramount. Ingestion can be quickly recognized by the appearance of brown stains in the mouth or on the lips, or of brown-colored vomitus.

Iodine ingestion should still be antidoted to assure that damage will be kept at a minimum. Gastric lavage with soluble starch should be undertaken to absorb iodine. Then, a 1 to 5% solution of sodium thiosulfate can be instilled to convert remaining iodine to iodide. Glucocorticosteroids should be administered as quickly as possible to reduce the chance of esophageal fibrosis, a complication that may occur later.

Death from massive ingestions usually occurs within 48 hr from circulatory collapse due to shock, or from aspirations during emesis which causes pulmonary edema.

Quaternary Ammonium Compounds

Quaternary ammonium compounds (QACs) are cellular cationic surfactants used in a wide variety of products such as disinfectants, bactericides, deodorants, and sanitizers. QACs are all potentially toxic, although the toxicity varies with the specific compound, the concentration of the product, dose ingested, and the rate of administration. All QACs produce similar symptoms through a similar mechanism.

Strong aqueous compounds produce superficial necrosis of mucous membranes with which they come into contact. Internally, they cause gastrointestinal tract erosion, ulceration, and hemorrhage throughout the entire intestine. Edema of the glottis and brain has been reported, as has damage to the heart, liver, and kidney.

All QACs cause disinfection only to chemically clean areas. In the presence of any traces of soap, they are inactivated. Thus, soap serves as the best means for antidoting QAC poisoning.

Following skin contamination, the area should be thoroughly cleaned with soap. Following ingestion, a weak soap solution will inactivate any QAC and reduce its toxicity. Ordinary bar soap or dishwashing liquids are sufficient.

SUMMARY

In some respects, this chapter did not need to be written. The majority of household products that are ingested or cause poisoning by any manner fall into one of the general categories of poisons found elsewhere in this book. But since a large number of poisonings occur in or around the home, the time we spent reviewing these items was to our benefit.

Case Studies

CASE STUDY: INTOXICATION WITH MOUTHWASH

History

A 33-month-old, otherwise healthy girl was found by her parents in a stuporous state. Beside her was a partially filled bottle of mouthwash. A summoned paramedic team began intravenous therapy, then transported her to the emergency room.

On admission, the victim was comatose, and nonresponsive to all stimuli except deep pain. The pulse rate was 125 beats/min, respirations were 28/min, and blood pressure 88/50 mm Hg. Her temperature was 35.4°C.

Laboratory data showed a blood alcohol level of 306 mg/100 ml (approximately 3½ hr postingestion). Blood electrolyte measurement showed an anion gap of 28.

It was estimated that the girl had ingested 11 ounces of 18.5% (v/v) ethanol (48.2 g absolute alcohol).

Treatment. The child received nasogastric lavage; intravenous fluids supplemented with bicarbonate were continued. By 8 hr postingestion, blood alcohol concentration was reduced to 128 mg/100 ml. Eighteen hours after admission, all blood values had returned to normal, symptoms had disappeared, and she was discharged several hours later.

Mouthwash ingestions are commonplace; this probably relates to the pleasing taste and odor that many of these products have. During an 18-month period, 422 cases in children under the age of 6 were reported to the National Poison Control Network. Ethanol content and the approximate lethal dose for five leading brands of mouthwash are listed in Table 6.

Our learning objective for this case study is to show that some household products that otherwise seem to be innocuous may not be. This point is well illustrated by the case study. (See ref. 23.)

Discussion

1. If the identity of the poison this victim ingested had not been known, of what value would it have been to know the anion gap value (refer back to Chapter 4)?

TABLE 6. *Ethanol concentrations of leading mouthwashes*

Mouthwash	Ethanol (% v/v)	Approximate lethal dose (oz/12-kg child)
Cepacol	14.0	10.9
Listerine	26.9	5.7
Listermint	14.2	10.7
Scope	18.5	8.2
Signal	14.5	10.5

From ref. 23.

2. Comment on the girl's blood alcohol level versus clinical symptoms. Was there a proper correlation?

3. To prevent future cases like the one illustrated here from occurring, what specific steps should be undertaken by manufacturers of these products and by people who purchase them?

CASE STUDIES: CHLORINE BLEACH POISONINGS

History: Case 1

A 2-year-old female drank several ounces of household bleach (5.4% sodium hypochlorite). She vomited almost immediately, then was given milk and olive oil. She presented to the emergency room with burns of the lips, tongue, and hard and soft palate. An esophagoscopy was delayed because the child had pneumonia. The course of treatment consisted of antibiotics and corticosteroid therapy.

It was necessary to begin parenteral feeding because of increased difficulty in swallowing. Hematemesis and fecal occult blood were noted on the fourth hospital day. It was not until 3 weeks after admission that an esophagoscopy could be performed, at which time it revealed a severely burned esophagus with a 4 to 5 cm area of narrowing. At the end of 1 month there was no change in the size of stricture, despite several attempts at dilation. The following week a gastrostomy was performed. She was discharged 2½ months after admission. (See ref. 11.)

History: Case 2

An 83-year-old female diabetic was cleaning her bathtub with undiluted Clorox® (5.2% sodium hypochlorite). The stain was "stubborn" to remove, even with soap, so she added almost a full can of Sani-Flush® (80% sodium bisulfate). Almost immediately she experienced an intense burning sensation around the mouth, nose, throat, and eyes. Even though she began coughing, she persisted in cleaning the area. She finally left the small unventilated room when her breathing became extremely difficult, approximately 3 to 4 min after coughing began.

She presented at the emergency room with symptoms of severe, near-fatal pulmonary edema.

Treatment. Treatment consisted of oxygen, morphine, rotating tourniquets, prednisone, and a diuretic. She completely recovered within 10 days and was discharged. (See ref. 16.)

Discussion

1. Is a solution of sodium hypochlorite acidic or basic?

2. Is the site of injury consistent with the chemical classification of this poison?

3. What happens when bleach is mixed with the gastric juices?

4. What is a gastrostomy, and why was it performed on the patient in Case 1?

CASE STUDY: CARBON TETRACHLORIDE-INDUCED LIVER DAMAGE

History

The patient was a 48-year-old woman who was brought to the hospital 2 hr after drinking 2 ounces of carbon tetrachloride. At the time of admission her liver was neither enlarged nor tender. She experienced nausea over the next 4 days and vomited once, but, otherwise, her condition was symptom-free and nonremarkable.

Treatment, which began upon admission, consisted of intravenous fluids. Nitrofurantoin was administered after a week of hospitalization, because of a minor urinary tract infection.

Liver function. Liver function tests showed abnormalities from the first day. Albumin and cholesterol synthesis were depressed. Organic ion clearance by the liver decreased and serum bilirubin increased.

Serum levels of liver enzyme rose dramatically, with a peak shown by 3 days postingestion. Afterwards, they began a downward trend, except for a smaller upward peak at Day 7 which was short-lived. By the end of 30 days postingestion, most parameters had returned to normal. (See ref. 3.)

Discussion

1. From what is stated in this case study, and also based upon your knowledge of physiology, what were the probable reasons for the increased blood levels of bilirubin?

2. Are you surprised that no treatment other than intravenous fluids was administered? If so, what procedures could have been used?

CASE STUDY: CHRONIC BORAX INTOXICATION

History

A 4½-month-old male had been experiencing seizures since the age of 2 months. At 3 months of age,

he was diagnosed as having epilepsy and given phenobarbital. The seizures continued despite the barbiturate. On admission to the hospital, he appeared pale and irritable and had patchy, dry erythema over the scalp, trunk, and limbs. The results of a physical examination were generally unremarkable.

Laboratory values were mainly within normal limits, but a hypochromic normocytic anemia was detected.

During the examination the patient was quite irritable and began to cry. In order to appease the child, his mother dipped a pacifier into a small brown bottle she carried in her purse. When she gave the baby the pacifier coated with this thick yellow-brown liquid, he immediately stopped crying.

The bottle was examined and found to be labeled "Borax and Honey." The ingredients listed were: Borax 10.5 g, glycerin 5.25 g, and honey to 100 g. Apparently she had learned this practice from her own mother who had used this preparation on all her children. The child had received approximately 1 ounce per week since he was 1 month old.

When this information was obtained, blood and urine samples were analyzed for boric acid content. The results were:

	Blood	Urine
Borax	14.5 mg%	12.3 mg%
Boric acid	9.44 mg%	7.95 mg%

After the borax-honey-pacifier "therapy" was discontinued the child had no further seizures, and the EEG recording returned to normal after 1 week. Phenobarbital therapy was also discontinued.

The infant was discharged, but therapy with iron supplements was initiated. After several months, the blood profile became normal. (See ref. 13.)

Discussion

1. A fatal dose of acute borax ingestion ranges from 4.5 to 14 g. What was the weekly amount of borax ingested by this patient?

2. How does acute borax intoxication differ from chronic intoxication as seen in this case study?

CASE STUDY: BENZALKONIUM CHLORIDE POISONING

History

Two and one-half month old twins (one male, one female) were brought to a hospital. They had fever, dehydration, circumoral erythema, and numerous oral and pharyngeal grayish-white lesions. Both infants also had a red, dry, scaly diaper rash. The male twin had been diagnosed the day before as having candidiasis and benzalkonium chloride (1:50,000) was prescribed to be applied topically.

The mother had a prescription filled and had been applying the medication to the mouth of both children. But whenever the drug was applied to the mouth of either child, immediately the child would salivate profusely and cry. This was followed by a period of anorexia, irritability, and fever. It was at this point the twins were brought to the hospital.

Direct laryngoscopy showed no lesions. Drooling and an intermittent cough were noted. The male also had evidence of pneumonitis which cleared within 4 days.

The following laboratory results were obtained:

	Male infant	Female infant
WBC	22,700 cu mm	24,800 cu mm
Serum uric acid	12 mg%	9.2 mg%
Alkaline phosphatase	350 IU/L	240 IU/L
SGOT	40 IU/L	20 IU/L

Information was later obtained from the pharmacist who dispensed the benzalkonium prescription that a 17% stock solution had been incorrectly diluted to its prescribed concentration. Instead, it was diluted two parts to one part water (resulting in an 11% solution) and was dispensed.

The female patient stayed 1 week, but the male remained in the hospital for 2 weeks. (See ref. 24.)

Discussion

1. How is benzalkonium chloride classified, and what is its toxicity rating?

2. What toxic effects are produced by this type of product?

3. What is considered a "safe" or recommended dose of benzalkonium chloride for topical use?

4. How would the clinical manifestations of an acute ingestion of this compound differ from the present case study?

5. On admission, the male had a fever; the female did not. What was the probable cause?

Review Questions

1. "Automatic toilet bowl cleaner" product ingestion should be treated the same as would ingestion of any other:

A. acid
B. base

2. Laundry bleach contains a 3 to 6% concentration of:
A. sodium hypochlorite
B. carbon tetrachloride
C. oxalic acid
D. carbolic acid

3. Oven and drain cleaners that contain ammonia are:
A. acidic
B. alkaline

4. Liquid hard-surface cleaners may contain pine or petroleum distillates. Discuss the total ramifications of swallowing, then vomiting one of these products.

5. Which of the following is a true statement?
A. Soap causes emesis through stimulation of the chemoreceptor trigger zone (CTZ).
B. On the average, detergents are more toxic than soap.
C. Enzymes in some soap and detergent products are of toxic concern.
D. Shampoo ingestion should be treated as a toxic emergency.

6. Discuss the toxic potential for dishwasher granules.

7. If a child under the age of 3½ years ingests one "swallow" of a liquid product, about how many milliliters has he actually ingested?

8. Differentiate between soaps and detergents as sources of toxicity.

9. Why does ethanol enhance the toxicity of carbon tetrachloride on the (a) liver and (b) CNS?

10. Radiographic examination of the gastrointestinal tract will reveal the presence of carbon tetrachloride.
A. True
B. False

11. Carbon tetrachloride-induced hepatotoxicity is believed to occur through free radical formation. Explain how this comes about, and what the toxic problems are.

12. Describe the expected toxic consequences of mixing bleach with strongly acidic or alkaline

cleaning agents. How should this problem be treated?

13. Outline the procedures to follow when antidoting bleach ingestion.

14. Of naphthalene and paradichlorobenzene, which is the more toxic?

15. Symptoms, including hyperglycemia and ketonemia, that resemble diabetic coma may be expected following intoxication with which of the following?
    A. Boric acid
    B. Paradichlorobenzene
    C. Acetone
    D. Carbon tetrachloride

16. Persons with a glucose-6-phosphate dehydrogenase deficiency are at high risk of poisoning from a substance found in the household. What is this substance? What is the special risk?

17. Erythema, reported as a "boiled lobster rash," is a symptom reported to occur following ingestion of:
    A. phenol
    B. boric acid
    C. acetone
    D. benzalkonium chloride

18. Most nail polish remover products contain:
    A. naphthalene
    B. carbon tetrachloride
    C. phenol
    D. acetone

19. Glucocorticoids are recommended for a specific purpose following iodine ingestion. What is the reason?

20. Discuss the specific action of sodium thiosulfate in antidoting iodine ingestion.

21. What types of household products contain phenol? Name as many as you can.

22. Describe the symptoms produced by ingestion of phenol. How is this substance antidoted?

23. The usual cause of death following an acute toxic ingestion of boric acid is:
    A. CNS depression
    B. renal damage
    C. hepatic necrosis
    D. red blood cell hemolysis

24. Describe symptoms that would follow from topical application of a strong (toxic) solution of benzalkonium chloride.

25. Ingestion of a household product containing which of the following would be met as a greater toxic emergency?
    A. Cationic detergent
    B. Anionic detergent

References

1. Aupperle, D. J., Darmstadt, R., Kuemmel, A. G., Booman, K. A., Gilman, M. R., and Yam, J. (1980): *Cleaning Products and Their Accidental Ingestion.* The Soap and Detergent Association, New York.
2. Bagnasco, F. M., Stringer, B., and Muslim, A. M. (1978): Carbon tetrachloride poisoning—radiographic findings. *NY State Med. J.*, Vol. 78, 4:646–647.
3. Campbell, C. B., Collins, D. M., and Van Tongeten, A. (1980): Serum bile acids and other liver function tests in hepatocellular damage from carbon tetrachloride ingestion. *NZ Med. J.*, 91:381–384.
4. Carter, R. O., Griffith, J. F., and Weaver, J. E. (1969): The household products manufacturer's role in poison prevention. *Clin. Toxicol.*, 2:289–294.
5. Clark, M. N. (1981): A fatal case of iodine poisoning. *Clin. Toxicol.*, 18:807–811.
6. Cornish, H. H. (1980): Solvents and vapors. In: *Toxicology: The Basic Science of Poisons*, 2nd ed., edited by J. Doull, C. D. Klaassen, and M. O. Amdur, pp. 468–496. Macmillan, New York.
7. DiVincenzo, G. O., Yanno, F. J., and Astill, B. D. (1973): Exposure of man and dog to low concentrations of acetone vapor. *Am. Ind. Hyg. Assoc. J.*, 34:329–330.
8. Doull, J. (1980): Factors influencing toxicology. In: *Toxicology: The Basic Science of Poisons*, 2nd ed., edited by J. Doull, C. D. Klaassen, and M. O. Amdur, pp. 70–83. Macmillan, New York.
9. Dreisbach, R. H. (1983): *Handbook of Poisoning*, 11th ed. Lange Medical Publications, Los Altos.
10. Fogel, R. P., Davidman, M., Poleski, M. H., and Spanier, A. H. (1983): Carbon tetrachloride poisoning treated with hemodialysis and total parenteral nutrition. *Can. Med. Assoc. J.*, 128:560–561.
11. French, R. J., Tabb, H. G., and Rutledge, L. J. (1970): Esophageal stenosis produced by ingestion of bleach. *Southern Med. J.*, 63:1140–1143.
12. Goldstein, A., Aronow, W. L., and Kalman, S. M. (1978): *Principles of Drug Action*, 2nd ed. John Wiley, New York.
13. Gordon, A. S., Pritchard, J. S., and Freedman, M. H. (1973): Seizure disorders and anemia associated with chronic borax intoxication. *CMA Journal*, 108:719–724.
14. Harvey, S. C. (1975): Antiseptics and disinfectants;

fungicides; ectoparasiticides. In: *The Pharmacologic Basis of Therapeutics*, 5th ed., edited by L. S. Goodman and A. Gilman, pp. 987–1017. Macmillan, New York.

15. Harvey, S. C. (1980): Antiseptics and disinfectants; fungicides; ectoparasiticides. In: *The Pharmacologic Basis of Therapeutics*, 6th ed., edited by A. G. Gilman, L. S. Goodman, and A. Gilman, pp. 964–987. Macmillan, New York.

16. Jones, F. L. (1972): Chloride poisoning from mixing household cleaners. *JAMA*, 222:1312.

17. Klaassen, C. D. (1980): Nonmetallic environmental toxicants: Air pollutants, solvents and vapors, and pesticides. In: *The Pharmacologic Basis of Therapeutics*, 6th ed., edited by A. G. Gilman, L. S. Goodman, and A. Gilman, pp. 1638–1659. Macmillan, New York.

18. Krenzelok, E. P., and Clinton, J. E. (1979): Caustic esophageal and gastric erosion without evidence of oral burns following detergent ingestion. *J. Am. Coll. Emerg. Phys.*, 8:194–196.

19. Lehner, E. R. (1935): Acute CCl_4 poisoning. Report of a case. *Arch. Int. Med.*, 56:98.

20. Lichtman, S. S. (1969): *Diseases of Liver, Gallbladder and Bile Ducts*. Lea & Febiger, Philadelphia.

21. Rumack, B. H. (1983): *Poisindex*. Rocky Mountain Poison Center, Denver.

22. Truss, C. D., and Killenberg, P. G. (1982): Treatment of carbon tetrachloride poisoning with hyperbaric oxygen. *Gastroenterology*, 82:767–769.

23. Weller-Fahy, E. R., Berger, L. R., and Troutman, W. G. (1980): Mouthwash:A source of acute ethanol intoxication. *Pediatrics*, 66:302–304.

24. Wilson, J. T., and Burr, I. M. (1975): Benzalkonium chloride poisoning in infant twins. *Am. J. Dis. Child.*, 129:1206–1207.

Plants

12

Ingestion of plants currently ranks as the most common cause of poisoning in children under 5 years of age in America, and is a significant cause of toxicity in adults (10). The incidence of plant-induced poisoning is also reported to be increasing. As more and more adults forage through the countryside in search of "nature's foods," too frequently poisonous plants are mistaken for edible ones. Also, as the nation's awareness for self-care and self-medication grows, many people are looking to herbs and natural products for prevention or self-treatment of various ailments. Studies have shown that many products of plant origin are available in numerous retail outlets, and these are potentially toxic if misused (2). Children see the bright berries of many plants and, perhaps believing they are fruits or confections, consume them. Sometimes they associate plant greens with salads, or with other nontoxic food items growing in the family garden plot.

In some cases, an actual plant part may not need to be ingested. For example, drinking the water from a vase containing plant stems may cause serious toxicity; or sticks holding meat for roasting may poison an individual who consumes this meat.

Although plant ingestions are commonplace, they are rarely the cause of serious toxicity or death. At most, the victim experiences localized disturbances such as pain or irritation in and around the mouth. But more serious toxicity and numerous fatalities do occur and, for this reason, any ingestion of a plant of unknown identity must be treated as a potential poison until it can be classified otherwise.

Of the approximately 30,000 species of plants growing in North America, both cultivated and wild, only a surprisingly few are responsible for most poisonings. In 1976, 12 species represented over 30% of all toxic ingestions (9). Fewer than 50 species, of the approximately 700 to 1,000 toxic plants growing in the United States, cause over 95% of all poisonings.

Therefore, in this chapter we will first discuss plant toxicity in general terms, then consider a few of those plants that are most commonly ingested.

Defining exactly what constitutes a poisonous plant is not easy, as almost any plant can cause nausea and vomiting or intestinal cramping if enough of it is ingested. When it concerns plant toxicity, separating scientific realities from folklore and myth is extremely difficult. However, a definition suitable for our purpose is that poisonous species are those that contain specific components capable of causing specific biochemical or physiological symptoms when small quantities are ingested. Thus, Jimson weed and foxglove are poisonous plants because very small quantities of their components will produce significant effects on the body, with death likely if enough is ingested. Thousands of such toxic constituents known to be poisonous exist in the plant kingdom. Many others are suspected, but have not yet been positively identified.

Not all parts of some poisonous plants are toxic, and the poisonous principles may only be present in the plant during certain seasons or at certain stages of growth. Slight variations in methods used to prepare plants for consumption may also make a tremendous difference in whether or not the final substance is safe or poisonous (see the Case Studies that follow). Thus, the specific plant portion that was ingested must be identified before antidotal treatment begins. To subject a youngster to the rigors of chemically-induced emesis when rhubarb stalk, but not the leaf, was ingested, imposes an unnecessary risk for possible aspiration and choking. On the other hand, this is considered to be the standard procedure for ingestion of rhubarb leaf, which contains dangerous quantities of oxalic acid that must be eliminated from the gastrointestinal tract before the poison can be absorbed.

MANAGEMENT OF THE PLANT-POISONED PATIENT

Several important rules dictate what should be done when a person is the victim of a plant ingestion. Figure 1 serves as a guide to the procedures to follow.

All ingestions must be considered to be potentially toxic until shown to be otherwise.

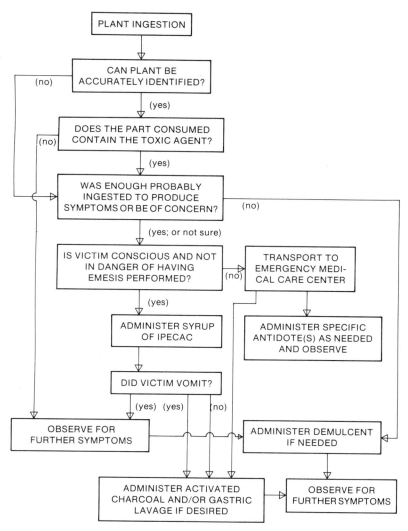

FIG. 1. Flow chart illustrating the steps involved in assessment and management of a victim of poisoning by a plant.

Identification of the plant is often the most difficult task. The parent of a child who has ingested a plant part may be completely unaware as to the plant's identity, or where the child found it, or may not be able to describe it accurately. People frequently use "nicknames," family, or trivial names for plants and do not know the correct botanical names. On a regional basis, different names may also be applied to the same plant. In certain areas, poison dogwood refers to a species of *Cornus*, whereas in other regions it refers to poison sumac. The

name "elephant's ears" may refer to *Caladium, Colocasia,* or *Dieffenbachia* species, to mandrake, or to several other plants.

So, the first task at hand is to try and identify the plant (Table 1). Fortunately, time is usually on the victim's side. Since the toxic principles of most plants must first be leached out of the plant leaf, stem, etc., there is usually sufficient time to make a proper identification.

The Poison Control Center should first be contacted. If the Poison Control Center cannot positively identify the plant, it may suggest other

TABLE 1. *Aids to help identify a potentially poisonous plant*

Specific site where plant was growing, including whether in sunny or shady area, moist or dry soil. Is this a house plant, cultivated variety, or wild growing weed?

Shape and texture of leaves including description of edges, and arrangement on stalk, and vein structure.

Color, size, texture and shape of seeds, fruits, berries or flowers, including their arrangement and grouping.

Plant's dimensions, both above and below the soil.

Nature of plant (e.g., free-standing plant, bush, or tree, vine, groundcover, etc.)

Common and botanical names.

---

centers elsewhere in the country that specialize in plant toxicology. These centers can be quickly contacted by phone and often a positive identification of the plant can be made. If identification is still not positive, as much of the plant as possible should be taken to a local florist. Wild plants are best taken to a botanist, high school or university biology/botany teacher, or local agricultural extension agency. Many libraries also have reference books which can be used to help identify the plant.

Following positive identification of the plant material as toxic, or if it cannot be identified and the victim is conscious and emesis is not specifically contraindicated, syrup of ipecac should be administered. All regurgitated material should be carefully examined for assessment as to the nature of parts of the plant that were ingested, as well as to estimate the approximate time of ingestion.

Frequently, all that is needed from this point is demulcent therapy. Many plants contain constituents that are extremely irritating to mucous membranes in the mouth and throat, but not damaging to other tissues. Ice cream, milk, or a frozen confection will soothe most irritations. Milk should not be given prior to ipecac for reasons explained in Chapter 3. The victim should be watched closely over the next 12 to 24 hr to assure that no additional symptoms appear as a result of delayed absorption.

Many plants have a powerful emetic action of their own and this may cause profuse spontaneous vomiting. If this occurs, the vomitus should be examined as above, and if it appears that the part ingested is not toxic, no further action is necessary. Demulcents may be given at this time, if needed.

Occasionally, an antidote chart or text will state that emesis should not be performed because the plant is highly corrosive or irritating to mucous membranes. This warning, however, is without merit because no plant is sufficiently corrosive as to cause further irritation to the esophagus if it is vomited.

If the plant was poisonous or, if after vomiting, the victim displays symptoms that cause suspicion for further toxicity, he should be taken to a physician without delay. The victim may require more specific antidotal measures.

Activated charcoal is generally not an acceptable alternative to syrup of ipecac to rid the gastrointestinal tract of a poisonous plant. Adsorption of the toxic principles onto charcoal is dependent on these components existing as a fine powder or solution. A leaf, berry, or other coarse plant part that contains these toxic principles will not release them until the part is digested sufficiently. It is far better to remove the entire plant part, if at all possible. Activated charcoal may be given following emesis to adsorb any residual poison not removed by emesis.

Gastric lavage is normally not a useful procedure to rid the stomach of an ingested plant. Most plant parts will not fit through the opening of even the largest orogastric tube. Still, following emesis, gastric lavage may be performed to wash out any remaining poison. Activated charcoal washes can be used at this time. When the patient is unconscious, gastric lavage, with or without activated charcoal, is indicated as long as ingestion occurred within the past 5 to 6 hr. It serves to withdraw toxic constituents as they are released from the plant, before they can be absorbed.

Saline cathartics may also be given to hasten removal of ingested plants.

COMMON POISONOUS PLANTS

As pointed out earlier, there are many poisonous plants. However, most poisonings occur from a relatively small number.

Arum Family Plants

Of all the houseplants, those of the arum family (Fig. 2,**a–d**) are the most frequently ingested by curious youngsters. These plants include caladium or "fancy leaf" *(Caladium)*, dumbcane *(Dieffenbachia sequine)*, elephant's ear *(Colocasia antiquorum)*, and philodendron *(Philodendron scandus)*.

These plants all possess large leaves that contain tiny needle-sharp crystals of calcium oxalate, arranged parallel in compact bundles called raphides, or in star-like clusters called druses (Fig. 3). When a victim bites into a leaf, he frequently cries out in pain as these crystals pierce the sensitive membranes of the mouth and lips. Because of this intense pain and stinging, a second bite is usually avoided and, thus, serious systemic poisoning is rare.

Symptoms include localized edema, with pain and irritation in and around the mouth. A localized dermatitis may appear if the plants are handled and the skin comes into contact with the sap from within the plant. Occasionally, the

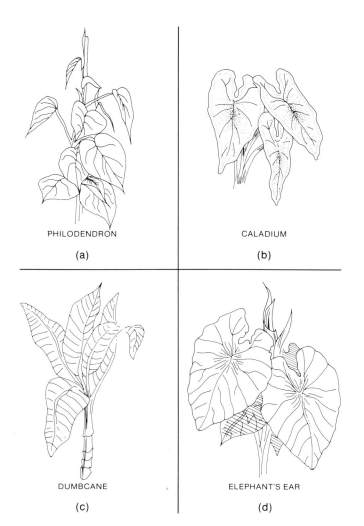

PHILODENDRON

(a)

CALADIUM

(b)

DUMBCANE

(c)

ELEPHANT'S EAR

(d)

FIG. 2. Common houseplants that cause poisoning.

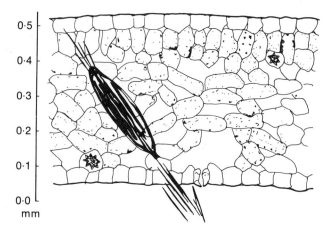

FIG. 3. Section of a Dieffenbachia leaf illustrating calcium oxalate raphides (long, clusteral structure), and druses (star-like structures).

tongue swells to the point that swallowing and speaking become difficult (hence, the origin of the term "dumbcane"). If swelling of the tongue, pharynx, or larynx becomes so severe as to hamper breathing or induce choking, the victim should be taken to a physician at once. One case report describes a victim whose tongue swelled so large that it protruded through his mouth for 3 days (16).

For treating most cases of poisoning by arum family plants, demulcent therapy is all that is required.

Christmas Plants

The other group of houseplants that children frequently ingest includes poinsettia, holly, mistletoe, and Jerusalem cherry (Fig. 4,**a–d**). Jerusalem cherry *(Solanum pseudocapsicum)*, also known as the natal cherry, contains the extremely toxic substance solanine in its red berries. Solanine, also found in the nightshades, may induce intense gastrointestinal symptoms, respiratory distress, weakness, mental confusion, bradycardia, tremors, abnormal pulse, unconsciousness, and shock. It is frequently lethal if not antidoted, with death due to hypothermia, coma, or respiratory paralysis. Solanine is also a toxic principle found in the vines and leaves of the tomato plant; and in the vine, tuber, and sprouts of the potato plant. Thus, ingestion of any of these plant parts may induce serious toxicity.

All ingestions of Jerusalem cherry or any other plant in the Solanaceae family must be

treated as an emergency. Spontaneous vomiting should occur. If it does not, however, the victim should receive syrup of ipecac, then be transported at once to a physician for care.

Most nurserymen and many health practitioners believe that poinsettia leaves are toxic. This consensus can be traced back to 1919 when a report described them as such. The report is often quoted, unfortunately, but its conclusion is not true. While the leaves, stems, and flowers do contain a milky sap that can cause mucous membrane irritation, this sap is not lethal. Discomfort to the mouth from a first bite usually prevents a second bite.

Victims should be given a demulcent, if necessary, to reduce mouth pain. If any of the sap touches the skin, it should be washed off with soap and water. Vomiting may be intense following ingestion, and this will usually rid the gastrointestinal tract of any swallowed plant.

White mistletoe berries *(Phorandendrop flavescens)* or the bright red berries of Christmas holly *(Ilex)* are potentially toxic. Rarely does toxicity occur, since both berries cause intense gastrointestinal irritation with nausea and vomiting.

Mistletoe's toxic principles, β-phenethylamine and tyramine, cause direct stimulation of smooth muscle, including that of the vasculature, urinary bladder, intestines, and uterus. Ilicin, the toxic principle of holly, is responsible for intense gastrointestinal symptoms which on occasion have included blood in the vomitus and

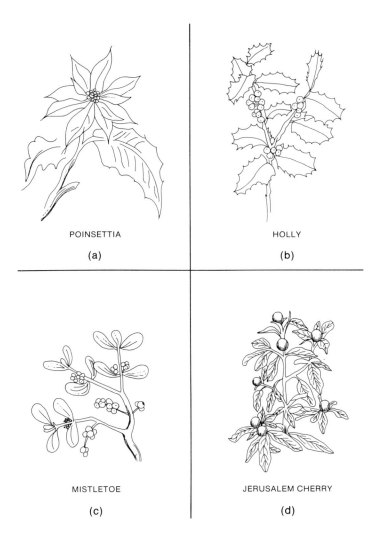

POINSETTIA

(a)

HOLLY

(b)

MISTLETOE

(c)

JERUSALEM CHERRY

(d)

FIG. 4. Common "Christmas" plants that cause poisoning.

bile, indicating that gastric hemorrhage has occurred.

Cardiotoxic Plants

Numerous plants cultivated in gardens and displayed as houseplants contain toxic principles that produce digitalis-like actions on the heart (Fig. 5,**a–d**). These plants include foxglove *(Digitalis purpurea)*, oleander *(Nerium oleander)*, lily-of-the-valley *(Convallaira majalis)*, and star-of-Bethlehem *(Ornithogalum umbellatum)*. The ornamental hedge, yew *(Taxus)*, also contains a potent cardiotoxic principle, taxine.

Ingestion of small quantities of these plants must be treated as an emergency. Syrup of ipecac should be given, with emesis followed by treatment of any specific symptoms. Constant monitoring of cardiovascular functions is necessary for at least 24 hr.

The greatest concern for cardiotoxic plant ingestions is with yew, since it is the most common of these plants. Yew is a favorite ornamental evergreen shrub that grows in most areas of the midwest and northeast. The tiny red berries that adorn the stems are especially attractive and enticing to children. All portions of these berries, except the fleshy part, contain taxine. A single chewed berry (containing the seed which contains concentrated toxin) is potentially lethal to a child.

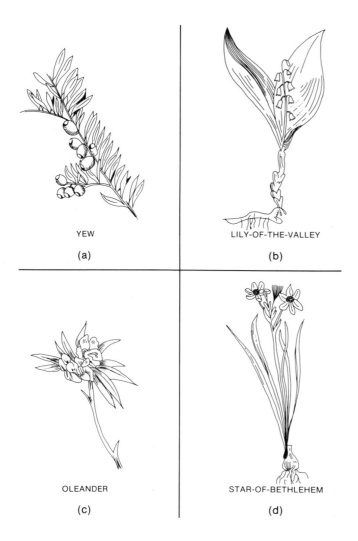

YEW

(a)

LILY-OF-THE-VALLEY

(b)

OLEANDER

(c)

STAR-OF-BETHLEHEM

(d)

FIG. 5. Common outdoor ornamental plants that cause poisoning.

Symptoms include intense irritation of the gastrointestinal tract, with muscular weakness, convulsions, and respiratory and cardiovascular depression leading to coma. Even the remotest suspicion that ingestion of one or more seeds occurred is reason for expedient antidotal measures. To withhold treatment for even an hour or more when an ingestion has actually occurred may significantly reduce the chances for the victim's recovery.

Castor Bean

Seeds of the castor plant *(Ricinus communis)* are among the most toxic of all the cultivated plants that grow in the United States. The castor plant (Fig. 6,**a**) is grown for its oil and as an ornamental shrub. Castor beans (seeds) are quite attractive to children and ingestion of a single chewed seed may prove to be fatal. Unchewed seeds usually pass through the gastrointestinal tract without causing clinical problems.

Castor beans contain the deadly phytotoxin substance, ricin. Ordinarily inactivated by heat during production of castor oil, ricin in its pure form may cause gastrointestinal hemorrhage. Hemolysis, liver and kidney damage, convulsions, and shock also occur. *In vitro*, solutions as dilute as 1:1,000,000 can produce erythrocytic damage.

Symptoms of poisoning include intense gastrointestinal irritation, with burning in the mouth and throat. Muscle weakness, general malaise, reduced reflexes, convulsion, and dyspnea are also reported. The blood pressure remains normal until 2 to 3 hr before death, at which time it falls (4). The cause of death is usually depression of cardiovascular and respiratory functions. Onset of all symptoms, other than localized irritation, may be delayed for 12 to 18 hr or more. Consequently, close observation of the victim throughout this period is absolutely required.

Ingestion of castor beans, even if not chewed, or of any part of the castor plant, must be treated as a potential emergency. Again, spontaneous vomiting may remove most of the plant parts from the gastrointestinal tract. Activated charcoal and cathartics should follow emesis, and the child must be observed in a hospital for at least 24 hr. Symptoms appearing over this period should be treated appropriately (e.g., convulsions with diazepam). Urinary alkalinization with sodium bicarbonate may aid in elimination of absorbed ricin. Blood transfusions or treatment of anemia may be required if these problems occur.

Rhubarb

The leaf, but not the stem, of the rhubarb plant *(Rheum rhaponticum)* (Fig. 6,**b**) contains oxalic acid. The leaf is occasionally used to embellish salads, or is cooked as a side dish. Heating does not destroy the toxic principle. Once absorbed, it combines with calcium from the blood to form the insoluble substance, calcium oxalate, which may crystalize in the renal tubules. If severe, this precipitate may block the tubules to cause acute renal failure. A single bite of rhubarb leaf is usually not sufficient to cause systemic toxicity, but multiple bites may be.

Symptoms of oxalic acid poisoning include nausea and vomiting, weakness, and muscle cramps.

Ingestions should be treated by emesis, followed with milk (a source of calcium) or calcium hydroxide solution (lime water) to combine with oxalic acid in the gastrointestinal tract and form insoluble calcium oxalate. This is not absorbed and passes out of the body. Calcium salts may be administered intravenously to replace calcium which might be lost from the blood. Intravenous fluids are given to help prevent accumulation of the precipitate in the renal tubules.

Nightshade

Three nightshade species, bittersweet or woody nightshade *(Solanum dulcamera)*, black or common nightshade *(Solanum nigrum)*, and the deadly nightshade *(Atropa belladonna)* all contain deadly toxic alkaloids, although in different proportions (Fig. 6,**c**). The woody nightshade is reported to be one of the most commonly ingested plants in the United States. It is not considered lethal in quantities usually ingested, and usually produces little more than gastrointestinal irritation. Ingestion of several berries may be serious. Berries of the black nightshade are, likewise, as noxious as those of the woody nightshade.

The deadly nightshade is the plant to avoid. Atropine, at a concentration of 0.25 to 0.5%, is found in this species, and it can be lethal if ingested in sufficient quantity.

Symptoms of poisoning and their management are the same as for Jimson weed. Fortunately, intoxication with deadly nightshade is rare in the United States because the plant does not grow well here.

Jimson Weed

Jimson weed *(Datura stramonium)*, also known as thorn apple, locoweed, and angel's trumpet, is commonly encountered throughout most of the United States (Fig. 6,**d**). It is often seen growing wild among rows of crops. Unilateral mydriasis has been reported in farmers working with harvesting equipment (14), indicating poisoning. Children have been fatally poisoned by eating the flowers, and teenagers have suffered the consequences from ingesting a "tea" made by infusing the seeds in water.

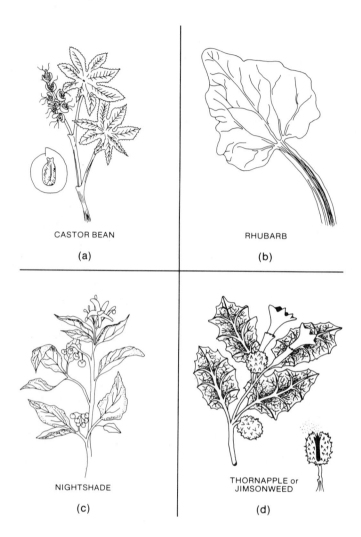

CASTOR BEAN

(a)

RHUBARB

(b)

NIGHTSHADE

(c)

THORNAPPLE or
JIMSONWEED

(d)

FIG. 6. Common outdoor plants that cause poisoning.

The fruit pods that appear in the fall each contain 50 to 100 brown-black seeds. It is these seeds that are most toxic, with each 10 seeds containing approximately 1 mg atropine. Other alkaloids include hyoscyamine, scopolamine, and hyoscine, present throughout the plant in varying proportions. As little as 4 to 5 g of the leaves or seeds are fatal (19).

Intentional ingestions of Jimson weed concoctions have increased in frequency over recent years (12,17). This incidence will undoubtedly increase even more in future years, as licit drugs that are commonly abused, and illicit drug items become more difficult to obtain.

Symptoms of Jimson weed poisoning include all of the typical manifestations of anticholinergic drug poisoning (Chapter 19). These include blurred vision, CNS stimulation, euphoria, delirium, terrifying hallucinations, tachycardia, hyperthermia, and coma. A study involving 29 patients who had ingested Jimson weed revealed the composite symptoms noted in Table 2. Especially vivid were the hallucinations seen in all patients. Most were visual; e.g., insects appearing on a wall, persons being chased by sharks, etc. Disorientation to time, place, or person was also prevalent.

Jimson weed intoxication must be antidoted quickly. Following removal of as much of the

TABLE 2. *Symptoms and signs of Jimson weed ingestion[a]*

Signs and symptoms	No. of patients	% of patients	Not recorded
Hallucinations	26	100	3
Disorientation	27	100	2
Mydriasis	29	100	—
Dry mucous membranes	16/17	94	12
Flushed face	11/13	85	16
Combative state	20	74	2
Tachycardia	21	72	—
Blood pressure			
Systolic	8	28	—.
Diastolic	7	24	—
Temperature > 38.2°C	3	10	—

[a]Total number of patients = 29.
From ref. 17.

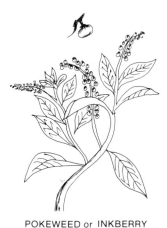

POKEWEED or INKBERRY

FIG. 7. Pokeweed.

poison from the stomach as is possible, physostigmine salicylate is given intravenously. Physostigmine is a reversible cholinesterase inhibitor that promotes accumulation of endogenous acetylcholine. This neurotransmitter competes with the poison for the body's muscarinic receptor sites, and reverses the toxic symptoms. While other cholinesterase inhibitors (e.g., neostigmine) may benefit the victim by raising acetylcholine levels at peripheral sites, they are quaternary amines and, consequently, do not enter the CNS in sufficient concentration. Thus, they are without antidotal effect on the central component of poisoning. Physostigmine, a tertiary amine, does penetrate into the CNS. (This will be explained in more detail in Chapter 18.)

Hospitalization of the poisoned patient is indicated, since a deranged mental state and sensorium may persist for several days. Even days after an apparent recovery, victims of poisoning have been known to wander aimlessly into a remote area and die of exposure, or into a lake or pond and drown.

Pokeweed

Boiled shoots of the pokeweed *(Phytolacca americana)* (Fig. 7) are considered delicacies and, in fact, are processed and canned for the table. However, pokeweed can be extremely dangerous if it is improperly prepared. Its clumps of shiny purple berries ("inkberries") are attractive to children who may associate them with grapes or other fruits. The berries, while poisonous in large numbers, do not usually cause severe toxicity in the amounts normally ingested unless they are macerated into "grape juice" and this liquid is consumed. Pokeweed roots are occasionally mistaken for horseradish or parsnips. They contain high concentrations of the extremely toxic substances, saponin and glycoprotein.

Pokeweed induces a variety of symptoms that include burning in the mouth, nausea and vomiting, visual disturbances, weak pulse, and respiratory difficulties.

Poisoning is best antidoted by removing all traces of the plant from the stomach, then administering follow-up doses of activated charcoal and a saline cathartic. Specific symptoms are treated as necessary.

Mushrooms

Five hundred or more people each year in America are poisoned by mushrooms, with over a hundred fatalities reported (8). Poisoning by mushrooms is unpredictable, since the dozens of different mushroom species may produce variable symptoms and require various treatment. Some are poisonous only if eaten raw;

some others only if ingested during certain stages of growth. Even differences in soil composition may significantly influence the potential to cause toxicity. The problem is compounded still further because poisonous mushrooms may grow immediately next to the nonpoisonous varieties. The rule of thumb is that no wild mushroom should ever be consumed unless an accurate identification is possible.

Almost all cases of mushroom poisoning in this country are caused by members of the *Amanita* genus, especially *A. muscaria* and *A. phalloides* (toadstools) (see Fig. 8,**a,b**). As little as one-third of a cap of *A. phalloides* has been fatal to a child. Most fatal poisonings are from *A. phalloides*, and it is responsible for over 95% of all deaths (3).

Amanita mushrooms contain a mixture of toxic principles including phalloidin, phalloin, and α-, β-, and γ-amanitin. Muscarine is the toxic principle of *A. muscaria* and certain other species. While muscarine provokes symptoms of toxicity within a few minutes to hours, onset of symptoms from phalloidin, phalloin, or amanitin is usually delayed for up to 24 hr.

Symptoms of Mushroom Poisoning

Symptoms of poisoning vary widely among various species of mushrooms (Table 3). Severe poisoning from muscarine results in symptoms characteristic of acetylcholine-like (muscarinic) stimulation and culminates in death from cardiac or respiratory failure if a large quantity was ingested and not antidoted. Poisoning by the other phytotoxins previously mentioned is characterized by actual damage caused to cells throughout the body, with the heart, liver, kidney, and brain at the greatest risk of danger. Thus, poisoning by the latter is of the greatest concern. Because the patient often remains asymptomatic for up to 24 hr following ingestion, the parent or physician may not suspect that damage is occurring. Eventually, though, muscarinic-like symptoms appear. These are followed later by liver damage, oliguria, and anuria. Circulatory failure manifests even later, with the victim usually lapsing into a coma within a week.

Treatment of Mushroom Poisoning

All cases of suspected poisonous mushroom ingestion should be treated and the victims must be closely observed. Active emesis, followed by gastric lavage with tannic acid or potassium permanganate, then followed by activated charcoal and saline catharsis, is the first order of business. This should then be followed with atropine sulfate, a specific muscarinic antagonist, with doses repeated as often as necessary.

In severe poisonings, hemodialysis or peritoneal dialysis can be undertaken. Both proce-

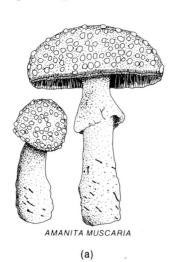

AMANITA MUSCARIA

(a)

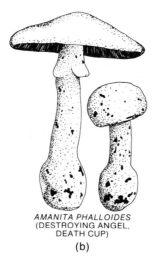

AMANITA PHALLOIDES
(DESTROYING ANGEL,
DEATH CUP)

(b)

FIG. 8.   Toxic mushroom species.

TABLE 3. *Signs and symptoms of mushroom poisoning[a]*

Muscarine type
    May onset within minutes; no chronic
      poisoning; fatalities rare
    "SLUD" syndrome (salivation, lacrimation,
      urination, diarrhea)
    Bradycardia
    Hypotension
    Miosis
    Bronchospasm
    Cardiac arrhythmias
Amanitin type
    Latent period of 12–24 hr or more before onset;
      fatality rate approximately 50%
    Muscarinic symptoms
    Headache
    Painful tenderness and enlargement of the liver
    Jaundice
    Oliguria and anuria
    Mental confusion and depression
    Hypoglycemia
    Convulsions, coma

---

[a]Signs and symptoms are extremely variable. In addition to those shown above, other species of mushrooms may induce symptoms that are disulfiram-like, while others are highly hallucinogenic.
From ref. 8.

dures have been successfully used to reduce the chance for renal damage. Vitamin K administration may help control hemorrhage. Diazepam will reduce convulsions. The death rate from poisoning by *A. phalloides* is reported at 50% of untreated victims. With good antidotal therapy, however, this rate may be reduced to less than 5% (9).

Thioctic acid (α-lipoic acid) is an investigational agent being studied for treatment of poisoning by *Amanita*, or the rare *Galerina* species. The substance exerts a direct protective effect against hepatocellular damage by a yet unknown mechanism. It must be given early after ingestion of the toxic mushroom, although in some studies, where it was given after definite hepatic damage was apparent, it has shown positive results.

Cyanogenic Plants

Several plants contain cyanogenic glycosides such as amygdalin, prulaurasin, and prunasin in their leaves, stems, bark, and seed pits, but not in their pulpy, edible fruits. Common examples of such plants are listed in Table 4. When ingested, the glycosides hydrolyze in an alkaline medium to produce hydrocyanic acid. Cyanide may induce all of the effects illustrated in Chapter 6.

Herbal Intoxication

Herbal remedies were once the mainstay of treating most illnesses of colonial Americans. But with the development or importation, and eventual refining of commercial remedies, the use of herbs in health care began to decline. This apparent decrease in the use of home remedies persisted until fairly recently when the emphasis once again began to change. Americans now seem to have a resurgence of interest in herbal remedies. Hardly a week goes by without one or more reports appearing in the literature that stress the potential these substances have for causing toxic reactions. While many herbal remedies are safe, and may even be pharmacologically worthwhile, many others can be lethal if misused.

The Food and Drug Administration has evaluated the safety of many herbs offered for sale in brewing teas (1). While many were shown to be safe, others are known to be toxic, and a large number are classed as "undefined" in their safety (Table 5). It should be pointed out that the herbs shown in this table represent only a sampling.

The range of potential toxic action is widespread. One specific toxic concern involves the psychoactive effects that are well known to occur with a large number of herbs. Many of these herbs are rolled into cigarettes, boiled into tea, or taken in capsulated form. Table 6 lists a

TABLE 4. *Common cyanogenic plants*

Apple (*Pyrus sylvestris*)
Apricot (*Prunus armeniaca*)
Cherry (*Prunus cerasus*)
Peach (*Prunus persica*)
Wild black cherry (*Prunus serotina*)
Cherry laurel (*Prunus caroliniana*)
Choke cherry (*Prunus virginiana*)

TABLE 5. *Herb ratings by the Food and Drug Administration*

Unsafe herbs		
Common names	Botanical name	Remarks
Arnica, arnica flowers, wolf's-bane, leopard's bane, mountain tobacco, *Flores arnicae*	*Arnica montana*	Aqueous and alcoholic extracts of the plant contain, besides choline, two unidentified substances which affect the heart and vascular systems. Arnica is an active irritant which can produce violent toxic gastroenteritis, nervous disturbances, change in pulse rate, intense muscular weakness, collapse, and death.
Belladonna, deadly nightshade	*Atropa belladonna*	Poisonous plant which contains the toxic solanaceous alkaloids, hyoscyamine, atropine, and hyoscine.
Bittersweet twigs, *dulcamara*, bittersweet, woody nightshade, climbing nightshade	*Solanum dulcamara*	Poisonous. Contains the toxic glycoalkaloid, solanine, also solanidine and dulcamarin.
Calamus, sweet flag, sweet root, sweet cinnamon, sweet cane	*Acorus calamus*	Oil of calamus. Jammu variety is a carcinogen.
Hemlock, *Conium*, poison hemlock, spotted hemlock, spotted parsley, St. Bennet's herb, spotted cowbane, fool's parsley	*Conium maculatum*	Contains poisonous alkaloid, coniine, and four other closely related alkaloids. Often confused with water hemlock (*Cicuta maculata*). Not to be confused with hemlock, hemlock spruce, etc. (*Tsuga canadensis*).
Henbane, *Hyoscyamus*, black henbane, hog's bean, poison tobacco, devil's eye	*Hyoscyamus niger*	Contains alkaloids, hyoscyamine, hyoscine (scopolamine), and atropine. A poisonous plant.
Wormwood, absinthium, absinth, absinthe, madderwort, wermuth, mugwort, mingwort warmot, magenkraut, *Herba absinthii*	*Artemisia absinthium*	Contains a volatile oil which is an active narcotic poison. Oil of wormwood is in absinthe, a liqueur which can produce absinthism.
Herbs of undefined safety		
Boneset, *Eupatorium*, thoroughwort, vegetable antimony, feverwort, sweating plant, Indian sage	*Eupatorium perfoliatum*	Has diaphoretic effect. Emetic and aperient in large doses. Household remedy never prescribed by the medical profession.
Horsetail, *Equisetum*, scouring rush	*Equisetum hyemale*	Infusion of whole plant used sometimes in renal diseases but the diuretic action is very feeble.
Mormon tea, Brigham tea, teamaster's tea, Mexican tea, mountain tea, whorehouse tea, desert tea, Mormon plant, Brigham weed, joint fir, mountain rush, shrubby horsetail, herb of the sun, *Popotillo*	*Ephedra antisyphilitica* and other species of *Ephedra* of the western U.S. (e.g., *Ephedra nevadensis*)	Used as an antisyphilitic, also as an astringent. A chinese species. *Ephedra sinica*, called mahuang in China, contains the alkaloid ephedrine, a powerful decongestant.
Poke root berries, poke root, *Phytolacca*, poke, pocan, scoke, American nightshade root	*Phytolacca americana; Phytolacca decandra*	Contains an acidic steroid saponin. Emetic action is slow but of long duration. Narcotic effects have been observed. Has been employed internally in chronic rheumatism but is not therapeutically useful and is no longer prescribed. Overdoses have sometimes been fatal.
Senna, senna leaves, Alexandria senna, Tinnevelly senna, India senna	*Cassia acutifolia; Cassia augustfolia*	Cathartic. The usual dose of senna leaf is 2 g. Used as a drug.

From ref. 1.

TABLE 6. *Psychoactive substances used in herbal preparations*

Labeled ingredient	Botanical source	Pharmacologic principle	Reported effects
African yohimbe bark; yohimbe	*Corynanthe yohimbe*	Yohimbe	Mild hallucinogen
Broom; Scotch broom	*Cytisus* spp	Cytisine	Strong sedative-hypnotic
California poppy	*Eschscholtzia californica*	Alkaloids and glucosides	Mild euphoriant
Catnip	*Nepeta cataria*	Nepetalactone	Mild hallucinogen
Cinnamon	*Cinnamomum camphora*	?	Mild stimulant
Damiana	*Turnera diffusa*	?	Mild stimulant
Hops	*Humulus lupulus*	Lupuline	None
Hydrangea	*Hydrangea paniculata*	Hydrangin, saponin, cyanogenes	Stimulant
Juniper	*Juniper macropoda*	?	Strong hallucinogen
Kavakava	*Piper methysticum*	Yangonin, pyrones	Mild hallucinogen
Kola nut; gotu kola	*Cola* spp	Caffeine, theobromine, kolanin	Stimulant
Lobella	*Lobella inflata*	Lobeline	Mild euphoriant
Mandrake	*Mandragora officinarum*	Scopolamine, hyoscyamine	Hallucinogen
Mate	*Ilex paraguayensis*	Caffeine	Stimulant
Mormon tea	*Ephedra nevadensis*	Ephedrine	Stimulant
Nutmeg	*Myristica fragrans*	Myristicin	Hallucinogen
Passion flower	*Passiflora incarnata*	Harmine alkaloids	Mild stimulant
Periwinkle	*Catharanthus roseus*	Indole alkaloids	Hallucinogen
Prickly poppy	*Argemone mexicana*	Protopine, bergerine, isoquinilines	Narcotic-analgesic
Snakeroot	*Rauwolfia serpentina*	Reserpine	Tranquilizer
Thorn apple	*Datura stramonium*	Atropine, scopolamine	Strong hallucinogen
Tobacco	*Nicotiana* spp	Nicotine	Strong stimulant
Valerian	*Valeriana officinalis*	Chatinine, velerine alkaloids	Tranquilizer
Wild lettuce	*Lactuca sativa*	Lactucarine	Mild narcotic-analgesic
Wormwood	*Artemisia absinthium*	Absinthine	Narcotic-analgesic

From ref. 18.

variety of such psychoactive substances, along with their reported effects. Any one of them may be the cause of serious toxic harm. Unfortunately, many of the users may be unprepared for these effects. They may not even suspect that they can occur, since herbs are often viewed as food items rather than as drugs.

SUMMARY

To date, few medical problems have been reported from ingesting herbal remedies. However, the "medicinal" teas and other crude dosage forms of commerce are, for the most part, neither uniformly prepared nor assayed for purity. Rather, they consist of crudely prepared mixtures containing plant fibers, crystalline oxalates, and often pollen, mold spores, insect parts, and other allergy-causing substances. Thus,

the potential for a toxic or allergic response to these preparations is always present.

Poisonings do occur due to plant ingestions. But as we learned early in the chapter, most ingestions cause little more harm than simply burning the mouth or stimulating nausea or vomiting. However, there are some very toxic plants and ingestion of these must be handled as any other toxic emergency.

Case Studies

CASE STUDY: *DIEFFENBACHIA* INGESTION

History

When brought to the emergency room, the 40-year-old female was experiencing dysphagia, excessive salivation, and pain of the mouth and tongue. Six hours previous to her admission to the emergency room, she had bitten into the stalk of a *Dieffenbachia* houseplant. She probably did not ingest any of the plant material because she reported that it caused her a great deal of oral pain and she quickly spat out the pulp and juices.

Physical examination revealed severe edema of the left side of the face, tongue, buccal mucosa, and palate. Salivation was profuse and she had an extremely difficult time speaking.

All laboratory findings were within the normal limits. She was admitted for observation.

Treatment. Treatment consisted of meperidine hydrochloride for pain, and then oral administration of 30 ml of aluminum-magnesium hydroxide every 2 hr. During the observation period, there was no evidence of respiratory distress, muscular hyperactivity, or gastrointestinal disturbance. The following day she could swallow soft foods and liquids, but the extent of inflammation was unchanged from her time of admission.

She was discharged 19 hr after admission even though inflammation and edema of the mouth remained unchanged. Pain continued in her face, and necrosis of the surface of the tongue and buccal mucosa was evident.

Eleven days afterwards, the lesions were still observable, but the facial edema was reduced. Dietary intake by this period was almost back to normal. (See ref. 7.)

Discussion

1. Although this patient had no systemic complications, what signs and symptoms are associated with ingestion of *Dieffenbachia*?

2. Why was aluminum-magnesium hydroxide given to this patient?

3. What drug is usually given to initially reduce the swelling?

CASE STUDY: JIMSON WEED POISONING

History

A 15-year-old male was found nude with a flushed face, incoherent behavior, and symptoms of hallucinations. On admission to the emergency room, he was comatose, responding only to deep painful stimuli. His pupils were dilated and equal, but only responded minimally to light. His skin was hot and

dry. Doll's eye movements were intact. Hyperactive deep tendon reflexes were noted, and positive Babinski responses were obtained. He occasionally displayed episodes of myoclonic jerks.

His vital signs changed within the first hour after admission and are noted below:

	Blood pressure (mm Hg)	Respirations/min	Pulse/min	Temperature (°C)
On admission	170/100	44	144	38.7
1 Hr after admission	140/50	60	160	39.8
15 Min after physostigmine (2.0 mg)	160/68	40	120	38.8

Within 1 hr after admission, the patient's vital signs began to diminish. Poisoning by an anticholinergic type substance was suspected so 2.0 mg physostigmine salicylate were administered i.v. Within 15 min he began to respond to this treatment. He became more alert and responsive to verbal commands. He then admitted to ingesting "loco seeds."

He was completely stabilized in 6 hr, although he still continued to experience hallucinations. His neurological status improved, and he was released by the eighth hospital day, without apparent neurological damage. (See ref. 13.)

Discussion

1. What is the alkaloid present in Jimson weed?

2. What is the botanical name for "locoweed"?

3. If physostigmine was not available, could neostigmine be given instead?

4. What do you suppose "Doll's eye movement" represents?

CASE STUDY: FATAL OLEANDER INGESTION

History

A 96-year-old female, with suicidal intentions, ingested an undetermined quantity of oleander leaf. She had previously taken no medication except for occasional aspirin. She was found at home by her family, weak and vomiting. She could barely talk, and within a few minutes after discovery her speech ceased.

On arrival at the emergency room 15 min later, she experienced a transient generalized tonic seizure which was followed by cardiopulmonary failure. Cardiopulmonary resuscitation was begun immediately.

She was given 5% dextrose in sodium bicarbonate, epinephrine, lidocaine, atropine, phenytoin, calcium chloride, and isoproterenol. Despite the vigorous treatment, she died 40 min after arrival at the emergency room.

The victim's laboratory findings were:

Na^+	= 161 mEq/L
K^+	= 8.6 mEq/L
Cl^-	= 111 mEq/L
CO_2	= 26 mEq/L
Digoxin level	= 5.8 ng/ml

On autopsy, all coronary vessels were patent and showed no signs of thrombotic occlusion. A quantity of green vegetative material was found in the stomach.

At first, the digoxin value noted above was thought to be in error since the patient was not previously taking a digitalis product. Additional laboratory studies confirmed it, however. Further studies later showed that the lethal dose of oleander glycosides swallowed by this patient was approximately 200 times higher than the lethal dose in several animal studies. (See ref. 15.)

Discussion

1. What is the toxic principle of oleander?

2. How does this toxic principle manifest its toxicity? Were the symptoms this patient displayed compatible with information described within the text?

3. Why was there a digoxin level of 5.8 ng/ml when the patient was not on any heart medication?

CASE STUDIES: POKEWEED POISONING

History: Case 1

A 43-year-old female purchased some powdered poke root from a local health food store. About a half-hour after consuming a cup of tea made from the powdered plant material (following mixing directions on the label), she became nauseated and vomited. She also experienced cramping, abdominal pains, and watery diarrhea. Later, she became very weak, and blood was found in the emesis and stool. She was brought to an emergency room by her husband.

She presented with hypotension and tachycardia. Gastric lavage was performed, followed by nasogastric suction.

Treatment. Treatment consisted of volume expansion and electrolyte balancing. Nasogastric suction of a bloody material continued, and the diarrhea

continued to reveal blood. She was stabilized in 24 hr and was discharged the following day. (See ref. 6.)

History: Case 2

On one summer afternoon, 52 campers and counselors of a "nature group" were offered a salad made with leaves from the pokeweed plant. The young leaves had been picked, boiled, drained, and boiled again, earlier that day.

Within a period of one-half to 5½ hr after consuming the salad, 21 people developed the following symptoms:

No. patients with symptoms	Symptom
18	Nausea, stomach cramps
17	Vomiting
11	Headache
10	Dizziness
8	Burning in stomach or mouth
6	Diarrhea

Symptoms lasted 1 to 48 hr, with a mean duration of 24 hr. Eighteen persons were seen by local physicians or in a hospital emergency room. Four of these were admitted to the hospital for 24 to 48 hr because of protracted vomiting and dehydration. All survived. (See ref. 11.)

Discussion

1. What are the active components of pokeweed?

2. What are the major toxic actions of these compounds? Do these case studies correlate with the expected signs and symptoms of toxicity?

3. Both of these reports of pokeweed toxicity would have never happened if certain obvious precautions would have been observed. What are these?

CASE STUDY: BURDOCK ROOT TEA POISONING

History

A 26-year-old female purchased a package of burdock root tea from a local health foods store. The tea was prepared by steeping the root product in water.

One morning, she drank one-half cup of tea which had been steeping for 1½ days. Within 5 min she began to experience blurred vision and a dry mouth. Her husband noted that her speech and actions were bizarre, and she appeared to be hallucinating.

She was brought to the emergency room with symptoms of dry mouth, blurred vision, urinary retention, and bizarre behavior. Physical findings revealed a blood pressure of 140/108 mm Hg, and pulse rate of 104 beats/min. Her pupils were equally dilated and minimally reactive to light. Chest and heart ausculatory examinations were unremarkable. There was a slight tenderness in the hypogastrum. Sensory and motor neuronal examination, as well as deep tendon reflexes, were normal.

Treatment with physostigmine salicylate was initiated since symptoms suggested poisoning by an anticholinergic substance. In addition, she was catheterized and 500 ml of urine were obtained and sent to the toxicology laboratory for screening. (See ref. 5.)

Discussion

1. The toxic principle in the burdock root tea which was responsible for the symptoms of this patient was atropine. Although we have not considered atropine toxicity, do the symptoms this victim displayed represent what you would expect, based on your knowledge of the drug's pharmacology?

2. What is the procedure used to establish or confirm an anticholinergic poisoning?

3. Name three other toxic plants that are commonly ingested that contain atropine-like alkaloids.

Review Questions

1. Gastric lavage may have limited value in poisoning by plants. State the reasons why.

2. A parent who states that his son was poisoned by dumbcane is referring to which of the following plants?
   A. Nightshade
   B. Poinsettia
   C. Dieffenbachia
   D. Jimson weed

3. What is the name that describes bundles of calcium oxalate crystals in a parallel arrangement?

4. Which of the following plants contain solanine: Jerusalem cherry (I), mistletoe (II), or poinsettia (III)?
   A. I only
   B. III only

C. I and II only
D. II and III only

5. Elimination of absorbed ricin may be hastened by administering:
   A. ammonium chloride
   B. sodium bicarbonate

6. Describe the toxic effects of ricin on the blood.

7. Which of the following plants contain β-phenethylamine and tyramine in its seeds?
   A. Oleander
   B. Castor bean
   C. Mistletoe
   D. Yew

8. The sap from poinsettia leaves, while not lethal, does cause a toxic effect. What is this response?

9. The vines and leaves of the tomato plant and vine, and the tuber and sprouts of the potato plant contain a poisonous principle. Name it.

10. Milk provides an antidotal effect on swallowed plant parts containing oxalic acid, for some reason other than its demulcent effect. What is it?

11. Poisoning by the nightshade plants is caused by which toxic component?

12. Symptoms of Jimson weed poisoning are:
    A. muscarinic
    B. antimuscarinic

13. Thioctic acid is under investigation as an antidote to treat poisoning by a certain plant.
    A. What is the plant?
    B. What specific toxic event does it protect against?

14. Distinguish between symptoms of poisoning by muscarine-type and amanitin-type mushrooms. For which type is poisoning usually more severe?

15. Which of the following is a true statement?
    A. Rhubarb stems and leaves both contain the toxic principle.
    B. Jimson weed seeds are also called "inkberries."
    C. Poisoning by oleander induces symptoms that are most closely descriptive of atropine.
    D. The poisonous principle of yew is taxine.

16. It has been stated that the incidence of poisoning

by plants is increasing. What are the reasons for this increased rate?

17. Intoxication by ingesting the toxic principle of rhubarb is most closely associated with dysfunction of the:
    A. brain
    B. liver
    C. heart
    D. kidney

18. All portions of the taxus berries are toxic except the fleshy part.
    A. True
    B. False

19. Intoxication with oleander causes symptoms most closely associated with dysfunction of the:
    A. brain
    B. liver
    C. heart
    D. kidney

20. All of the following belong to the arum family *except*:
    A. dieffenbachia
    B. poinsettia
    C. caladium
    D. philodendron

21. Plants that are considered to have a caustic component should not be vomited, if ingested.
    A. True
    B. False

22. Activated charcoal may be an effective adsorbent of the toxic principles of many plants. However, it is not considered to be a first-line "antidote" when one of these poisonous plants is ingested. Why?

23. Even in the absence of symptoms of toxicity following a plant ingestion, the victim should be carefully observed over the next 12 to 24 hr. Cite the reasons for this.

References

1. Anon (1978): *Health Food Business*, pp. 52–58.
2. Anon (1979): Toxic reactions to plant products sold in health food stores. *Med. Letter*, 21:29–31.
3. Anon (1980): Mushroom poisoning. *Lancet*, 2:351–352.
4. Balint, G. A. (1974): Ricin: The toxic protein of castor oil seeds. *Toxicology*, 2:77–102.
5. Bryson, P. D., Watanabe, A. S., Rumack, B. H., and Murphy, R. C. (1978): Burdock root tea poisoning. *JAMA*, 239:2157.
6. Centers for Disease Control (1981): Plant poisoning—New Jersey. *Morbidity and Mortality Weekly Report*, 30:65–66.
7. Drach, G., and Maloney, W. H. (1963): Toxicity of the common houseplant dieffenbachia. *JAMA*, 184:1047.
8. Dreisbach, R. H. (1980): *Handbook of Poisoning*. Lange, Los Altos.
9. Ellis, M., Robertson, W. O., and Rumack, B. (1979): Plant ingestion poisoning from A to Z. *Patient Care*, Vol 13, 12:86–140.
10. Kingsbury, J. M. (1980): Phytotoxicology. In: *Toxicology—The Basic Science of Poisons*, 2nd ed., edited by J. Doull, C. D. Klaassen, and M. O. Amdur, pp. 578–590. Macmillan, New York.
11. Lewis, W. H., and Smith, P. R. (1979): Poke root herbal tea poisoning. *JAMA*, 242:2759–2760.
12. Mahler, D. A. (1975): The jimson-weed high. *JAMA*, 231:138.
13. Mikolich, J. R., Paulson, G. W., and Cross, J. C. (1975): Acute anticholinergic syndrome due to jimson seed ingestion. *Ann. Int. Med.*, 83:321–325.
14. Mitchell, J. E., and Mitchell, F. N. (1955): Jimson weed poisoning in childhood. *J. Pediatr.*, 47:227–231.
15. Osterloh, J., Herold, S., and Pond, S. (1982): Oleander interference in the digoxin radioimmunoassay in a fatal ingestion. *JAMA*, 247:1596–1597.
16. Pohl, R. W. (1961): Poisoning by dieffenbachia. *JAMA*, 177:162–163.
17. Shervette, R. E., Schydlower, M., Lampe, R. M., and Fearnow, R. G. (1979): Jimson "Loco" weed abuse in adolescents. *Pediatrics*, 63:520–523.
18. Siegel, R. R. (1976): Herbal intoxication. *JAMA*, 236:473–476.
19. Weintraub, S. (1960): Stramonium poisoning. *Postgrad. Med.* Vol 28, 4:364–367.

Drug-Induced Poisoning: Relevance!

13

In previous chapters we have discussed poisoning caused by a wide variety of chemical products, plants, and other substances found in or around the home or workplace. Although these items are widely diverse in composition, source, and toxic actions, they do have one common trait. With only a few exceptions, they are not intended to be taken or used medicinally.

Starting with Chapter 14, however, the topics for consideration pertain to drugs or drug-related items. These are the substances people purposefully take or use to relieve their illnesses. In some instances (e.g., as with the illicit psychotomimetics), they are also the items intentionally taken to produce symptoms of pleasure and to cause dissociation from reality.

Toxicity related to therapeutic agents is a growing concern. Today, the incidence of adverse reactions related to drugs is variously reported at 6 to 30% of all hospitalized patients (5,11,12). From 2 to 9% of all admissions to medical clinics are due to adverse drug reactions (2,4,7). Not all of these reactions are life-threatening, and perhaps many could be managed outside a hospital. But the point is made that drug-related toxicity is more than a passing fancy, and its incidence is on the increase.

The reasons why people are poisoned by drugs are numerous and diverse in character (Table 1). Children accidentally ingest toxic doses from containers left carelessly unguarded. Or, they are innocently given doses of certain drugs that are inappropriate for them. For example, chil-

TABLE 1. *Common reasons why people are poisoned by drugs*

Accidental overdose by adult or child
Intentional overdose (for suicidal purpose)
Polypharmacy (drug interactions, potentiation, etc.)
Inappropriate or unsupervised drug use
    Thyroid hormone and ipecac syrup for weight reduction
    Adult drugs given to child
    Salicylates for children with high fever
    Mega doses of vitamins and minerals
Idiosyncratic reaction
    Genetic factors
    Hypersensitivity
Physician or pharmacist errors
    Wrong medication or dose, or treatment
    Insufficient directions to patient
Recreational uses
Poor compliance to medication use
Underlying disease states
Homicide

---

dren are not just small adults as far as how their physiological systems handle drugs (refer back to Chapter 2 for examples). Other times, therapeutic doses of drugs originally intended for the pediatric patient may accumulate in the body to cause lethal toxic symptoms. This will be illustrated in the next chapter when we study aspirin poisoning.

Adults are poisoned because they take overdoses accidentally or intentionally, or are given toxic doses by others, for homicidal reasons. Drugs are the most common means to commit suicide, with approximately 10,000 intentional drug-induced deaths reported each year in the United States (3). Part of the accidental (nonsuicidal) overdosing with drugs is no doubt due to patient noncompliance (not taking their drugs exactly as directed). Over half of all patients fail to comply, and this noncompliance frequently leads to hospitalization (7).

Then, there are numerous idiosyncratic (Chapter 2) and iatrogenic (technically, "doctor-induced," but we will use the term to mean any inappropriately recommended/prescribed drug) reasons. In the United States it is agreed that prescriptions for drugs are frequently given not in accordance to their actual need (8). This increased availability of drugs makes them a potential source of poisoning. Interactions between drugs, including ethanol, also account for a large number of poisonings.

Drug reactions have increased, both in number and severity, over the years because of an increased availability of potent prescription and over-the-counter drugs, and because of an increased number and variety of illicit drugs. Eighty-five percent of these reactions are due to the pharmacologic action of the drug, while the remaining 15% are due to immunologic mechanisms such as anaphylaxis, serum sickness, etc. (1). The annual cost of all drug-related toxicities is estimated to exceed a staggering 4.5 billion dollars for hospital rooms alone (8).

DRUGS THAT CAUSE POISONING

A recently published study sheds new light on the nature of the drugs that are common causes of poisoning (6). The investigation originated at one of the country's largest medical centers. The drugs that were most commonly responsible for poisoning are listed in Table 2.

Of special note is that the majority of the drugs that caused poisoning during the reporting period were legally manufactured and distributed, and legally obtained. This is consistent with our previous statement that prescriptions are often given for inappropriate purposes. Over the study period, poisoning by CNS depressants showed a steady decline, perhaps due to tighter regulatory controls, while stimulant-induced emergencies represented only a small percentage of the overall number. Heroin, cocaine, and marijuana all showed increases in poisoning incidence, while the use of hallucinogenic compounds declined. Solvent and inhalant abuse more than doubled. Problems with over-the-counter drug items (e.g., aspirin, sleep aids, diet aids, etc.) were down. But the precise pattern of drugs used for poisoning varies with time, so a similar survey conducted after another decade or so will no doubt list different figures and perhaps even different drugs.

We learned early in our pharmacology training that the first adage of drug therapy is, "No drug has a single effect." Stated in more elo-

TABLE 2. *Primary substance used by 11,287 drug emergency patients*[a]

Substance	1972		1973		1974		1975		1976	
Major tranquilizers	73	5.4%	133	6.2%	152	6.3%	207	7.8%	237	8.5%
Minor tranquilizers	169	12.5	260	12.2	368	15.4	396	15.0	341	12.2
Barbiturates	175	13.0	284	13.3	229	9.6	197	7.5	194	7.0
Nonbarbiturate sedatives	131	9.7	206	9.7	161	6.7	163	6.2	155	5.6
Antidepressants	25	1.8	59	2.8	59	2.5	57	2.2	62	2.2
Amphetamines	11	.8	53	2.5	30	1.3	34	1.3	35	1.3
Nonamphetamine stimulants	17	1.3	12	.6	21	.9	28	1.1	24	.9
Narcotics	15	1.1	46	2.2	69	2.9	56	2.1	46	1.7
Methadone	33	2.4	72	3.4	65	2.7	94	3.6	68	2.5
Analgesics	42	3.1	68	3.2	107	4.5	80	3.0	85	3.1
Heroin	170	12.6	164	7.7	209	8.7	379	14.4	387	14.0
Cocaine	12	.9	25	1.2	34	1.4	47	1.8	69	2.5
Miscellaneous Rx	49	3.6	100	4.7	139	5.8	165	6.3	210	7.6
Over-the-counter	102	7.5	148	7.0	178	7.4	149	5.6	142	5.1
Poisons	3	.2	8	.4	28	1.2	46	1.7	47	1.7
Hallucinogens	95	7.0	96	4.5	89	3.7	77	2.9	78	2.8
Marijuana	18	1.3	50	2.3	58	2.4	81	3.1	189	6.8
Inhalants	14	1.0	44	2.1	51	2.1	57	2.2	58	2.1
Unknown sedatives	11	.8	17	.8	8	.3	10	.4	6	.2
Unknown drug	189	14.0	284	13.2	342	14.2	314	11.9	337	12.2
Total	1,354	100.0	2,129	100.0	2,397	100.0	2,637	100.0	2,770	100.0

[a]Reported for the years 1972 to 1976.
From ref. 6.

quent terms, "Drugs are double-edged swords." With medical progress continuing to produce more and more drugs, we must expect more and more toxicities.

SPECIAL PROBLEMS

The clinical pattern of many drug-related poisonings is clear-cut and, in reality, most symptoms of poisoning are predictable extensions of the drugs' pharmacologic or therapeutic effect. However, some victims do not exhibit these expected symptoms. For example, many drug-poisoned patients have taken more than one drug, including ethanol. Too frequently, alcohol ingestion, concurrent with sublethal doses of a CNS depressant drug, has led to the patient's demise due to potentiation of the sedative effect. The problem is compounded even further because many people do not consider ethanol to be a drug, so they fail to observe the usual

cautions as they might with other drugs. Also, the ingestion of one drug may dull the senses to the point where the victim cannot remember how much of the drug he has taken, if any. Consequently, normal doses may be inadvertently doubled or tripled. Multiple drug therapy establishes an entirely new vista with new rules for handling clinical toxicology problems.

Occasionally, a victim of drug poisoning may have one or more diseases or disorders such as diabetic ketosis, respiratory or cardiovascular insufficiencies, head injuries, renal or liver disease, hypoglycemia, or epilepsy that are unknown to the examining physician. These disorders may complicate the clinical findings.

The pharmacokinetics of drugs taken in overdose are frequently assumed to be similar to those when the drugs are taken in normal therapeutic doses. However, this is not always the case (10). For example, following ingestion of a normal drug dose, the tablet dissociates in the stomach or intestine to yield the drug which is then absorbed to provide the expected onset and duration of effects. However, in a massive overdose involving many tablets, they may form concretions (tightly-packed masses) and dissociate at a much slower rate. Thus, a prolonged onset with delayed peak of effect is the outcome.

Or, some drugs, such as those with anticholinergic activity, will decrease the rate of gastrointestinal motility. This then may either increase or decrease another drug's absorption. For a drug that is poorly water-soluble, its absorption may be altered since the time the drug has to be absorbed is lengthened. Hence, the patient may continue to experience effects for many days, long after they would ordinarily have subsided. In another example, propoxyphene decreases the absorption of acetaminophen by delaying gastric emptying (9). This delays passage of acetaminophen into the small intestine from where it is normally absorbed.

The factors relating to toxicity that are discussed in Chapter 2 should be reviewed at this time. These hold true for drugs as well as for nondrug items.

TREATMENT

Treatment of most drug-related poisonings, as with nondrug-related intoxications, is largely supportive. For acute ingestions of a toxic dose, as much of the substance as possible should be removed from the gastrointestinal tract to reduce the chance for systemic absorption. A few specific antidotes are available for selected drugs (Table 3), but treatment is still largely supportive. At this point, a few minutes reviewing the important principles of antidoting poisoning that are discussed in Chapter 3 will help with our understanding of the next chapters.

As long as the patient receives medical assistance prior to onset of irreversible organ damage, most drug overdoses should not result in death.

It is often stated that the best treatment for any poisoning is prevention. While prevention is technically not a form of therapy, this advice

TABLE 3. *Specific antidotal therapy for drug overdoses and poisoning*

Acetaminophen	N-Acetylcysteine
Anticholinergics	Physostigmine
β-adrenergic blockers	Atropine; isoproterenol
Cholinergics, cholinesterase inhibitors	Atropine; pralidoxime
Coumarin	Vitamin K
Heparin	Protamine sulfate
Iron salts	Deferoxamine
Methotrexate	Tetrahydrofolic acid
Narcotics (including pentazocine and propoxyphene)	Naloxone
Oxidizing agents that cause methemoglobinemia	Methylene blue
Sympathomimetics	β-adrenergic blockers

is well stated. Safety-closure caps on prescription and many nonprescription medication containers have been shown to reduce the incidence of accidental drug poisonings in children.

SUMMARY

Most symptoms of drug-induced poisoning are actually extensions of their pharmacologic activities. Thus, the important principles we learned in pharmacology about drug activity should be reviewed at this time.

REFERENCES

1. Caranasos, G. J. (1978): Drug reactions. In: *Principles and Practice of Emergency Medicine*, Vol. II, edited by G. R. Schwartz, P. Safar, J. H. Stone, P. B. Storey, and D. K. Wagner, pp. 1309–1355. Saunders, Philadelphia.
2. Caranasos, G. J., Stewart, R. B., and Cluff, L. E. (1974): Drug-induced illness leading to hospitalization. *JAMA*, 228:713–717.
3. Holland, J., Massie, M. J., Grant, C., and Plumb, M. M. (1975): Drugs ingested in suicide attempts and fatal outcome. *NY State J. Med.*, 75:2343–2349.
4. Hurwitz, N. (1969): Admissions to hospital due to drugs. *Br. Med. J.*, 1:539–540.
5. Hurwitz, N., and Wade, D. L. (1969): Intensive hospital monitoring of adverse reactions to drugs. *Br. Med. J.*, 1:531–536.
6. Inciardi, J. A., Ruswe, B. R., Pottieger, A. E., McBride, D. C., Wells, K. S., and Siegel, H. A. (1979): Acute drug reactions in a hospital emergency room. *U.S. Department of Health, Education and Welfare, PHS Publication 79-806*, p 5.
7. McKenney, J. M., and Harrison, W. I. (1976): Drug-related hospital admissions. *Am. J. Hosp. Pharm.*, 33:792–795.

8. Melmon, K. L., and Morrelli, H. F. (1978): Drug reactions. In: *Clinical Pharmacology—Basic Principles in Therapeutics*, 2nd ed., edited by K. L. Melmon and H. F. Morrelli, pp. 951–981. Macmillan, New York.

9. Nimmo, W. S., Heading, R. C., Wilson, J., and Prescott, L. F. (1979): Reversal of narcotic-induced delay in gastric emptying and paracetamol absorption by naloxone. *Br. Med. J.*, 2:1189.

10. Rosenberg, J., Benowitz, N. L., and Pond, S. (1981): Pharmacokinetics of drug overdose. *Clin. Pharmacokinet.*, 6:161–192.

11. Seidl, L. G., Thornton, G. F., Smith, J. W., and Cluff, L. E. (1966): Studies on the epidemiology of adverse drug reactions: III. Reactions in patients on a general medical service. *Bull. Johns Hopkins Hosp.*, 119:299–315.

12. Smidt, N. A., and McQueen, E. G. (1972): Adverse reactions to drugs. A comprehensive hospital in-patient survey. *NZ Med. J.*, 76:397–401.

Nonnarcotic Analgesics

14

There are numerous nonnarcotic analgesic products that are used to treat a wide variety of clinical conditions, including pain and inflammation, and fever. Some are available without a prescription, while others require the patient to be under the care of a licensed medical practitioner. Despite this plethora of products, there are two nonnarcotic analgesics that emerge as being those which are most commonly used in the United States. They are, as might be expected, the two that produce the greatest incidence of serious toxicity: aspirin and acetaminophen.

Other commonly used nonnarcotic analgesics (e.g., the nonsteroidal antiinflammatory agents) may induce a variety of side-effects, but they are not usually associated with toxic reactions. Until recently, acetophenetidin (phenacetin) would have been included in our discussion of nonnarcotic agents that produce significant toxicity. However, manufacturers are in the process of removing it from their products. Phenacetin is no longer a major cause of toxicity in the United States.

Both aspirin and acetaminophen may produce a wide variety of adverse reactions. However, each causes one or two specific effects that are the most significant, as far as determining the patient's chance for survival. This chapter details only those most important actions.

SALICYLATES

Aspirin currently exceeds acetaminophen as a cause of acute toxic ingestions by nonnarcotic analgesics. Considering its widespread use and generalized disrespect by the public for its toxic potential, this should not be surprising.

Aspirin poisoning may affect people of all ages. However, children are most susceptible and are usually the victims of accidental ingestions. Whereas adult salicylate toxicity is normally due to chronic misuse or intentional ingestions of large quantities of salicylates, children present the greatest risk of developing serious toxic complications following salicylate poisonings.

The chance for a fatal outcome in children is enhanced if the child is febrile and/or dehydrated. Consider what often happens when a child with an upper respiratory tract infection or other minor affliction is given aspirin by a well-meaning parent. Since this child may also be lethargic and will not eat or drink adequately, the stage is now set for enhancement of the toxicity of salicylates. The child is given one dose followed by another and another. Within a couple days of continuous aspirin therapy, the tissues are completely saturated (2). At this point, serum levels increase geometrically. In other words, a 50% increase in the daily aspirin dose causes the serum level to rise by 300% (14). Before it is realized, the child has been accidently poisoned. Unfortunately, this scenario is repeated far too often every year.

Although the Poison Prevention Packaging Act of 1970 set guidelines which have contributed to a reduction by 40 to 55% in the incidence of accidental ingestions, aspirin is still listed by the National Clearinghouse for Poison Control Centers as being in the top five categories most frequently involved in ingestions by children under 5 years of age (6).

All too often, aspirin and acetaminophen are referred to as "candy" by the parent in order to encourage the child to ingest the necessary dose. The problem arises when a curious, unattended child finds a bottle or two of "candy-flavored" aspirin tablets, or even adult aspirin. The dose of aspirin for children at which symptoms of toxicity are likely to occur is 150 mg/kg. In an otherwise healthy 20-kg child, it would be necessary for the child to ingest approximately an entire bottle of 36 flavored baby aspirin (which contain 81 mg of salicylate/tablet). On the other hand, ingesting only 9 adult aspirin (325 mg) would place the child in the same jeopardy (see Table 1).

Another source of accidental salicylate intoxication in children is methyl salicylate, or oil of wintergreen. A child may find a bottle of methyl salicylate that smells like wintergreen candy, and the opportunity to taste some is difficult to refuse. Since it is a liquid, it can be easily ingested. It has been shown that as little as 4 ml of methyl salicylate may be lethal in an infant. One teaspoonful of methyl salicylate (5 ml) contains approximately 7 g salicylate. Therefore, one teaspoonful is equivalent to approximately 21 adult aspirin tablets (325 mg) or more than 2 bottles of 36 children's baby aspirin.

Mechanism of Salicylate Toxicity

The pathophysiology of salicylate toxicity can be explained by a central stimulation and interference with the uncoupling of oxidative phosphorylation within the electron transport system. It may be helpful to follow these events outlined in Fig. 1.

The respiratory center is stimulated by two mechanisms: direct stimulation, and indirectly by an increase in P_{CO_2} production. Salicylates increase oxygen consumption by increasing the cellular metabolic rate. This results in hyperthermia, as well as an accumulation of CO_2 which then causes hyperpnea.

Also, toxic doses of salicylate directly stimulate the respiratory center producing an increased depth (hyperpnea) and increased rate (tachypnea) of respiration. The increased respiration rate causes a greater than normal amount of CO_2 to be expired by the lungs. As a result, there is less plasma CO_2. Recall the following reactions of the bicarbonate buffer system for maintaining blood pH:

$$H_2O + CO_2 \rightleftharpoons H_2CO_3 \rightleftharpoons H^+ + HCO_3^-$$

Since there is less CO_2 available, less carbonic acid is formed. When this occurs, there is a

TABLE 1. *Toxicity profile for salicylate ingestions*

| Range of toxicity | Signs and symptoms | Blood level range | Single oral dose ingested | Approximate no. of tablets ingested by a child[a] | | Approximate no. of tablets (325 mg) ingested by an adult[b] |
				Baby aspirin (81 mg)	Adult aspirin (325 mg)	
Asymptomatic		<45 mg%				
Mild toxicity	Nausea					
	Gastritis	45–65 mg%	<150 mg/kg	up to 37	up to 9	>30
	Mild hyperpnea					
Moderate toxicity	Hyperpnea					
	Hyperthermia					
	Sweating	65–90 mg%	150–300 mg/kg	37–74	9–18	30–63
	Dehydration					
	Marked lethargy					
	Possible excitement					
Severe toxicity	Severe hyperpnea					
	Coma					
	Convulsions					
	Cyanosis	90–120 mg%	300–500 mg/kg	74–123	18–30	63–105
	Pulmonary edema					
	Respiratory failure					
	Cardiovascular collapse					
Lethal	Coma	>120 mg%	>500 mg/kg	>123	>30	>105
	Death					

[a]ASA tablets ingested by a 20-kg child.
[b]ASA tablets ingested by a 68-kg adult.
From ref. 7.

deficit of carbonic acid with a subsequent decrease in hydrogen ion concentration [H$^+$]. Also, the pH of the blood is dependent on the bicarbonate/carbonic acid ratio according to the Henderson-Hasselbalch equation:

$$pH = 6.1 + \log \frac{[HCO_3{}^-]}{[H_2CO_3]}$$

Normally, the concentration of $HCO_3{}^-$ in the plasma and extracellular fluid is 27 mEq/L, and the concentration of carbonic acid is 1.35 mEq/L. The pH of the plasma is dependent on the $HCO_3{}^-/H_2CO_3$ ratio of 27/1.35 or 20, and at this ratio the pH of the blood is 7.4. Therefore, as the P_{CO_2} and H_2CO_3 concentrations decrease, the $HCO_3{}^-$ concentration is the same, and the ratio of $HCO_3{}^-/H_2CO_3$ increases resulting in an increase in blood pH.

The kidney attempts to compensate for this abnormality in acid-base balance by excreting more $HCO_3{}^-$, and retaining H^+ and nonbicarbonate anions. Usually this mechanism operates to correct the acid-base imbalance and return the ratio to 20/1; but as can be seen in Fig. 1, in salicylate toxicity this may add to the latent metabolic acidosis.

The second action of salicylate intoxication results from the uncoupling of oxidative phosphorylation, which ultimately produces a metabolic acidosis with a high anion gap. Again, it may be useful to follow these events in Fig. 1.

We have previously discussed the electron transport chain and oxidative phosphorylation in response to cellular anoxia, as seen with cyanide (Chapter 6). It should be remembered that mitochondria are organelles whose preliminary function is the production of an energy source, ATP. Hydrogen atoms and electrons from glycolysis and the Kreb's cycle are transferred, via a series of oxidation-reduction reactions of the cytochrome system of the electron transport

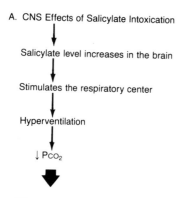

A. CNS Effects of Salicylate Intoxication

Salicylate level increases in the brain

Stimulates the respiratory center

Hyperventilation

↓ PCO₂

RESPIRATORY ALKALOSIS

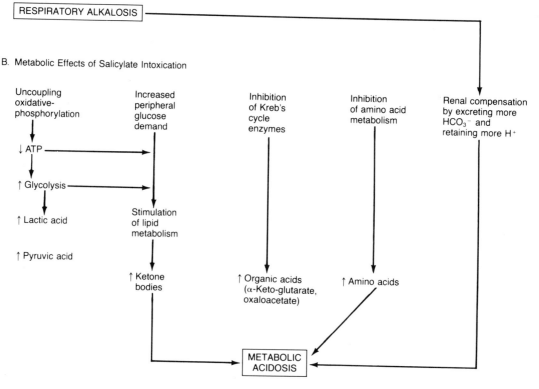

B. Metabolic Effects of Salicylate Intoxication

FIG. 1.   Pathophysiological consequences of salicylate intoxication.

chain, to molecular oxygen, forming water. During these reactions, inorganic phosphate becomes coupled with ADP to form ATP. The process of electron donor to acceptor with the resultant production of ATP is termed oxidative phosphorylation.

Uncoupling results in a decrease in ATP production. The cells try to compensate by increasing glycolysis. Only 2 moles of ATP are produced by substrate phosphorylation during glycolysis. In addition to a less efficient energy pathway, increased glycolysis also results in the production of lactic and pyruvic acids. The body also uses its glycogen stores to obtain energy. Eventually, these are also depleted and the body switches over to lipid metabolism to meet its demands for an energy source. Although this is an efficient energy mechanism, it leads to excess free fatty acid in the liver, producing an increase in ketone bodies which can cause ketoacidosis.

Another contributing factor to the metabolic acidosis, as a result of salicylate toxicity, is the inhibition of the dehydrogenase enzymes of the Kreb's cycle resulting in the accumulation of α-ketoglutarate and oxaloacetate, and the inhibition of amino acid metabolism results in the accumulation of amino acids. The end result of the uncoupling of oxidative phosphorylation is the production of metabolic acidosis with a high anion gap.

Salicylates also play havoc with the blood glucose concentration. Initially, there may be an increase in glucose because of the mobilization of fats to free fatty acids and ketones, and the utilization of muscle glycogen stores. Eventually, however, there is a depletion of glucose stores, and this causes hypoglycemia. Therefore, hypoglycemia may be of significance in chronic salicylism, or during the latter stages of acute salicylate intoxication.

Clinical Manifestations of Salicylate Poisoning

It has been estimated that in up to 50% of the suicide attempts which have involved aspirin, the medication was ingested in combination with other drugs such as anticholinergics, narcotics, isoniazid, or aluminum hydroxide (3). Consequently, the salicylate-intoxicated patient may present with a variety of signs and symptoms. The most commonly associated ones are listed in Table 1.

The major early toxic manifestations of salicylate poisoning result from stimulation of the CNS. These include nausea, vomiting, tinnitus, headache, hyperpnea, and neurological abnormalities such as confusion, hyperactivity, slurred speech, and generalized convulsions. The severity of the CNS toxic effects are closely related to the brain salicylate concentration. As previously pointed out, salicylate-induced CNS stimulation results in hyperventilation, decreased P_{CO_2}, and respiratory alkalosis. In sub-

toxic quantities, renal compensation proceeds to counteract the respiratory alkalosis. Compensated respiratory alkalosis is accomplished by renal excretion of bicarbonate, resulting in lowering of the blood pH toward normal. Adults and children older than 4 years of age, who have ingested a mild-to-moderate amount of salicylate (see Table 1) tend to correct the acid-base disturbance at this point. Young children rapidly develop metabolic acidosis.

In the discussion of the mechanism of toxicity of salicylate, we observed several metabolic abnormalities. Increased glycolysis, gluconeogenesis, and lipid metabolism result in depletion of glucose from the peripheral tissues, accumulation of organic acids in the blood, and an increase in ketone bodies (see Fig. 1). Two other factors also contribute to the metabolic acidosis related to salicylate poisoning. These include the vasomotor depressant effect related to toxic quantities of salicylate which impairs renal function, and the fact that salicylate dissociates at plasma pH and contributes to the lowering of the plasma pH. The severity of metabolic acidosis is dose-related and occurs more frequently in infants and very young children following chronic salicylate therapy for some febrile conditions. In adults, salicylate toxicity usually results from an accidental or intentional ingestion of a large single dose of salicylate and metabolic acidosis is usually delayed.

Another serious toxic effect of salicylates is dehydration. There are also several factors contributing to this problem. First, the increased heat production from salicylate-induced glucose and lipid metabolism results in hyperpyrexia and diaphoresis. Also, hyperventilation occurs as a result of CNS stimulation, and there is an increased pulmonary insensible water loss. Renal compensated respiratory alkalosis results in the loss of HCO_3^-, followed by sodium, potassium, and an equiosmolar quantity of water. Metabolic acidosis also adds to the increased urinary output and electrolyte loss. The severe dehydration described above is more common in children, and usually associated with moderate to severe levels of salicylate toxicity.

A useful means of evaluating the degree of potential toxicity following an acute oral ingestion of salicylate is to correlate the blood salicylate concentration with the clinical status of the patient. Several factors have been included in Table 1 to permit prediction of the extent of toxicity following an acute overdose of salicylate. For example, a 20-kg child would have to ingest the entire contents of one bottle of candy-flavored baby aspirin tablets, but only 9 to 18 adult aspirin tablets to produce moderate intoxication.

Blood salicylate concentration ranges were selected from the Done Nomogram (Fig. 2). This nomogram is valuable when evaluating an acute salicylate poisoning, provided the approximate time of ingestion is known and a single oral dose has been ingested. It is recommended that serial salicylate determinations be made, beginning at least 6 hr postingestion.

If a 6-hr postingestion blood salicylate level is less than 40 mg%, it is unlikely that any serious toxic effects will be observed. This cor-

relates to ingestions of less than 150 mg/kg of salicylate. The patient is generally asymptomatic and can be easily managed at home.

Poisoning by methyl salicylate proceeds in a manner similar to aspirin. However, symptoms are usually seen earlier, partly because methyl salicylate causes higher blood levels more rapidly. Prevalent early symptoms include CNS excitement, hyperpnea, and hyperpyrexia.

For salicylic acid, symptoms exhibit similarly to aspirin. However, it causes more intense gastrointestinal irritation. Salicylic acid is an infrequent cause of poisoning.

Treatment of Salicylate Poisoning

Salicylate poisoning from an acute oral ingestion of massive quantities requires prompt medical attention. Treatment is largely supportive and results are not always satisfactory. Generally, therapy involves the removal of aspirin from the gastrointestinal tract, and the correction of metabolic acidosis, dehydration, hyperthermia, hypoglycemia, and hypokalemia. The decision as to how rigorous a treatment should

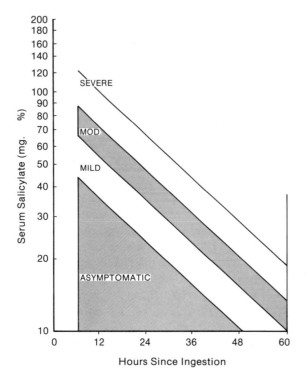

FIG. 2. Done nomogram for assessing the extent of salicylate poisoning. (From ref. 7.)

be is governed by the history of the ingestion. Unfortunately, this is usually complicated since, in children, the quantity ingested is seldom known, and, in adults, most salicylate poisonings involve a combination of other drugs as well.

The general sequence should begin with emesis or lavage. In children, emesis is easier to accomplish and may be more effective. Preferably, emesis should be induced at home or on the way to the hospital. Evacuation of the stomach should be followed by the administration of activated charcoal to adsorb any remaining aspirin. A saline cathartic may be given to hasten the passage of adsorbed salicylate through the gastrointestinal tract. Cathartics are usually repeated until a charcoal-laden stool is passed. Gastric evacuation may be omitted in cases where ingestion has occurred more than 12 hr previously, or in chronic salicylate poisonings.

Dehydration is a common finding in salicylate poisoning. This is managed by administering oral fluids. When toxicity is within the moderate-to-severe range, dehydration is usually treated with parenterally administered fluids. At this point rehydration, not correction of acid-base imbalance, is the only consideration. It is important to keep the patient hydrated so that kidney function is maintained, because salicylates are largely excreted by the kidneys.

Sodium bicarbonate is added to the intravenous fluids to help correct the metabolic acidosis associated with a moderate-to-severe salicylate toxicity.

Hyperthermia is a problem with moderate-to-severe salicylate toxicity. Fever can be reduced by cold or tepid water (*not* alcohol) sponging.

Glucose is added to correct the hypoglycemia and ketosis. Potassium chloride is added to correct the hypokalemia and help prevent alkalosis from sodium bicarbonate administration. Hypokalemia is sometimes a grave problem in children. Administration of sodium bicarbonate and forced diuresis can produce a severe hypokalemic state. Also, forced alkaline diuresis is only effective when potassium depletion is corrected. Furthermore, in older children and adults,

the presence of respiratory alkalosis aggravates the hypokalemic state. During potassium replacement, serum potassium levels should be closely monitored because either hypokalemia or hyperkalemia may cause cardiac arrhythmias.

Other symptomatic treatment includes diazepam for seizures, calcium supplements for hypocalcemic tetany, and vitamin K_1 (phytonadione) for coagulation defects.

Enhancing the elimination of salicylate can be accomplished by forced alkaline diuresis (15). Consequently, the correction of acidosis and alkalinization of urine with administration of sodium bicarbonate will promote the movement of salicylate from intracellular sites to the plasma, and then to the urine.

The use of forced alkaline diuresis is usually quite effective in cases of mild-to-moderate toxicity, but sometimes difficult in the case of severe salicylate intoxication.

Acetazolamide and tromethamine (THAM) have been advocated as alkalinizing agents, but their use is dangerous for the inexperienced, and can result in severe complications (8,25).

In cases of severe salicylate toxicity, consideration may be given to using an extracorporeal procedure to aid drug elimination. Some guidelines for using peritoneal dialysis, hemodialysis, or charcoal hemoperfusion include: salicylate blood levels greater than 130 mg% 6 hr postingestion, measured elimination half-life greater than 15 hr, and clinical manifestations indicating persistent CNS involvement, renal failure, and unresponsiveness to conventional therapy (24,26).

ACETAMINOPHEN

Acetaminophen (paracetamol in the British literature), also a nonnarcotic analgesic-antipyretic agent, follows aspirin as a major cause of poisoning. For many years acetaminophen was not generally recognized in the United States as an important source of toxicity. The British, on the other hand, had long ago acknowledged its toxic potential. Perhaps this was because the substance had been used in the United Kingdom much more extensively than by Americans.

With increasing use of acetaminophen in the United States over the past decade, an increasing number of toxic events have been reported. Unfortunately, acetaminophen does not cause an early neurologic signal or warning sign of toxicity (e.g., tinnitus) as does aspirin. Patients are frequently seen who are in otherwise good health and, by the time toxicity is realized (by either the victim or attending physician), irreversible damage may have already occurred. This damage is related primarily to fatal hepatocyte necrosis.

To understand what occurs during acetaminophen poisoning, some points need to be examined. First of all, acetaminophen, like aspirin, is considered to be safe when taken as directed. It is only when therapeutic doses are exceeded that toxicity occurs.

One reason why acetaminophen is causing an alarming increase in toxicity is that, as previously mentioned, there is no early warning sign that signals a poisoning has occurred. Early symptoms of poisoning are not specific (Table 2). Furthermore, there is a phase of apparent recovery when symptoms subside. If the victim interprets this as emergence from danger and fails to seek medical assistance, permanent hepatic damage may occur.

Mechanism of Acetaminophen Toxicity

The most serious and devastating toxic effect from acetaminophen is hepatic necrosis. The other problems are nonspecific. Events leading

TABLE 2. *Characteristics of acetaminophen toxicity*

Signs and symptoms	Laboratory values
Nausea	Increased serum transaminases
Vomiting	Increased bilirubin
Sweating	Prolonged prothrombin time
Anorexia	
Malaise	
Pain in right upper quadrant	
Jaundice	
Coma	

to hepatic necrosis occur in the following manner.

Acetaminophen is rapidly absorbed from the stomach and upper gastrointestinal tract, and is metabolized by conjugation with glucuronide and sulfate (Fig. 3). Another pathway, normally of minor importance, involves formation of a highly reactive and harmful electrophilic intermediate product. Approximately 4% of a therapeutic dose of acetaminophen is metabolized by this cytochrome P_{450}-dependent mixed-function oxidase system. This intermediate toxic metabolite can react with cellular proteins to cause hepatocellular death. Normally, before it produces toxic effects, glutathione inactivates it by conjugation and subsequent transformation to the nontoxic mercapturic acid. At therapeutic doses of acetaminophen, conjugation proceeds in its normal manner. However, when a massive overdose is ingested, the liver enzymes are saturated and the supply of glutathione is inadequate to meet its needs. The concentration of toxic metabolite then increases to toxic levels where it covalently binds to sulfhydryl groups of hepatic cellular proteins, resulting in centrilobular necrosis.

There are data which show that the P_{450} microsomal enzyme system is more active in children than adults. If this is so, it would logically follow that more of the toxic metabolite would be formed in children. However, there are too many unanswered questions remaining. Thus far, any differences in P_{450} activity have not shown significant influences on hepatotoxic reactions (17).

A dose of 15 g for adults, or 4 g for children, is normally sufficient to cause fatal liver damage. Drugs such as phenobarbital and ethanol, which stimulate the cytochrome P_{450} system, enhance formation of the electrophilic (toxic) metabolite. A patient in such a condition who ingests acetaminophen may, thus, experience lethal toxicity to a dose of acetaminophen as low as 10 g. Many physicians will begin antidotal treatment when the dose ingested is 6 g or more.

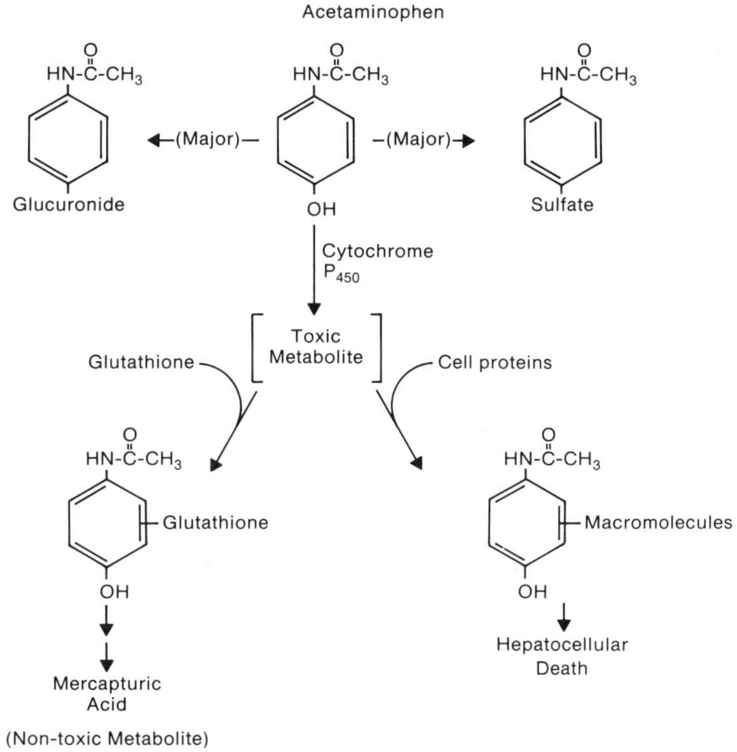

FIG. 3. Scheme for acetaminophen metabolism.

Clinical Manifestations of Acetaminophen Poisoning

Except for signs of hepatotoxicity that often do not manifest for days after ingestion, acetaminophen does not cause many other signs or symptoms. Those which have been reported are summarized in Table 2.

Stages of Poisoning

Acetaminophen poisoning occurs according to three distinct stages. The ultimate outcome is not correlated with the intensity of the initial symptoms.

For example, as can be seen in Table 3, acute acetaminophen toxicity usually begins with symptoms of gastrointestinal distress. Stage I may be seen within 14 hr of ingestion, and these nonspecific symptoms may persist for 24 hr or more. If acetaminophen alone was ingested, it is not likely that there will be serious CNS

depression. The real danger is that these symptoms may subside quickly and the patient then is in Stage II, which is a period of relative quiescence with apparent recovery. If the individual fails to seek medical assistance during this period, thinking that the serious event is past and that no further damage is occurring, the prognosis may be quite grave. The events that will eventually bloom into full scale hepatotoxicity are underway. As shown by the increase in serum glutamic acid oxalacetic transaminase (SGOT) levels in Fig. 4, liver damage has begun. The figure also shows the anticipated outcome of acetaminophen toxicity. That is, during Stage I (nausea, vomiting, etc.) blood SGOT levels are within the normal range. However, during Stage II these levels begin to rise, and other laboratory abnormalities may also be concurrently detected (e.g., bilirubin and prothrombin time abnormalities). The *solid line* in Fig. 4 represents the natural course of

TABLE 3. *Clinical stages of acetaminophen poisoning*

Stage	Time	Clinical characteristics
Stage I	Within 24 hr	Abdominal pain Anorexia, nausea, vomiting Malaise Diaphoresis Drowsiness
Stage II	24–48 hr	Period of "apparent recovery" Patient feels better Possibly pain in right hypochondrium Hepatic necrosis develops Urine output slightly decreased
Stage III	3–5 days	Marked hepatotoxicity Jaundice Coagulation defects Hypoglycemia Hepatic encephalopathy Renal failure Myocardiopathy Coma Death

toxicity, the *dotted line* shows the outcome when the antidote acetylcysteine is given, and the *dotted-dashed line* shows expected outcome for patients with a severe course of toxicity. If the results of liver function tests are still normal after the second day, there probably will not be significant liver damage. If survival is to be assured, treatment with the antidote acetylcysteine must be initiated before Stage II begins.

The third stage (III) may manifest within 3 to 5 days of poisoning. It is characterized primarily by elevated plasma levels of lactic de-

hydrogenase (LDH) and SGOT, as well as bilirubin. The prothrombin time may be increased and those case reports that describe hemorrhagic tendencies following acetaminophen toxicity more than likely relate to this mechanism.

Eventually the liver damage that occurs may cause jaundice and the other sequelae depicted in Table 3. Myocardial tissue has also been reported to be depressed in some instances, and renal damage may appear. These effects are less predictable, and overall, less devastating than the hepatic effects.

Acetaminophen occasionally causes clinically significant methemoglobinemia. In therapeutic doses, the concentration of methemoglobinemia is not of clinical importance. On the other hand, during periods of chronic abuse, or in acute overdosing situations, the levels may be significant. As stated in Chapter 5, the tendency toward formation of clinically important methemoglobinemia is enhanced in persons who are genetically inclined to do so.

Plasma acetaminophen levels play an important role in assessing the acetaminophen-intoxicated patient's probability of developing hepatic damage. Some feel that the acetaminophen concentration is a more accurate indicator of the likelihood of hepatic damage than the actual amount of drug ingested (1). Therapeutic, toxic, and lethal acetaminophen serum concentrations are listed in Table 4. Significant damage is likely with levels greater than 20 mg% at 4 hr after ingestion, or above 5 mg% at 12 hr postingestion. These values were obtained from the Ru-

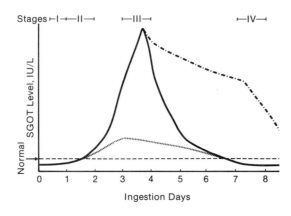

FIG. 4. Hepatotoxicity, as shown by an elevation of SGOT following toxic acetaminophen ingestion. The *solid line* is acetaminophen alone, the *dotted line* shows protection of liver damage with acetylcysteine, and the *dotted-and-dashed line* shows those individuals with a severe course. Notice that the *solid line* begins to rise early and peaks by Stage III. (From ref. 20.)

TABLE 4. *Serum acetaminophen concentrations*

Therapeutic	Toxic	Lethal
0.5–2.0 mg%	<12 mg%—no hepatic problems 12–30 mg%—50% develop hepatic necrosis >30 mg%—hepatic necrosis	150 mg%

From ref. 13.

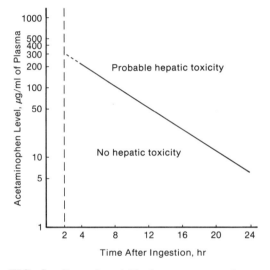

FIG. 5. Rumack and Matthew nomogram for assessing the extent of acetaminophen toxicity. (From ref. 20.)

mack-Matthew nomogram for acetaminophen poisoning (Fig. 5). Like the nomogram for salicylate poisoning, this graph should be used only in relation to a single acute ingestion, and only when the approximate time of ingestion is known. Blood samples for the analytical determination of acetaminophen should be drawn at least 4 hr postingestion to allow for complete absorption and peak serum concentration. Then the patient's serum acetaminophen concentration can be plotted on the nomogram to assess the possibility of hepatic damage. Of course, the time of ingestion of all accidental or intentional acetaminophen overdoses cannot always be determined.

One way to possibly overcome this obstacle is to determine the patient's plasma half-life of acetaminophen. This is accomplished by determining at least three plasma levels and plotting them to obtain a $t_{1/2}$ value. The approximate normal serum acetaminophen half-life is 1 to 3 hr, and is prolonged following an overdose. Using this method as an indicator for potential liver toxicity, it is generally assured that if the plasma $t_{1/2}$ exceeds 4 hr, liver damage is likely to occur; and if the half-life is greater than 12 hr, hepatic coma will probably ensue.

Treatment of Acetaminophen Poisoning

Prompt diagnosis and early treatment are extremely essential for assuring recovery from the toxic agent. Many of the early reports on acetaminophen stated that activated charcoal was ineffective for reducing absorption. However, in more recent studies it has been shown that activated charcoal will effectively adsorb acetaminophen and reduce the amount eligible for absorption. Early in the treatment protocol, as soon as poisoning has been realized, methods should be undertaken to reduce the quantity of acetaminophen present within the gastrointestinal tract, and thereby reduce the amount that will be absorbed. Activated charcoal or syrup of ipecac can be used to achieve these purposes. However, a problem may emerge if activated charcoal is chosen, and it is mentioned here to illustrate that sometimes an "antidote" may create more problems than it helps solve.

Activated charcoal is a nonspecific adsorbent and will adsorb almost any chemical in the gastrointestinal tract, including the specific antidote for acetaminophen, acetylcysteine (21). If acetylcysteine is adsorbed onto the activated charcoal, it cannot be absorbed into the blood, and its antidotal potential will be lost.

This interaction between two treatment procedures means that activated charcoal may be of more theoretical than practical importance. In most instances, by the time acetylcysteine is administered, several hours have usually elapsed since the dose of activated charcoal was given. As long as the first dose of acetylcysteine is

TABLE 5. *Effect of* N-*acetylcysteine on blood SGOT levels at different times after acetaminophen ingestion*

Initiation of treatment (time)	No. of patients	Means maximum SGOT level (IU/L)
<10 hr	57	229
10–16 hr	52	1,557
16–24 hr	39	2,695

From ref. 20.

given within the first 16 hr of ingestion of acetaminophen, the regimen should still be beneficial. Also, not all studies show that activated charcoal significantly reduces acetylcysteine blood levels (16). Thus, most of the activated charcoal will have already passed into the small intestine, far enough away from the initial dose of acetylcysteine.

To be on the safe side, syrup of ipecac is still considered to be the initial antidote of choice as a means to reduce the quantity of poison in the stomach. An exception to this rule is activated charcoal given by lavage. In this instance, it is placed in the stomach and then removed.

The same reasoning holds for cathartics. They should not be administered prior to or concurrent with acetylcysteine, since the antidote may be removed before it has a chance to be completely absorbed.

As stated earlier, hepatotoxicity is not due to acetaminophen, per se, but to a chemically reactive toxic metabolite which accumulates when the body's own glutathione is inadequate to convert all of the toxic metabolite to a nontoxic form. This point is reached when blood levels of acetaminophen fall in the area above the line in the nomogram shown in Fig. 5. The logical response would be to administer glutathione to the poisoned patient. Unfortunately, glutathione will not enter the hepatocyte, so it is useless as an antidote. The next choice is to administer a substance which will penetrate into the hepatocyte and substitute for glutathione. Experi-

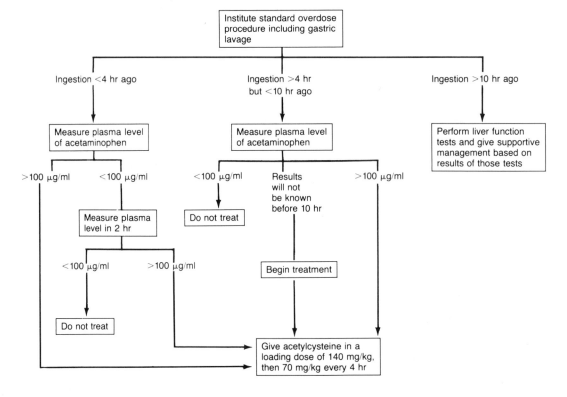

FIG. 6. Flow chart for management of acetaminophen poisoning. (From ref. 22.)

ence has shown that several substances with sulfhydryl groups will serve this purpose.

Acetylcysteine is one substance that will antidote acetaminophen. Others include L-methionine, L-cysteine, and even dimercaprol and D-penicillamine. Cimetidine (Tagamet®) inhibits the cytochrome P_{450} mixed-function oxidase system and offers the possibility of an interesting (at least theoretical) alternative approach to antidoting acetaminophen (19). However, at this time, acetylcysteine remains as the first choice. It is best tolerated, has little inherent toxicity of its own, and can be given orally. It also can be administered later than the others, following an acetaminophen overdose, and still provides antidotal activity (20).

Besides enhancing the synthesis of glutathione, acetylcysteine also serves as a source of inorganic sulfur. This may promote an increased conversion of acetaminophen to its sulfate metabolite, as well as reduce the formation of other metabolites including the toxic intermediate metabolite (9).

Just as blood acetaminophen levels assess the likelihood for developing hepatic damage, the patient's serum acetaminophen level is the best guide to therapy. Within the first 10 to 16 hr following poisoning, a loading dose of 140 mg/kg of acetylcysteine is given orally, followed by 70 mg/kg every 4 hr for 17 to 18 doses (72 hr total). In the event that the individual vomits the loading or maintenance doses within 1 hr of administration, a replacement dose is immediately given and the patient is continued on the same dosing schedule. When persistent vomiting occurs, acetylcysteine can be instilled through a nasogastric tube directly into the duodenum. Oral administration is at least theoretically better than intravenous dosing (18). Recall that substances which are absorbed from the gastrointestinal tract are immediately transported to the liver. If injected intravenously, a smaller quantity will be delivered to the liver because it is distributed throughout the body.

The importance of beginning acetylcysteine therapy early cannot be overemphasized. Table 5 summarizes data obtained from a study which examined the effect on blood SGOT levels of acetylcysteine given at different times following acetaminophen ingestions. The data clearly show that there is a correlation between the time treatment is initiated and the increases in SGOT levels, which should indicate a relative degree of hepatotoxicity.

Throughout the antidoting period, the patient is constantly monitored for vital signs, blood chemistry, and hepatic function. Decisions as to further therapy are decided at these times (Fig. 6). Blood levels of liver enzymes (e.g., SGOT, SGPT, alkaline phosphate) indicate the probable extent of toxic hepatic injury. However, these levels are not used to prescribe the quantity of acetylcysteine to be given. This is a fixed quantity (see above).

At present, the use of acetylcysteine to antidote acetaminophen is still considered experimental in the United States, and the user must follow an established protocol for "experimentation" with an unproven drug. On the other hand, it is generally recognized that acetylcysteine must be given quickly after the poisoning event. Administration of the antidote is initiated, then the official personnel are notified. If the protocol is followed, there should be few fatalities due to hepatic damage.

SUMMARY

Many of us will take a dose of an analgesic within the next few weeks. Normal therapeutic doses are not causes of poisoning. Rather, poisoning occurs when massive quantities that are far greater than those intended for pain relief are ingested.

Also, acetaminophen poisoning is a fairly new phenomenon in the United States. However, poisoning with it is a serious event and unless the victim receives quick treatment, irreversible hepatotoxicity may occur.

Case Studies

CASE STUDIES: SALICYLATE TOXICITY

History: Case 1

An 18-month-old male weighing 10 kg was brought to a local hospital because of fever, irritability, hyperventilation, and hematemesis. It was reported that he had been treated for the past 2 days for an upper respiratory infection. The parents said they gave him only one baby aspirin tablet every 4 to 6 hr. Aspirin poisoning was nevertheless suspected, so a salicylate level was ordered. When the salicylate level was found to be 55 mg%, he was transferred to a larger medical center for further assessment.

On arrival at the second hospital, the patient was lethargic, but arousable. Physical examination revealed signs of moderate dehydration and a temperature of 40.5°C. The systolic blood pressure was 90 mm Hg, pulse 220/min, and respirations were 70/min.

Laboratory findings are listed below:

Na^+	= 148 mEq/l
K^+	= 7.2 mEq/L
HCO_3^-	= 11 mEq/L
Glucose	= 87 mg%
BUN	= 158 mg%
Creatinine	= 3.9 mg%
WBC	= 16,600/cu mm
PT	= elevated
PTT	= elevated
Arterial blood gasses	= 20 mm Hg (Pco_2) 7.34 pH
Blood salicylate	= 168 mg%

Treatment. Treatment consisted of volume expansion with saline, dextrose, and $NaHCO_3$. Fifty grams of albumin per liter were added to the intravenous fluid. The patient was lavaged with normal saline, and activated charcoal and magnesium sulfate were added by means of the nasogastric tube. He was given 100% oxygen and placed on a ventilator.

Due to the onset of renal failure and persistence of elevated serum salicylate levels, peritoneal dialysis was initiated using 1.5% Impersol solution containing 5% albumin. Twenty-four hours later the salicylate level had decreased to 40 mg% and the BUN was down to 34 mg%. After 48 hr, the salicylate level was only 4 mg% and kidney function was markedly improved. Dialysis was discontinued, and he was showing signs of improvement until 12 hr later when he became hypotensive, and signs of septic shock appeared (WBC = 5,400 cu mm with a severe shift to the left). A diagnosis of disseminated intravascular coagulation (DIC) was made. Blood cultures grew *Escherichia coli*. The victim died on the 4th hospital day, despite antibiotics and additional supportive measures. (See ref. 5.)

History: Case 2

Twelve hours prior to admission to an emergency room, an otherwise healthy 5-year-old male com-

plained to his mother of stomach pain and vomited. This was later followed by difficult, rapid breathing. He complained further of a "ringing" in his ears. His mother found an empty bottle of adult aspirin tablets and brought him to the emergency room.

On arrival, he was lethargic, but arousable. There were signs of dehydration. Physical examination revealed a rectal temperature of 102°F, the blood pressure was 110/65 mm Hg, the pulse rate was 120 beats/min, and respiratory rate was 45/min.

Laboratory findings are listed below:

Serum salicylate	= 61 mg%
Blood glucose	= 160 mg%
Pco_2	= 25 mm Hg
pH	= 7.30
HCO_3^-	= 15 mEq/L
Urine	= scanty; pH 5.3, 3+ ketonuria

Overall, this patient's condition was largely unremarkable and he survived following supportive therapy. (See ref. 23.)

Discussion

1. Patient 1 was given albumin by intravenous infusion. What was its purpose?

2. Comment on the dose of aspirin the victim in Case 1 supposedly received. Is this most likely all the aspirin he ingested? If it was, what were the complicating factors that caused his salicylate level to rise so high?

3. The victim in Case 2 may have taken a larger dose of salicylates than the other victim, but his blood salicylate was lower. Is this possible?

4. Was either patient in metabolic acidosis?

5. Patient 1 had a normal blood glucose level while patient 2 had a blood glucose reading that was above normal. What are the factors that influence this value, and why was there a difference in values?

CASE STUDY: SALICYLATE POISONING

History

A 22-year-old female who was feeling depressed the night before she was admitted to an emergency room consumed a full glass of vodka. She vomited throughout the night. The following morning her husband tried unsuccessfully to awaken her. He even immersed her in a cold bath.

At this time, he brought her to the emergency room where a physical examination revealed an unresponsive female with a blood pressure of 128/90 mm Hg, pulse 140 beats/min, temperature 102°F, and respiration rate of 40/min. She occasionally exhibited spontaneous movements of her extremities. Other physical findings were unremarkable.

The laboratory findings are included in Table 6. Information was later obtained to reveal that the patient had ingested approximately 250, 5-g (325 mg) aspirin tablets during the previous night.

Treatment. Treatment consisted of hydration and forced alkaline diuresis. As shown in Table 6, the serum salicylate concentration had decreased to below the toxic level after approximately one day. (See ref. 10.)

Discussion

1. Does the initial blood salicylate level correspond to the amount of aspirin tablets reportedly ingested as listed in Table 6? If not, can you give some reasons for the discrepancy?

2. Would the glassful of vodka have caused her clinical states? If she weighed 125 pounds, what would her maximum BAC have been? (See Chapter 4.)

3. Explain why this patient presented to the emergency room in an alkalotic state.

CASE STUDY: SALICYLIC ACID OINTMENT INTOXICATION

History

A 42-year-old male suffering from psoriasis used a 40% salicylic acid ointment to cover his hands and feet, and covered it with an occlusive polyethylene covering. A 2% salicylic acid ointment was used to treat affected areas on the rest of his body.

After the fourth application, all of which occurred within 24 hr, he developed malaise associated with deafness, flushing, and sweating. The serum salicylate concentration was 72%, and other laboratory results revealed metabolic acidosis. He had used a total of 300 g of 40% and 150 g of 2% salicylic acid.

The patient received forced alkaline diuresis and recovered without further incident. (See ref. 2.)

Discussion

1. List the substances that could be used to promote forced alkaline diuresis. How does alkalinization of the urine assist in promoting salicylate excretion?

CASE STUDIES: POISONING WITH ACETAMINOPHEN

History: Case 1

A 19-year-old female ingested a bottle of 30 Tylenol® Extra Strength tablets (500 mg acetaminophen). Sixteen hours after ingestion she was brought to the emergency room. She presented there with nausea, vomiting, and dizziness while standing. Her physical examination was unremarkable. She indicated she had taken no other medicine and her health was good. The serum acetaminophen concentration was 32 μg/ml. Other laboratory findings are shown in Table 7.

At this point, approximately 20 hr postingestion, the acetylcysteine protocol was initiated. Liver enzyme levels rapidly returned to normal. She continued to complain of abdominal discomfort and cramping.

Four days later, there were signs of kidney failure (see Table 7). She became lethargic, and her urine

TABLE 6. *Serum salicylate levels and state of consciousness, blood gases, and pH*

Hr after admission	Level of consciousness	Serum salicylate level (mg/100 ml)	P_{O_2}[a]	P_{CO_2}[a]	HCO_3^-[b]	pH
0	Comatose	140	113	21	17.5	7.54
4	Semicomatose	110	162	20	22	7.65
9	Awake-drowsy	94	121	22.5	19	7.55
15	Awake-drowsy	68	82	26	21	7.52
23	Awake-drowsy	46	91	29	24	7.53
32	Awake-alert	34				

[a]Expressed as mm Hg.
[b]Expressed as mEq/L.
From ref. 10.

TABLE 7. *Laboratory values associated with an acute acetaminophen overdose*

	Days after ingestion								
	1	2	3	4	5	6	8	13	18
Prothrombin time (sec, patient/control)	15/12	24/12	47/12	29/12	17/12	14/12	13/12	11/12	11/12
SGOT (U/ml)	197	910	3,000				50	30	40
SGPT (U/ml)	190	800	11,720	5,500			1,170	178	64
Alkaline phosphate (U/ml)	97								
LDH (U/ml)	261								
Bilirubin (mg/dl, total/direct)	2.5/1.5	4.2[a]	4.9[a]		3.6				
Creatinine (mg/dl)		0.7	1.0	N.D.[b]	6.0	8.1	11.3	3.5	1.2
BUN (mg/dl)	7	5	7		46	59	79	31	23
Sodium (mEq/L)	145					134	138	145	151
Potassium (mEq/L)	4.2					2.8	3.4	4.4	4.5
Chloride (mEq/L)	109					92	104	110	112
CO$_2$ (mEq/L)	12					13	9	20	23
Hemodialysis performed(X)							X		

[a]Total bilirubin only.
[b]Quantity of blood not sufficient for test.
From ref. 11.

output was diminished. Dialysis was started on the seventh hospital day because of signs of increased metabolic acidosis and azotemia. Two days later she entered the diuretic phase of acute tubular necrosis. Serum creatinine levels decreased over the next few days.

The patient was discharged about 2 weeks after hospitalization. (See ref. 11.)

History: Case 2

A 3-year, 4-month-old female was in otherwise good health except for a slight cough. Her mother administered a single oral dose of a cough preparation containing dextromethorphan hydrobromide. The next day the child told her mother she had taken some acetaminophen (Tylenol® tablets). She appeared in good health except for a slight weakness and unsteadiness while walking, and went to bed as usual. No other medications were given to the child.

The next morning the child awakened and complained of a headache. She vomited four times. She was pale and very lethargic.

On admission to the emergency room she was described as "shaky," lethargic, and sleepy. She also had decreased consciousness, was vomiting, and had hepatomegaly. There were no signs of liver disease, jaundice, or hepatitis. Physical examination revealed a normal pulse rate, blood pressure, and temperature. A presumptive diagnosis of Reye's syndrome was made and she was transferred to a larger medical center.

Physical examination revealed the same findings. Laboratory results revealed a hemoglobin content of 10.5 g% and WBC count of 10,800/cu mm with 80% banded neutrophils. Serum electrolytes, BUN, calcium, phosphate, and albumin levels were all within the normal limits. Blood glucose was 150 mg% and the ammonia concentration was 88 μg%.

A drug toxicology screen showed the presence of salicylate at 4.8 mg% and acetaminophen at 94 μg/ml. Table 8 lists the significant effects observed with the liver enzymes and prothrombin time for this patient until she was released on the seventh hospital day.

It was estimated, by the parents, that she had probably ingested about 35 acetaminophen tablets (325 mg each).

Treatment. The patient received intravenous fluids with glucose and hydrocortisone added. Acetylcysteine was not given.

This case is especially interesting from two standpoints. First, the enzyme levels (Table 8) were reported to be the highest ever reported by the hospital. Second, the young girl did not receive the standard antidotal protocol, but survived without apparent sequelae. Upon further examination, approximately 7 weeks after discharge, all hepatic enzyme levels were within normal limits. (See ref. 4.)

Discussion

1. In Case 1, there seemed to be more kidney toxicity than hepatic toxicity. The antidote was not

TABLE 8. *Laboratory values indicating the degree and time course of toxicity associated with acute acetaminophen intoxication*

Time after ingestion (days)	Acetaminophen (μg/ml)	SGOT (IU/ml)	SGPT (IU/ml)	LDH (IU/ml)	Prothrombin time (min)	Total bilirubin (mg%)
1	96	617	557	497	1.3	1.0
2	26	—	—	—	—	—
3		20,376	13,303	11,640	1.6	1.3
4		2,967	5,772	533	1.3	1.1
5		761	4,093	300	0.8	0.9
50		52	30	234		

From ref. 4.

even begun for 20 hr after ingestion. Is there any special reason for this?

2. Were the blood levels for acetaminophen in the two cases within the toxic or nontoxic range?

3. Would you have suspected hepatic coma in Case 2?

4. Based on the information presented in the history portion of these case studies, did both of these cases show signs and symptoms of all three phases of acetaminophen toxicity?

Review Questions

1. At what dose, expressed in mg/kg of body weight, are symptoms of toxicity following aspirin ingestion most likely to appear?

2. All of the following statements about aspirin-induced toxicity are true *except*:
   A. Salicylates increase oxygen consumption by increasing the cellular metabolic rate.
   B. Metabolic acidosis occurs, in part, when oxidative phosphorylation is uncoupled.
   C. Hyperglycemia is the usual outcome of chronic salicylism.
   D. The kidney attempts to compensate for decreasing H_2CO_3 levels by excreting HCO_3.

3. Define the terms hyperpnea and tachypnea.

4. Give the reasons why some attendant physicians recommend that activated charcoal is *not* to be given to a victim of toxic acetaminophen ingestion.

5. Following ingestion of a toxic acetaminophen

dose, at which of the following periods does hepatocellular toxicity begin?
   A. Stage I
   B. Stage II
   C. Stage III

6. Activated charcoal will effectively reduce absorption of acetaminophen.
   A. True
   B. False

7. Give the reasons why children are considered to be at greater risk than adults for aspirin toxicity.

8. Explain why a patient is in greater danger of serious toxicity from a toxic dose of acetaminophen if he has been using alcohol or barbiturates.

9. The Poison Prevention Packaging Act of 1970 has:
   A. Reduced the incidence of accidental aspirin poisoning.
   B. Had no influence on the incidence of accidental aspirin poisoning.

10. Which of the following is true about oil of wintergreen?
    A. One teaspoon contains approximately 4 g of salicylate
    B. One teaspoon is a potentially lethal dose to a child
    C. Both A and B are true
    D. Neither A nor B are true

11. Which of the following is contraindicated in treating acetylsalicylic acid toxic ingestion?
    A. Syrup of ipecac
    B. Oral fluids

C. Saline cathartics

D. None of the above

12. Blood levels of salicylate are detected more rapidly following ingestion of methyl salicylate than after aspirin.
    A. True
    B. False

13. Salicylate blood levels are considered to be lethal at the point when which of the following concentrations is exceeded?
    A. 45–64 mg%
    B. 65–90 mg%
    C. 90–120 mg%
    D. Greater than 120 mg%

14. Tinnitus is an early warning signal of aspirin and acetaminophen toxicity.
    A. True
    B. False

15. What drug treatment is given to the aspirin-intoxicated patient to treat acidosis?

16. To hasten elimination of salicylate from the blood, forced diuresis should be coupled with making the urine:
    A. Acidotic
    B. Alkaline

17. Discuss the reasons why potassium chloride is sometimes given to persons being treated for aspirin intoxication.

18. Which of the following can be given to antidote acetaminophen toxicity: glutathione (I), acetylcysteine (II), or L-methionine (III)?
    A. I only
    B. II only
    C. I and II only
    D. II and III only
    E. I, II, and III

19. What are the single, acute toxic doses of acetaminophen in children and adults?

20. It has been stated that acetaminophen is more toxic in children than adults, because children have a *more active* drug metabolizing system than adults. What is this system, and how significant is the above statement?

21. Cite at least two reasons why the chance for lethal toxicity is more potentially severe with acetaminophen than with aspirin.

22. At which of the following blood levels of salicylate are most patients considered to be asymptomatic?
    A. 45 mg%
    B. 55 mg%
    C. 65 mg%
    D. 75 mg%

23. Discuss the physiological event known as "compensated respiratory alkalosis" which occurs following a toxic ingestion of aspirin.

24. Discuss the factors which lead to salicylate-induced ketoacidosis. Would you expect the anion gap to be normal or increased?

25. The early toxic manifestations of salicylate poisoning are due to an action on the:
    A. CNS
    B. Heart
    C. Liver
    D. Kidney

References

1. Ambre, J., and Alexander, M. (1977): Liver toxicity after acetaminophen ingestion. Inadequacy of the dose estimate as an index of risk. *JAMA*, 238:500–501.
2. Anderson, J. A. R., and Ead, R. D. (1979): Percutaneous salicylate poisoning. *Clin. Exp. Dermatol.*, 4:349–351.
3. Anderson, R. J., Potts, D. E., Gabrow, P. A., Rumack, B. H., and Schrier, R. W. (1976): Unrecognized adult salicylate intoxication. *Ann. Int. Med.*, 85:745–748.
4. Arena, J. M., Rourk, M. H., and Sibrack, C. D. (1978): Acetaminophen: Report of an unusual poisoning. *Pediatrics*, 61:68–72.
5. Bender, K. J. (1975): Salicylate intoxication. *Drug Intell. Clin. Pharm.*, 9:350–360.
6. Clarke, S., and Walton, W. W. (1979): Effect of safety packaging on aspirin ingestion by children. *Pediatrics*, 63:687.
7. Done, A. K. (1960): Salicylate intoxication: Significance of measurements of salicylate in blood in cases of acute ingestion. *Pediatrics*, 26:800–807.
8. Feurstein, R. C., Finberg, C., and Fleishman, E. (1960): The use of acetazolamide in the therapy of salicylate poisoning. *Pediatrics*, 25:215–227.
9. Galinsky, R. E., and Levy, G. (1979): Effect of N-acetylcysteine on the pharmacokinetics of acetaminophen in rats. *Life Sci.*, 25:693–700.
10. James, S. H., and Martinak, J. F. (1975): Recovery

following massive self-poisoning with aspirin. *NY J. Med.*, 75:1512–1514.

11. Jeffery, W. J., and Lafferty, W. E. (1981): Acute renal failure after acetaminophen overdoses: Report of two cases. *Am. J. Hosp. Pharm.*, 36:1355–1358.

12. Keller, E. L. (1979): Poisoning in children—An approach for the primary physician. *Postgrad. Med.*, 65:177–186.

13. Koch-Weser, J. (1976): Acetaminophen. *N. Engl. J. Med.*, 295:1297–1300.

14. Levy, G., and Tsuchiya, T. (1972): Salicylate accumulation kinetics in man. *N. Engl. J. Med.*, 287:430–432.

15. Morgan, A. G., and Polak, A. (1971): Excretion of salicylate in salicylate poisoning. *Clin. Sci.*, 41:475–484.

16. North, D. S., Peterson, R. G., and Krenzeick, E. P. (1980): Effect of activated charcoal administration on acetylcysteine serum levels in humans. *Am. J. Hosp. Pharm.*, 38:1022–1024.

17. Peterson, R. G., and Rumack, B. H. (1981): Age as a variable in acetaminophen overdose. *Arch. Intern. Med.*, 141:390–393.

18. Prescott, L. F. (1981): Treatment of severe acetaminophen poisoning with intravenous acetylcysteine. *Arch. Intern. Med.*, 141:366–369.

19. Ruffalo, R. L., and Thompson, J. F. (1982): Cimeti-dine and acetylcysteine as antidote for acetaminophen overdose. *South. Med. J.*, 75:954–958.

20. Rumack, B. H., and Peterson, R. C. (1981): Acetaminophen overdose: 662 cases with evaluation of oral acetylcysteine treatment. *Arch. Intern. Med.*, 141:380–385.

21. Schwartz, W., and Oderda, G. M. (1981): Adsorption of oral antidotes for acetaminophen poisoning (methionine and *N*-acetylcysteine) by activated charcoal. *Clin. Toxicol.*, 18:283–290.

22. Sellers, E. M., and Freedman, F. (1981): Treatment of acetaminophen poisoning. *CMA Journal*, 125:827–829.

23. Snodgrass, W., Rumack, B. H., Peterson, R. G., and Holbrook, M. L. (1981): Salicylate toxicity following therapeutic doses in young children. *Clin. Toxicol.*, 18:247–259.

24. Spritz, N., Fahey, T., and Thompson, O. D. (1959): The use of extracorporeal hemodialysis in the treatment of salicylate intoxication in a 2-year-old child. *Pediatrics*, 23:540–543.

25. Strauss, J., and Nahas, G. G. (1960): The use of amine buffer (THAM) in treatment of acute salicylate intoxication. *Proc. Soc. Exp. Biol. Med.*, 105:348–351.

26. Temple, A. R. (1981): Acute and chronic effects of aspirin toxicity and their treatment. *Arch. Intern. Med.*, 141:364–369.

Narcotics

15

Generally, when we refer to overdoses of a narcotic, heroin (diacetylmorphine) is the first drug that comes to mind, and the victims are pictured as teenaged habitual abusers, of low socioeconomic status. This association is, of course, unjustified since victims of a narcotic overdose may be any age, represent all social and economic levels, and the drug may be illicit or legally obtained by prescription.

It does appear that even though the number of narcotics abusers (estimated at 500,000 Americans) (15) is high, the overall frequency of Emergency Department visits involving narcotic agents has leveled off in recent years. But this reversal has been somewhat offset by other semisynthetic and synthetic opiates which have gained popularity on the streets as illicit drugs of abuse. For example, we could cite the surge of "T's and Blues" abuse which began in the late 1970s, with the combining of pentazocine (Talwin®) and tripelennamine (Pyribenzamine®). Another example of "street" pharmacology is the combination of glutethimide (Doriden®) and codeine, commonly referred to as "loads." By combining narcotics and other centrally acting drugs, victims suffering from acute toxicity will definitely experience a greater array of symptoms than from typical heroin overdoses alone. Additionally, propoxyphene, diphenoxylate, codeine, and methadone continue to be encountered in acute narcotic intoxication, both from accidental ingestion of legitimate use, as well as from illicit use. An overdose involving any one of these "soft" narcotics can be just as life-threatening as an over-dose of morphine or heroin, and victims must receive the same heroic measures to assure their recovery.

Over the years, many attempts have been made to develop an analgesic compound that was just as potent and effective as morphine but without having significant depressant action on respiration, and one that was less likely to produce physical dependence. It was first anticipated that drugs such as methadone, pentazocine, propoxyphene, and meperidine would not be as addictive as morphine. Unfortunately, today these synthetic analgesics pose a significant national problem with chemical dependence and acute narcotic intoxication. Also, there is always the danger of accidental ingestion of these compounds. This is especially true for children of parents who are participating in a methadone maintenance program (2).

Another menace related to the street use of pharmaceutical preparations is the increase in fraudulent prescriptions for narcotics and an increase in thefts and burglaries of pharmacies and physicians' offices. The increased use of these narcotics seems to be related to the supplies and potency of heroin. In 1978, the purity of heroin on the street plunged to a concentration reported as low as approximately 2%. Although this is not the all-time low for street heroin potency, there was definitely an increase in the use of other narcotics such as pentazocine, hydromorphone, and meperidine.

The differences between the naturally occurring opiate alkaloids, semisynthetic, and synthetic opioids are minimal when dealing with an acute toxic episode. They are primarily related to the individual pharmacokinetic properties of the different narcotics. There are very few differences in the characteristic signs and symptoms of an acute narcotic overdose. When significant differences exist, these will be pointed out for that particular drug. As far as treatment is concerned, naloxone (Narcan®), a pure antagonist, will reverse the effects of all narcotic-related intoxications. The variability of the effectiveness of this antagonist is a function of the pharmacokinetic properties of the narcotic, and these differences will also be pointed out.

The naturally occurring and semisynthetic opiate alkaloids are derivatives of phenanthrene. Structural differences are noted in Table 1. The natural opium alkaloids have been used many centuries. The familiar dried exudate of the unripened seed pod of the Asian poppy plant, *Papaver somniferum*, contains at least 25 different alkaloids. The phenanthrene derivatives, morphine and codeine, are the two major naturally occurring opiates.

Acetylation of morphine at the C-3 and C-6 position will produce one of the most potent semisynthetic opiate alkaloids, heroin. Other semisynthetic derivatives of morphine include the morphones, e.g., hydromorphone (Dilaudid®); oxymorphone (Numorphan®); codones, e.g., hydrocodone (Hycodan®), and oxycodone (Percodan®) formed by oxidation of the alcoholic hydroxyl at the C-3 position to a keto group and saturation of the double bonds between C-7 and C-8 (7–8). It is interesting to note that by substituting an allyl group at the C-17 position to produce *N*-allyl-normorphine, an antagonist to morphine and other opiates is formed.

CODEINE

Codeine, or methylmorphine (Fig. 1), possesses analgesic and antitussive properties. It is less potent than morphine, i.e., 120 mg of injected codeine produces the same degree of analgesia as 10 mg of morphine. Also, tolerance does not develop as rapidly with codeine as compared to morphine. Therefore, codeine is less addictive.

Deaths, and even toxicity, due to codeine alone are infrequently encountered. The lethal dose is between 500 mg and 1.0 g. Codeine is usually taken in combination with other drugs, including analgesics, antihistamines, expectorants, or sedatives. Besides the legitimate pharmaceutical preparations available, users of illicit medications have also found that the combination of codeine with glutethimide taken orally may produce a euphoria comparable to heroin,

TABLE 1. *Naturally occurring and semisynthetic opiate alkaloids and antagonists*

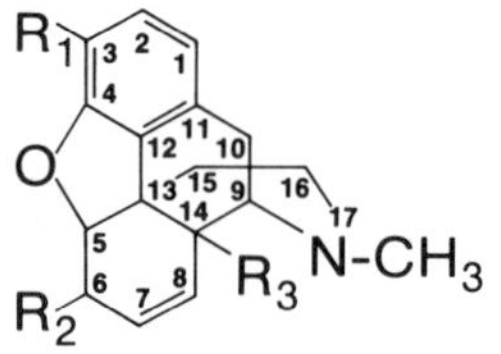

Phenanthrene Nucleus

	R_1	R_2	R_3	7,8
Morphine	$-OH$	$-OH$	$-H$	Present
Methylmorphine (Codeine)	$-O-CH_3$	$-OH$	$-H$	Absent
Hydrocodone (dihydrocodeinone)	$-O-CH_3$	$=O$	$-H$	Absent
Oxycodone	$-O-CH_3$	$=O$	$-OH$	Absent
Oxymorphone	$-OH$	$=O$	$-OH$	Absent
Hydromorphone	$-OH$	$=O$	$-H$	Absent
Diacetylmorphine (heroin)	$-O-\overset{\overset{O}{\|}}{C}-CH_3$	$-O-\overset{\overset{O}{\|}}{C}-CH_3$	$-H$	Present
Naloxone[a]	$-OH$	$=O$	$-OH$	Absent

[a] $C_{17}-CH_2-CH_2=CH_2$.

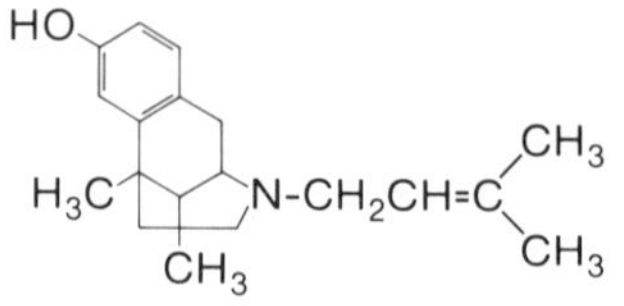

FIG. 1. Pentazocine structural formula.

lasting about 6 to 8 hr. Typically, two gluteth-imide tablets (1 g) and four codeine No. 4 tablets (240 mg) are referred to as "loads." Unlike "T's and Blues," "loads" are usually not injected, but taken orally. Street use of "loads" is increasing; thus, this combination should be added to the list of drugs commonly abused.

Acute intoxication may result in ataxia, slurred speech, nystagmus, and seizures. The more important consideration in ingestion of toxic quantities is the presence of glutethimide and its toxic manifestations, as will be discussed in Chapter 16.

Acute toxic ingestion of codeine causes the typical triad as seen with morphine: coma, pinpoint pupils, and respiratory depression.

DIPHENOXYLATE

Diphenoxylate (Table 2) is a meperidine congener that is used in combination with atropine in an antidiarrheal preparation (e.g., Lomotil®). The adult therapeutic dose is 20 mg daily, and 3 to 10 mg daily in children. Despite the fact that this preparation is not indicated for children under age 2, accidental and therapeutic intoxications from its ingestion continue to be a problem (20). Unfortunately, most people do not view diphenoxylate products as extremely toxic, so they leave them carelessly unattended on bedroom tables, bathroom shelves, or elsewhere where children have easy access to them.

There appears to be an extremely narrow dose range between therapeutic and toxic blood levels in children. While part of the toxicity problem with diphenoxylate products in children is due to the narcotic component, a large portion is due to the anticholinergic component, atropine. This is discussed in further detail in Chapter 17.

Acute intoxications, especially in children, are characterized primarily by the anticholinergic effects of atropine. These consist of hyperpyrexia, flushing of the skin, lethargy, hallucinations, urinary retention, and tachycardia. This phase is followed by miosis, respiratory depression, and coma due to the narcotic activity. Symptoms are highly variable and dose-dependent. The quantity of atropine contained in each

TABLE 2. *Synthetic opiates: phenylpiperidine type*

	R_1	R_2
Meperidine	−H	−CH₃
Alphaprodine	−CH₃	−CH₃
Diphenoxylate	−H	$-CH_2-CH_2-C-C{\equiv}N$

Lomotil® dose unit is considered to be subtherapeutic, although it will cause anticholinergic side effects. But these effects differ qualitatively depending on the dose ingested (see Chapter 17). Thus, a definitive statement about them cannot be made unless the dose is specified.

PENTAZOCINE

Pentazocine (Fig. 1), a benzomorphan derivative that is 3 to 4 times less potent than morphine as an analgesic, was expected to possess little or no abuse potential when initially studied and first marketed. Like so many other drugs that are marketed with the same hope, today there is little question of the abuse potential of pentazocine. Reports of addiction and abuse among narcotic addicts began to appear shortly after it was introduced into therapy (11). Its illicit use has continued to increase over the years (14). The manufacturer of Talwin® tablets introduced a new form of this oral medication early in 1983. Called Talwin-NX®, pentazocine is combined with naloxone, a narcotic antagonist. The objective is to inhibit the action of pentazocine if the tablets are dissolved and then injected. Naloxone is not normally absorbed from the gastrointestinal tract, so when taken orally, naloxone exerts no antagonistic pharmacological activity. However, when injected parenterally, they will cause withdrawal symptoms in narcotic-addicted abusers. Time will be the judge of how effective this new dosage formulation will deter pentazocine abuse.

A parenteral dose of 30 to 45 mg has the same analgesic actions as 10 mg of morphine or 75 to 100 mg of meperidine. The onset of clinical effects is 15 to 20 min following an intramuscular or subcutaneous injection, but only 2 to 3 min after an intravenous injection.

Pentazocine exerts its major actions on the CNS and smooth muscles. CNS effects include analgesia, sedation, and respiratory depression at doses of 20 to 30 mg. Parenteral doses of 60 to 90 mg may produce psychiatric disturbances including dysphoria, depression, confusion, and hallucinations (13). One report has shown a higher incidence of perceptual disturbances associated with the use of pentazocine than with other narcotic analgesics (1). The cardiovascular responses to pentazocine differ from those seen with opiates in that high doses cause an increase in blood pressure and heart rate, flushing, chills, and sweating. These effects may be because pentazocine causes an increase in blood concentrations of epinephrine and norepinephrine (23). Both tolerance and physical dependence have been reported with frequent and repeated use of pentazocine (12).

Chronic parenteral use of pentazocine may result in skin ulcerations which appear as deep and woody indurations distinguishable from skin lesions commonly seen resulting from other abused drugs. Severe cellulitis, ulcerations, abscesses, and muscle necrosis are commonly found among users of "T's and Blues" (7,21).

Combination With Tripelennamine

The antihistamine tripelennamine has had a long history of use among street addicts. It was therefore not unexpected to see it combined with paregoric, heroin, or morphine in mixtures known on the street as "blue velvet." Today, the practice of combining tripelennamine with pentazocine in a 2:1 or 3:1 ratio has gained popularity. The use of more than one or two antihistamine tablets increases the risk of seizures. This combination was first observed when heroin supplies were scarce and the purity of street heroin was low.

The tablets are dissolved in water, strained through cotton, and injected intravenously. There is an immediate "rush" similar to that of heroin which lasts about 5 to 10 min, and is followed by dysphoria which usually results in the person injecting a second dose. After three or four injections, the "rush" may be followed by a feeling of well-being lasting about 4 to 6 hr (7,21).

PROPOXYPHENE

Propoxyphene is a synthetic analog of methadone (Fig. 2) and, if taken in overdose, causes all the classic signs of narcotic poisoning. Both salt forms, the hydrochloride and napsylate, cause similar toxic problems. As with diphenoxylate-containing products, most people do not con-

sider propoxyphene to be dangerous. Physicians too frequently prescribe, and pharmacists dispense, large quantities for trivial pain without advising the recipient of the potential for toxicity. It is, however, estimated that approximately 5,000 cases of overdosing with propoxyphene occur in the United States each year, the same number as for codeine. Unlike codeine, the majority of its victims are adults, and it is a frequent means of committing suicide. Toxic doses for adults are stated to be 800 mg of the hydrochloride salt and 1,200 mg of the napsylate form. Cardiac and respiratory arrest have been reported with doses of 35 mg/kg (3,9).

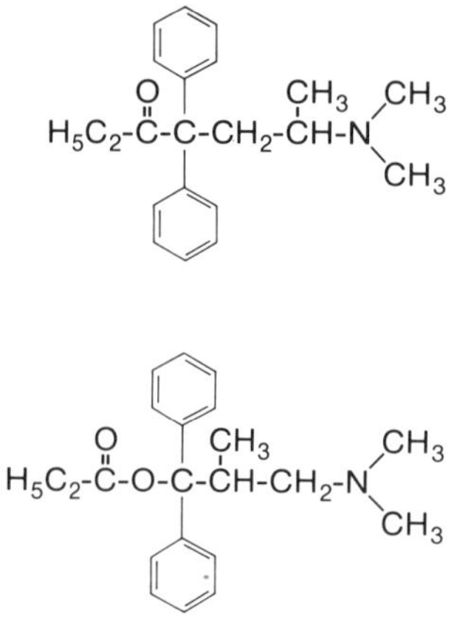

One special concern is when there is a toxic ingestion involving a product that also contains acetaminophen. Clinical symptoms caused by propoxyphene overdose may completely overshadow those of a toxic acetaminophen ingestion, leading to the sequel of events discussed in the previous chapter. The problem is magnified even more when the victim has previously taken ethanol, barbiturates, or other CNS depressants. This is frequently the case, especially when suicide is the intent (6,26). These agents stimulate the hepatic mixed-function oxidase enzymes responsible for converting acetaminophen to its toxic intermediate metabolite. They also potentiate the CNS sedative action of propoxyphene. The influence that ethanol exerts on propoxyphene toxicity, as shown by blood levels of propoxyphene at the time of death, is illustrated in Table 3. In this study, fatalities associated with ethanol consumption occurred

FIG. 2. Methadone *(above)* and propoxyphene *(below)* structural formulae.

TABLE 3. *Blood levels of propoxyphene with and without concurrent ethanol ingestion[a]*

Group	No.	Mean (mg/dl)	SD[b]
With ethanol	13	0.48	0.36
Without ethanol	22	0.72	0.39

[a]Blood levels represent total of drug plus its major metabolite, norpropoxyphene.
[b]SD = standard deviation.
From ref. 25.

at significantly lower blood levels of propoxyphene than when the alcohol was not present.

Propoxyphene is reportedly responsible for 30% of all drug overdose deaths in Britain, more than the total caused by all barbiturates combined (25). Over 90% of all deaths occurred outside the hospital, from 1 to 5 hr after ingestion of the fatal dose. Ethanol was present in the blood of 54% of the fatalities.

MECHANISMS OF TOXICITY AND CLINICAL MANIFESTATIONS OF ACUTE NARCOTIC POISONING

Although we have discussed a variety of narcotic analgesics in this chapter, they all have the potential for producing a toxic effect which is dependent on dose and route of administration. The mechanisms by which narcotics produce their toxic effects are similar, no matter if it is an overdose of morphine, codeine, propoxyphene, methadone, etc. In order to understand the reasons why these toxic effects occur, it is necessary to briefly review how narcotics produce their pharmacologic effects.

It has been postulated that the toxic effects of narcotics are related to the drugs' different actions at the various opiate receptors in the CNS. A listing of some narcotics with the receptor sites they are thought to affect is shown in Table 4 (10,17,18). The clinical responses of

analgesia, euphoria, respiratory depression, and miosis are believed to result from occupation of the μ-receptors. A different type of analgesia results when the κ-receptors are involved, and the psychogenic effects, such as dysphoria, delusions, and hallucinations, result from narcotic action at the σ-receptor.

Acute opiate toxicity may result from accidental overdosage in a heroin-dependent individual, or as the result of therapeutic overdosage from prescribed narcotic medications. Whatever the reason, the results and effects are basically the same. Trying to generalize the effects observed from acute opiate overdoses is a difficult task because of different people's individual variability to these drugs, and the rapid production of tolerance that occurs with the opiates. The most common characteristics are listed in Table 5.

The signs and symptoms associated with acute narcotic overdose usually begin within 20 to 30 min after oral ingestion, and within minutes following a parenteral route of administration.

The most significant effects observed with an acute opiate overdose involve its action on the CNS. Nausea and vomiting are also among the first symptoms noted. Vomiting results from stimulation of the chemoreceptor trigger zone and is less likely to occur if the victim is kept in the recumbent position.

The most obvious and severe toxic effect of narcotic overdose is central depression. The victim is usually asleep or in a stuporous condition following an acute overdose. The extent of CNS depression and its duration will vary according to the class of narcotic that is involved, the quantity of drug that has been taken,

TABLE 4. *Opioid receptors for possible toxic action*

Receptor	Narcotic	Clinical effect
μ	Morphine-like analgesics	Analgesia Euphoria Respiratory depression Miosis
κ	Pentazocine Nalorphine Cyclazocine (morphine-like analgesics may have some K activity) Levallorphan	Analgesia Sedation Miosis
σ	Pentazocine Cyclazocine Nalorphine	Dysphoria Delusions Hallucinations

From refs. 10, 17, and 18.

TABLE 5. *Characteristics of narcotic toxicity*

CNS depression—coma
Respiratory depression
Pulmonary edema
Hypothermia
Miosis
Bradycardia
Hypotension
Decreased urinary output
Decreased gastrointestinal motility

and the route of administration. For a large overdose, the victim will rapidly lapse into a coma and will not be arousable by verbal or painful stimuli.

It is believed that when narcotics bind to the specific opiate receptors, there is an alteration in the release of central neurotransmitters from afferent nerves, which are sensitive to noxious stimuli. The highest concentration of these receptors appears to be in the limbic system (22). This interaction on the limbic system with narcotics produces the euphoria, tranquility, and other mood alterations. On the other hand, the site of the sedative/hypnotic action is the sensory area of the cerebral cortex.

In an acute narcotic overdose, respiration will be severely depressed to a rate as low as 2–4/ min. Cyanosis will become apparent and many victims will have a frothy pulmonary edema. In humans, death from an acute narcotic overdose is almost always the result of respiratory arrest. When there is a high concentration of narcotic analgesics in the medulla and brainstem, there is a decrease in the sensitivity of the brainstem respiratory centers to increases in carbon dioxide, and, in the medulla, there is depression of the rhythmicity of respiration (8,24).

The respiratory depression observed with acute narcotic overdoses is further complicated by bradycardia and hypotension. There are two possible explanations for the decreased heart rate. One theory suggests that the narcotic analgesics stimulate the vagal centers. The other suggests that there is a selective depression of the supramedullary centers which can lead to suppression of autonomic reflexes. During an acute narcotic poisoning, blood pressure is normally not greatly affected. Hypotension usually occurs in the later stages of poisoning and is the result of hypoxia (8).

Pin-point pupils (miosis) are usually considered to be a classical sign of narcotic poisoning. Tolerance to miosis does not occur. In some narcotic overdoses, however, the pupils may not be constricted, due to asphyxial changes resulting from the decrease in pulmonary oxygen exchange. Therefore, they relax and become dilated.

The body temperature usually decreases and the skin feels cold and clammy. This is due to suppression of the hypothalamic heat-regulatory mechanisms. The skeletal muscles also become flaccid and sometimes the jaws relax, and the tongue may even fall back to block the airway. There is a decrease in urinary output which can be related to the release of antidiuretic hormone (ADH).

If a large overdose has been ingested rapidly, convulsions may occur due to stimulation of the cortex.

Gastric motility and tone of both the small and large intestines may be decreased, so severe constipation results.

Death, even in an addict, is almost always due to respiratory failure, complicated by such factors as pneumonia, shock, and pulmonary edema. The usual triad of coma, pin-point pupils, and depressed respiration strongly suggests an opiate overdose, but an accurate diagnosis also depends on the history of the individual and evidence of prior narcotic misuse.

TREATMENT OF NARCOTIC TOXICITY

Narcotic ingestion frequently delays gastric emptying. Thus, in an acute overdose situation, as long as the patient is alert, emesis should be performed. If symptoms of CNS depression or seizures are apparent, however, emesis should not be undertaken. Lavage is indicated for such persons, followed by a saline cathartic.

Since victims of narcotic overdoses are often comatose with depressed respiration when brought to the emergency department, the major objective in treatment of the narcotic-intoxicated patient is to maintain and support the vital functions. Therefore, the first step is to provide for adequate respiratory assistance and cardiovascular support.

Treatment of narcotic overdoses shows an example of a situation where a direct antagonist is available. The use of an antagonist brings about dramatic improvement in respiration within minutes after it is administered. Overall, the antagonist will reverse the depressant, analgesic, convulsant, psychotogenic, and dysphoric actions of narcotics (10).

Naloxone was the first pure antagonist discovered, and it is considered to be the drug of choice for treatment of all narcotic intoxications. It also reverses euphoria associated with narcotics and is generally safe even in large doses.

Levallorphan is an antagonist, but also a partial agonist. It can also reverse the respiratory depressant effects of the narcotic analgesics, with the exception of pentazocine. The major disadvantage, however, is that if it is given to a semicomatose or comatose individual, in whom the CNS depression is not due to a narcotic analgesic, or in whom depression is partially due to some other agent such as alcohol or barbiturates, it may produce additive effects that are similar to the narcotic analgesics. Consequently, it can further decrease the depressed respiration. Mixed poisonings are extremely common in many clinical settings. For this reason, naloxone is the preferred treatment.

The recommended initial dose of naloxone is 0.4 mg for adults and 0.01 mg/kg for children. Several doses may be given at 2- to 3-min intervals. If the CNS depression is due to a narcotic, coma and respiratory depression will be resolved within 1 to 2 min. If it is not due to a narcotic, naloxone will not worsen the existing condition. Since it has a short half-life of 60 to 90 min, and usually causes no ill effects in a patient without an opiate overdose, a 2-mg bolus may be given and, if necessary, repeated within 5 min. Twenty to 24 mg may be required for certain cases of opiate intoxication.

Table 6 lists the half-lives of the narcotics. It should be pointed out that for those narcotics with a long half-life, larger doses of naloxone are frequently required. For example, acute oral ingestion of toxic quantities of methadone or propoxyphene will be better antidoted by continuous infusion of naloxone rather than by bolus administration. The reasoning for continuous infusion of naloxone is based on the fact that respiratory depression may recur because of the short half-life of naloxone.

Comatose patients must be aroused as quickly as possible. If hypoxia persists and adequate tissue oxygenation is not achieved quickly, capillary damage followed by shock will occur.

Patients with pulmonary edema are at special high risk. Diuretics, digitalis, steroids, and antihistamines have all been recommended as supportive therapy. However, all are of doubtful efficacy.

Respiratory depression lasts much longer than the antagonistic effects of naloxone. Therefore, the patient must be closely monitored for at least the next 24 to 48 hr. If depressed respiration reappears, additional naloxone is necessary. Naloxone should ideally be used only to return respiration to normal. Other symptoms can usually be managed by other means. A victim of overdose who is breathing normally does not need naloxone.

SUMMARY

Narcotic use is centuries old, and shows few signs of becoming less popular. A significant number of Americans are involved in using these substances. Because of this popularity, poisoning occurs at a high rate. Symptoms are characteristic and death is common in persons who have taken a large quantity. But important symptoms of poisoning can and often do appear because the victim has ingested a normal dose of narcotic, but has also taken another drug or chemical that potentiates its effects. A specific antagonist is available to antidote narcotics. No similar item exists for symptomatic treatment of nonnarcotic depressants.

Case Studies

CASE STUDIES: NARCOTIC OVERDOSES

History: Case 1

A 19-year-old female with a history of psychiatric illness, weighing 70 kg, ingested 200 tablets of Codenal® (British dosage form) which contained a total dose of 2.3 g codeine base and 1.7 g phenobarbital.

TABLE 6. *Comparison of narcotic agents*

Narcotic	Equianalgesic dose (mg)	Plasma half-life (hr)	Blood levels		
			Therapeutic μg%	Toxic μg%	Lethal
Morphine	10	2.5–3	1–7	10–100	>400 μg%
Codeine	120	3–4	1–12	20–50	>60 μg% +>
Heroin	3–4	2.5–3	—	10–100	>400 μg%
Methadone	8–10	15 single dose 22–25 maintenance	30–100	200	>400 μg%
Propoxyphene	240	~12	5–20	30–60	80–200 μg%
Meperidine	80–100	3–4	30–100	500	1–3 mg%
Pentazocine	30–50	2–3	10–60	200–500	1–2 mg%
Hydromorphone	1.5	2–4	0.1–3	10–200	>300 μg%
Oxycodone	15	—	1–10	20–500	—

She arrived at an emergency facility in a deep coma with pin-point pupils and shallow respirations.

Treatment. The patient was given two intravenous injections of naloxone, 0.4 mg each dose, after which there was significant improvement in her respiratory status, and a slight dilation of the pupils. The gastric contents were found to contain large amounts of codeine. There was no quantitative codeine analysis reported for blood or urine.

The patient was further treated by a continuous drip of nalorphine, 0.7 μg/kg/min, but after 36 hr there was still no improvement in her neurological status. Naloxone was not available in sufficient quantity, which accounts for the change in medication. A 6-hr hemodialysis was unsuccessfully tried.

The nalorphine drip was discontinued 5 days later and her respiratory condition remained satisfactory. There were signs of brainstem damage, and the patient suddenly died during a convulsive crisis 10 days after admission. (See ref. 2.)

History: Case 2

A 2-year-old female was found playing in her father's briefcase about 4:00 p.m. He usually kept a container of Lomotil® (diphenoxylate) tablets in the case. The tablets were prescribed for him because of spastic colitis. At this point there were no indications that the child had tampered with her father's medication or that ingestion had actually occurred.

The child went to bed for the evening at 7:00 p.m., and at that time appeared to be "dopey." She awoke at 11:30 p.m., staggered into the living room with her arms and hands in a stiffened position, and collapsed. She turned blue, and it appeared as if she stopped breathing.

She arrived at the emergency room cyanotic with shallow, irregular respirations. Her temperature was normal, pupils constricted, reflexes brisk, and she displayed some catatonic-like behavior.

Treatment. Since there was the possibility that she had ingested some of the Lomotil®, she was given 1 mg nalorphine, after which she began to respond with normal respirations and the disappearance of the cyanosis. She later relapsed back into a comatose state and developed cyanosis. She was then given oxygen, and three additional 1-mg doses of nalorphine every half-hour. Again, she became conscious. A chest X-ray showed a mild infiltrate in the right lower lobe, and she developed a fever of 102°F. She was placed on antibiotic therapy. The patient was discharged the second hospital day.

It was later determined that the girl probably ingested about 25 Lomotil® tablets. Lomotil® contains 2.5 mg diphenoxylate hydrochloride and 0.025 mg atropine sulfate per tablet. (See ref. 4.)

History: Case 3

A 2-year-old female ingested 20 mg methadone hydrochloride which she had found in her baby sitter's purse. She was brought to the emergency room 3 hr after ingestion.

Physical examination revealed irregular respirations of 12/min, heart rate of 100 beats/min, and systolic blood pressure of 100 mm Hg. She was comatose and her pupils were constricted.

Laboratory findings included:

	On admission	2 hr later
P_{CO_2}	37 mm Hg	33 mm Hg
P_{O_2}	72 mm Hg	40 mm Hg
O$_2$ saturation	92%	70%
pH	7.31	7.29

Treatment. Treatment consisted of intravenous nalorphine hydrochloride and gastric lavage. Over an 8-hr period, the patient was given the antagonist seven times following bouts of CNS and respiratory depression. Each time nalorphine hydrochloride was given, there was prompt improvement in her respiration rate.

Eight hours after admission to the hospital, the child had spontaneous respirations. However, she then had respiratory problems and her breathing rate fell to 10/min. Again, she was given nalorphine hydrochloride and placed on a respirator. She was responsive within 10 min and her breathing rate increased to 18/min.

Bilateral infiltrates were noted on a chest X-ray. A tracheal aspirate sample was cultured and grew a coagulase-positive *Staphylococcus aureus*. Antibiotic therapy was initiated.

The victim was alert and respirations were stabilized by the third day. Because of legal problems (her father was a known addict currently serving a jail term because of assault on her mother; the mother was also serving a jail term because of contempt of court), she was not discharged until 15 days after admission. The child was readmitted 2 weeks later for lead poisoning. (See ref. 5.)

History: Case 4

A 21-year-old female with a history of heroin abuse and a participant in a methadone maintenance program was comatose when admitted to the emergency room. On admission she was covered with vomitus, there were needle marks present on both arms, and her pupils were pin-point but responsive to light. Respirations were shallow, the blood pressure was 86/30 mm Hg, the pulse 144 beats/min. A chest X-ray revealed pulmonary edema.

Laboratory results were as follows:

Na^+	= 130 mEq/L
K^+	= 5.1 mEq/L
Cl^-	= 97 mEq/L
CO_2 combining power	= 20 mEq/L
Glucose	= 409 mg%
P_{CO_2}	= 49 mm Hg
P_{O_2}	= 47 mm Hg
O_2 saturation	= 75%
pH	= 7.24

Treatment. Treatment consisted of oxygen, fluid replacement, insulin, and two ampules of naloxone hydrochloride (total of 0.8 mg) intravenously. The patient was alert almost immediately after injection of the antidote, but over the next 3 hr it was necessary to administer three additional bolus injections in order to maintain her responsiveness.

She was then started on naloxone intravenous infusion, 2.5 μg/kg/hr. It was necessary to continue this infusion for 30 hr. There was great improvement by the fifth hospital day at which time she was discharged. (See ref. 20.)

Discussion

1. Does the necessity for repeated or continuous doses of narcotic antagonist correlate to the type of narcotic involved?

2. What signs of narcotic intoxication were evident in all the case studies? Give a pharmacological reason for each of these signs.

3. In Case 2, what was the approximate quantity of narcotic ingested? What effect would the atropine have on the gastrointestinal tract? How does this affect the poisoned patient?

4. In Case 4, why was it especially necessary to administer naloxone by continuous intravenous infusion? Besides methadone, what other narcotic overdoses might need to be treated in this manner?

5. Patient 1 had a large amount of codeine in her stomach. Why was this not absorbed into the blood? Is it likely that her respiratory depression was due more to the phenobarbital rather than to the codeine she ingested? Why or why not?

CASE STUDIES: PROPOXYPHENE POISONING ALONE AND COMBINED WITH ACETAMINOPHEN

History: Case 1

A 19-month-old female ingested an unknown quantity of 65-mg-propoxyphene capsules. She was brought to a local emergency room 40 min later. On arrival the child was lethargic, rigid, and staring; her pupils were miotic. She experienced a generalized seizure and was given 2.5 mg diazepam, intramuscularly. She then had a respiratory arrest which required intubation. When she was administered 0.2 mg naloxone, she awoke from the coma.

She was transferred to a larger medical center; at this time propoxyphene was detected in the urine, but not in the blood. From time to time there were signs of increasing CNS depression, but this was easily overcome by giving another intramuscular dose of naloxone (0.2 mg). Within 10 min of each dose, she showed clinical improvement in vital signs, and her pupils returned to normal. She showed complete recovery 12 hr after ingestion. (See ref. 16.)

History: Case 2

In the previous chapter we learned that intoxication by multiple drugs was commonplace. This case study illustrates such a problem: poisoning by propoxyphene complicated by acetaminophen.

A 48-kg, 28-year-old female currently on a methadone maintenance program (80 mg methadone/day) stated that she had ingested about 90 tablets, each containing 100 mg propoxyphene napsylate and 650 mg acetaminophen. The patient went to bed but awoke 10 hr later and vomited five times. Nine hours later she was unresponsive and was brought to a local emergency room.

On admission, she was comatose but could move her extremities in response to painful stimuli. Her blood pressure was 100/70 mm Hg, her pulse was 60/min, and a rectal temperature of 88°F was recorded. Pupil size was 8 mm, and they were responsive to light. Coarse rhonchi were detected in both lungs.

Laboratory evaluation revealed the following drugs in a urine sample: propoxyphene, methadone, phenobarbital, secobarbital, pentobarbital, methaqualone, and salicylic acid.

Treatment. A bolus (2.8 mg) of naloxone was given without response. The stomach was lavaged with activated charcoal, followed by a magnesium citrate solution.

Acetylcysteine dosing was initiated 24 hr after drug ingestion, and repeated five additional times.

Hemodialysis was initiated at 36 hr and continued for 4 hr. Following this period, the patient awoke, appeared oriented, and was able to follow instructions. She was discharged 2 weeks after admission with no apparent residual hepatic or CNS involvement.

The admitting physician stated that the patient most likely absorbed the contents of the ingestion, because she did not vomit for 10 hr after ingestion. Also, her blood levels of acetaminophen and propoxyphene were consistent with the massive ingestion reported by the patient. (See ref. 19.)

Discussion

1. When respiratory depression is complicated by seizures (i.e., as the victim in Case 1 experienced), what is the additional problem encountered? Why was diazepam given to control seizures rather than a barbiturate?

2. Patient 2 survived in spite of all the reasons she should have succumbed. Comment on these (i.e., the dose, presence of barbiturates, 24-hr lapse before acetylcysteine was given, lack of response to initial naloxone dose, etc.). Why do you suppose she lived?

3. Which of Patient 2's symptoms were caused by acetaminophen, and which were caused by propoxyphene?

4. Is it probable that propoxyphene reduced the absorption of acetaminophen, or vice versa? If you answer yes, state why you arrived at that conclusion.

Review Questions

1. Discuss the major theories that attempt to explain why the heart rate is depressed following an acute narcotic overdose.

2. The most significant toxic effect from a narcotic overdose is an action on the CNS.
   A. True
   B. False

3. Explain why naloxone is sometimes given as an intravenous bolus and other times as an infusion. List each of the major narcotic derivatives and indicate the method the antidote would be given in case of overdose.

4. Emesis may or may not be indicated as a means to antidote a narcotic overdose. What is the major criterion used to determine this?

5. Ideally when naloxone is used to antidote narcotic poisoning, it is intended to bring about a single physiological response. What is that response?

6. All of the following symptoms are characteristic of narcotic overdose *except*:
   A. ataxia
   B. hypertension
   C. euphoria
   D. miosis

7. A victim of narcotic toxicity is reported to have dilated pupils. What is the origin of this response, and what is the person's probable prognosis?

8. Identify the expected contents of each of the following:
   A. "Loads"
   B. "T's and Blues"
   C. "Blue Velvet"

9. Signs and symptoms of acute narcotic overdose vary significantly depending on the specific agent responsible for the effect.

A. True
B. False

10. Several drugs have been available during previous years which have been advocated as narcotic antagonists. However, only naloxone has persisted and is still used. Discuss why this is so.

11. A victim of severe narcotic toxicity may receive diuretics and steroids as part of the antidoting process. Cite the reasons why each would be given.

12. Which of the following is true about the narcotic receptor sites? I. Respiratory depression results from stimulation of the κ (kappa)-receptor. II. Hallucinations result from stimulant action on the μ (mu)-receptor. III. Dysphoria is an outcome of narcotic action of the σ (sigma)-receptor.
    A. II only
    B. III only
    C. I and II only
    D. II and III only
    E. I, II, and III

13. Discuss why toxic ingestions of propoxyphene-acetaminophen combination products present a greater health hazard than ingestion of the same dose of either drug alone.

14. The reported toxic dose of propoxyphene hydrochloride is 500 mg.
    A. True
    B. False

15. Cite a reason why the toxic action of high doses of pentazocine on the cardiovascular system differs from other narcotics.

16. Pentazocine for oral administration is now marketed with naloxone combined into the tablet formulation. Discuss why a manufacturer would market an oral narcotic agent combined with a narcotic antagonist.

17. An acute toxic ingestion of Lomotil® causes symptoms of poisoning that are not generally seen with most other narcotic drugs. What are the reasons for these symptoms?

18. Which of the following is a true statement?
    A. Deaths due to codeine toxicity from overdose are a common occurrence.
    B. The synthetic narcotic derivatives are, as a general rule, less toxic than natural opiates.
    C. Propoxyphene is most closely related chemically and toxicologically to pentazocine.
    D. Pentazocine produces a lower incidence of perceptual disturbances than other narcotics.

References

1. Adverse Drug Reactions Advisory Committee (1980): Pentazocine and hallucinations. *Aust. Prescriber*, 5:22.
2. Aronow, R., Paul, S. D., and Woolley, P. V. (1972): Childhood poisoning—An unfortunate consequence of methadone availability. *JAMA*, 219:321–324.
3. Bogartz, L. J., and Miller, W. C. (1971): Pulmonary edema associated with propoxyphene intoxication. *JAMA*, 215:259.
4. Bradberry, J. C., and Roebel, M. A. (1981): Continuous infusion of naloxone in the treatment of narcotic overdose. *Drug. Intell. Clin. Pharm.*, 15:945–950.
5. Cardan, E. (1981): Fatal case of codeine poisoning. *Lancet*, 2:1313.
6. Carson, D. J. L., and Carson, E. D. (1977): Fatal dextropropoxyphene poisoning in Northern Ireland. *Lancet*, 1:894–897.
7. DeBard, M. L., and Jagger, J. A. (1981): "T's and B's"—Midwestern heroin substitute. *Clin. Toxicol.*, 18:1117–1123.
8. Eckenhoff, J. E., and Dech, S. V. (1960): The effects of narcotics and antagonists upon respiration and circulation in man: A review. *Clin. Pharmacol. Ther.*, 1:483–524.
9. Gary, N., Maher, J. F., DeMyttevaere, M. H., Liggero, S. H., Scott, K. G., Matusiak, W., and Schriener, G. E. (1968): Acute propoxyphene hydrochloride intoxication. *Arch. Intern. Med.*, 121:453.
10. Gilbert, P. E., and Martin, L. R. (1976): The effects of morphine and nalorphine-like drugs in the nondependent, morphine-dependent and cyclazocine-dependent chronic spinal dog. *J. Pharmacol. Exp. Ther.*, 196:66–82.
11. Inciardi, J. A., and Chambers, C. D. (1971): Patterns of pentazocine abuse and addiction. *NY State J. Med.*, 71:1727–1733.
12. Jasinski, D. R., Martin, W. R., and Hoeldtke, R. D. (1970): Effects of short- and long-term administration of pentazocine in man. *Clin. Pharmacol. Ther.*, 11:385–403.
13. Kand, F. J., and Pokorny, A. (1975): Mental and emotional disturbances with pentazocine (Talwin) use. *South. Med. J.*, 68:808–811.
14. Lahmeyer, H. W., and Steingold, R. G. (1980): Medical and psychiatric complications of pentazocine and tripelennamine abuse. *J. Clin. Psychiatry*, 41:275–278.
15. Levine, D. G. (1978): Alcohol and drug abuse. In: *Principles and Practice of Emergency Medicine*, Vol.

II, edited by G. R. Schwartz, P. Safar, J. H. Stone, P. B. Storey, and D. K. Wagner, pp. 1257–1272. Saunders, Philadelphia.

16. Lovejoy, F. H., Mitchell, A. A., and Goldman, P. (1974): The management of propoxyphene poisoning. *J. Pediatr.*, 85:78–100.

17. Martin, W. R. (1976): Naloxone. *Ann. Intern. Med.*, 85:765–768.

18. Martin, W. R., Jasinski, D. R., and Mansky, P. A. (1973): Naltrexone, an antagonist for the treatment of heroin dependence. *Arch. Gen. Psychiatry*, 428:784–791.

19. Pond, S. M., Tong, T. G., Kaysen, G. A., Menke, D. J., Galinsky, R. E., Roberts, S. M., and Levy, G. (1982): Massive intoxication with acetaminophen and propoxyphene: Unexpected survival and unusual pharmacokinetics of acetaminophen. *J. Toxicol. Clin. Toxicol.*, 19:1–16.

20. Rumack, B. H., and Temple, A. R. (1974): Lomotil poisoning. *Pediatrics*, 53:495–500.

21. Showalter, C. V. (1980): T's and Blues: Abuse of pentazocine and tripelennamine. *JAMA*, 244:1224–1225.

22. Simon, E. J., and Hiller, J. M. (1978): The opiate receptor. *Ann. Rev. Pharmacol. Toxicol.*, 18:371–394.

23. Tammisto, T., Jaatela, A., Nikki, P., and Takki, S. (1971): Effect of pentazocine and pethidine on plasma catecholamine levels. *Ann. Clin. Res.*, 3:22–29.

24. Weil, J. V. (1975): Diminished ventilatory response to hypoxia and hypercapnia after morphine in normal man. *N. Engl. J. Med.*, 292:1103–1106.

25. Whittington, R. M., and Barclay, A. D. (1981): The epidemiology of dextropropoxyphene (Distalgesic) overdose fatalities in Birmingham and the West Midlands. *J. Clin. Hosp. Pharm.*, 6:251–257.

26. Young, R. J., and Lawson, A. A. H. (1980): Distalgesic poisoning—cause for concern. *Br. Med. J.*, 1:1045–1046.

Central Nervous System Depressants

16

There are large numbers of drugs that possess CNS-depressant activity. This includes the many sedative-hypnotic drugs (Table 1). Additionally, dozens of other drugs are used for purposes other than inducing sedation, and hundreds of nondrug chemicals cause drowsiness and sedation of the CNS as a major component of their

TABLE 1. *Representative CNS depressants*

Barbiturates
  Amobarbital
  Amobarbital/secobarbital
  Butabarbital
  Pentobarbital
  Phenobarbital
  Secobarbital

Nonbarbiturate sedative/hypnotics
  Chloral hydrate
  Paraldehyde
  Bromides
  Ethinamate
  Meprobamate
  Ethchlorvynol
  Methyprylon
  Glutethimide
  Methaqualone

Benzodiazepines
  Alprazolam
  Chlordiazepoxide
  Clorazepate dipotassium
  Clorazepate monopotassium
  Chlorazepam
  Diazepam
  Halazepam
  Flurazepam
  Lorazepam
  Oxazepam
  Prazepam

toxicity. Thus, the category of CNS depressants is massive.

In this chapter, we will limit our primary discussion to drugs which are used for their sedative (antianxiety) and hypnotic (sleep-producing) effects. We have already discussed the alcohols and narcotics as examples of drugs that have strong CNS depressant activity. The antipsychotic drugs (e.g., phenothiazines) and antidepressants (e.g., tricyclics) will be covered in Chapters 17 and 18.

The medical uses of sedative-hypnotic drugs have changed markedly over the years. At one time, sedative drugs were "the only game in town" to treat a wide variety of medical afflictions ranging from minor anxiety and pain to epilepsy, hypertension, and psychosis. The drugs initially included opium, bromides, and alcohol, and were followed in time by the barbiturates, chloral hydrate, and meprobamate. More recently, the benzodiazepine derivatives have largely replaced all of these older drugs as sedative-hypnotic agents.

Many of the older sedative-type drugs are now, at most, of historical interest only. Use of others, such as meprobamate, methyprylon, and ethchlorvynol, has declined over the past decade, but they are still occasional causes of toxic overdose. Today, most sedative-hypnotic drug-related poisonings are caused by barbiturates or benzodiazepines. Whereas poisoning with a barbiturate is an intense medical emergency, benzodiazepine intoxication does not normally require the same marathon treatment procedures, and the victim has a greater chance of surviving. But as will be discussed later, poisoning with benzodiazepine derivatives still carries with it a great potential for toxicity. Regardless of the exact nature of the drugs that are the most frequent causes of poisoning, it is still useful to our overall understanding of the principles of management of the patient who is intoxicated with a CNS depressant to discuss certain parameters of the older compounds.

It cannot be disputed that Americans love to be sedated. Sedative-hypnotic drugs account for hundreds of millions of prescriptions written annually in the United States. If we add to this figure the many millions of illicit doses of depressant medications that are taken, and the tens of millions of alcoholic drinks that are consumed each year, the magnitude of the potential toxic problem becomes obvious. In terms of toxic potential, toxic emergencies from CNS sedation occur too frequently.

Major differences in pharmacological effects among the various classes of sedative-hypnotic drugs can be measured. However, the same general principles hold true for management of toxicity caused by all of them. This is also true for management of poisoning caused by most other drugs and chemicals that are not classed pharmacologically as sedative-hypnotics but, nevertheless, cause CNS sedation as a major toxic event.

SEDATIVE-HYPNOTIC DRUGS

A sedative is defined as a compound that calms anxious and restless individuals. A hypnotic causes drowsiness and facilitates sleep which is close to the normal pattern. An anesthetic, on the other hand, produces deep sleep that is unlike natural sleep. Whereas a person who is asleep from a hypnotic can be aroused, this is not possible with anesthesia-induced sleep.

In a practical sense, the major difference between the actions of these three pharmacological classes is the degree of CNS depression they cause, and this is related to the dose of drug taken. However, large doses of antianxiety drugs can cause anesthesia, and smaller doses of a general anesthetic may produce little more than mild sedation.

All of these agents produce similar effects on mood and consciousness. The precise toxicity profile for the CNS depressants is variable and depends not only on the dose and duration of action of the drug, but also on the mental state of the individual and the physical setting involved with the poisoning.

Barbiturates

At the turn of the 20th Century, bromides were the most popular and widely used drugs to treat anxiety and insomnia. With the synthesis of barbituric acid, bromides were soon replaced with a new class of drugs, the barbiturates. The barbiturates were divided into three groups based on their latency of onset and duration of action. The short-acting barbiturates have a duration of action of 4 to 6 hr, and include pentobarbital and secobarbital. The intermediate-acting barbiturates last 8 to 10 hr, and include amobarbital and butabarbital. The long-acting barbiturates, such as phenobarbital and barbital, have a duration of action of 12 to 24 hr. Differences in potency of various barbiturates are minor.

This classification system is for convenience only. The shortness of action of certain barbiturates cannot be equated with decreased toxicity potential. In fact, just the opposite is true! The shorter-acting drugs are more lipid-soluble and, hence, reach higher levels in the CNS faster and cause greater depression than phenobarbital. Furthermore, toxic blood levels of phenobarbital are more readily reduced by hemodialysis and forced alkaline diuresis than are similar levels of a short-acting barbiturate.

Not long after these agents were introduced, their potential for abuse was realized and became widespread. At the same time, there was an increase in acute poisonings due to barbiturates. Today, barbiturate poisonings are common in intentional (suicidal) poisonings, but are less frequently encountered in accidental poisoning. In fact, over 70% of the suicides that occur annually are related to barbiturate overdoses, either alone or with ethanol (6,16). Barbiturate overdose currently ranks as one of the leading causes of drug-related hospital admissions and death in the United States, as well as in many other countries around the world.

One of the reported contributors to barbiturate poisoning is an event known as "drug automatism." The individual consumes a prescribed dose and becomes drowsy. Later, not remembering that a previous dose(s) has been taken, he swallows a subsequent dose. This act may be repeated again and again until a lethal quantity has been consumed.

An interesting speculation is that the term "automatism" is often used by the medical community as a convenient excuse to explain why a victim of barbiturate intoxication died, rather than admitting it was a suicide (17).

Mechanism of Barbiturate Intoxication

The most prominent toxic effect of barbiturate overdose mimics a classic, progressive CNS depression. Even when taken in large anesthetic doses, peripheral effects are minimal. However, if barbiturate-induced coma persists, toxic sequelae to the cardiovascular, pulmonary, and other systems may occur.

Barbiturates primarily depress polysynaptic neuronal pathways, with monosynaptic pathways affected to a lesser extent. This action is believed to be due to a direct γ-aminobutyric acid (GABA)-like effect, or to stimulation of GABA release. GABA is an inhibitory neurotransmitter within the CNS. When GABA is released, a central depressant effect is noted. The effect of barbiturates on GABA appears to be similar to those of the benzodiazepines, except not all actions can be explained by this mechanism. Other mechanisms of activity including an interaction with norepinephrine and acetylcholine have also been proposed. The evidence for these actions being significant is not as convincing as it is for an interaction with GABA.

Respiratory depression is the major toxic event that follows barbiturate ingestion, and is the usual cause of early death. At a dose approximately three times greater than that needed for hypnosis, the body's neurogenic driving force for breathing is eliminated (11). Hypoxic and chemoreceptor forces are also depressed, so that the driving force is diverted to carotid and aortic bodies. With increasing doses of barbiturates, the hypoxic driving force becomes even less responsive and the remaining forces eventually fail to operate. This then contributes to the acid-base imbalances that are characteristic of barbiturate poisoning.

Hypothermia is another potentially serious problem that follows toxic ingestions of barbiturates. It potentiates acidosis, hypoxia, and shock. Lowered body temperature results from a direct depressant action on the brain's thermoregulatory center.

Sympathetic ganglia are depressed with larger doses of barbiturates. This may help explain why toxic doses cause a fall in blood pressure. Normal doses of barbiturates do not cause a significant effect on cardiovascular function aside from a slight lowering of blood pressure and heart rate, as would be expected during sleep.

High concentrations also have a direct myocardial suppressant action that results in a negative inotropy with reduced cardiac output (23). This, along with the effect on the sympathetic nervous system and developing anoxia from depressed respiration, helps to explain the origin of shock that results from large doses.

Other significant clinical features of barbiturate intoxication include decreased gastrointestinal motility and tone, which may lead to an increased amount of drug absorbed; and bullous lesions on the fingers, buttocks, and around the knees are also reported with glutethimide and methaqualone overdoses. These vesicles are reported to be present in up to 6% of all patients with acute barbiturate intoxications, and may be helpful in the diagnosis of an unconscious patient.

Recovery from toxicity is usually complete following prescribed antidotal methods. However, complications including hypostasis pneumonia, bronchopneumonia, lung abscesses, pulmonary and cerebral edema, circulatory collapse, irreversible renal shutdown, and neurological lesions may result (21). Such complications are the usual cause of delayed death.

Manifestations of Barbiturate Poisoning

Barbiturates are capable of producing a wide range of CNS effects varying from sedation to hypnosis to anesthesia, and eventually to complete paralysis of central voluntary and involuntary functions. The extent of paralysis is dependent primarily on the dose. Consequently, the severity of CNS depression following a barbiturate overdose is also a function of dose.

Barbiturate intoxication can be expected to occur when ten or more times the normal hypnotic dose is ingested at once. Of course, the normal hypnotic dose, and therefore the toxic dose, for the different classes of barbiturates will vary because of their differences in duration of action and lipid solubility. For example, the short-acting barbiturates are highly lipid-soluble and potentially more toxic than the long-acting barbiturates, which are less lipid-soluble. Victims of lethal doses of short-acting barbiturates are frequently dead when found, whereas those intoxicated with a comparable dose of a long-acting barbiturate generally die in the hospital. The normal hypnotic doses for barbiturates, as well as some pertinent pharmacokinetic parameters and therapeutic, toxic, and lethal blood concentrations are given in Table 2. Also, whether or not tolerance to barbiturates or to other depressants is present will modify anticipated toxicity and should be taken into consideration.

Barbiturate blood levels. Great caution should be exercised when attempting to relate blood concentration data to the degree of poisoning. It must be remembered that these are not absolute values but, rather, represent a range of blood concentrations which indicate a therapeutic, toxic, or lethal level. The blood barbiturate concentration obtained from a barbiturate-poisoned patient should not be the sole criterion for establishing the severity of barbiturate intoxication. This is better determined by the victim's clinical features, and a barbiturate blood level is usually used only to confirm that an excessive quantity of barbiturate has been ingested. However, if the clinical features indicate signs of severe CNS depression, but the laboratory results still show a low level of barbiturates, then this may be an indication that there is one or more other CNS-depressant drug also involved. The most likely offender is ethanol.

In addition, blood levels can be used to identify the specific barbiturate involved, which will aid in predicting the duration of the toxic effects. The progress of the poisoned patient can also be monitored by using blood levels. For example, the elimination kinetics for barbiturates following an acute overdose or even chronic abuse is not the same as for therapeutic doses.

TABLE 2. *Barbiturate classification system*

	Short-acting		Intermediate-acting		Long-acting	
Characteristics	Pentobarbital	Secobarbital	Amobarbital	Butabarbital	Phenobarbital	Barbital
Trade name	Nembutal	Seconal	Amytal	Butisol	Luminal	Veronal
Duration of action (hr)	6–8	4–6	8–10	8–10	12–24	12–24
Plasma half-life (hr)	23–40	20–28	14–42	34–42	24–140	—
Detoxification	Hepatic	Hepatic	Hepatic/renal	—	Renal	Renal
Hypnotic dose	50–100	100–200	50–200	100–200	100–200	300–500
Therapeutic drug level (mg %)	0.01–0.10	0.01–0.10	0.10–0.50	0.10–0.50	1.5–3.9	1.0
Toxic drug level (mg %)	0.70–1.0	0.70–1.0	1.0–3.0	1.0–3.0	4.0–6.0	6.0–8.0
Lethal drug level (mg %)	1.0 and >	1.0 and >	3.0 and >	3.0 and >	8.0–15.0 and >	10.0 and >
pKa	7.85–8.03	7.90	7.75	7.7	7.24	7.8

Therefore, by making use of serial blood sampling and measuring the concentration of barbiturate in each sample, we can determine if the elimination kinetics have changed.

Table 3 lists the various states of consciousness and responses of the poisoned patient. The blood levels given generally parallel the clinical manifestations. Once again, the same precautions must be exercised when using these blood levels.

Benzodiazepines

Because of the inherent dangers common to therapeutic and toxic doses of barbiturate and older nonbarbiturate sedative-hypnotic drugs, medical scientists have been actively developing drugs that would be as pharmacologically effective as the barbiturates, but possess a wider margin of safety. One of the outcomes of this research was the development of the benzodiazepine derivatives.

Thousands of derivatives of benzodiazepine have been synthesized and hundreds tested for their CNS-depressant effects. Approximately a dozen are employed in various forms of therapy in the United States (Table 1) and, today, they represent the single most widely used group of sedative drugs. Current research efforts are directed toward further refinement of these drugs.

TABLE 3. *Clinical manifestations of acute barbiturate intoxication*

Stage of consciousness	Degree of intoxication	Short-acting barbiturate (blood concentration) μg/ml
Alert	No signs of CNS depression	<6
Drowsy	All degrees of CNS depression between alert and stuporous	8
Stuporous	Markedly sedated but responsive to verbal or tactile stimuli	14
Coma 1 (Stage 1)	Responsive to painful stimuli but not to verbal or tactile stimuli; no disturbance in respiration or blood pressure	18
Coma 2 (Stage 2)	Unconscious, not responsive to painful stimuli; no disturbance in respiration or blood pressure	22
Coma 3 (Stage 3)	Unresponsive or abnormally responsive to painful stimuli; slow, shallow, spontaneous respirations with low, but adequate, blood pressure	26
Coma 4 (Stage 4)	Unresponsive or abnormally responsive to painful stimuli; apnea and inadequate respirations; inadequate blood pressure	34

From ref. 18.

It is doubtful that they will be replaced as a group for many years into the future. New benzodiazepines will continue to be added to the list.

This is a worthwhile pursuit since the benzodiazepines have a wide therapeutic index (see Chapter 1) and are the safest of all the sedative-hypnotic drugs. In other words, the range in dosage between their therapeutic dose and toxic or lethal dose is extremely broad. Increasing their dosage, even to massive amounts, will not cause general anesthesia as is the case with other sedative drugs (11). This feature reduces their overall potential for toxicity and makes overdosing with benzodiazepines much less of a problem than with the barbiturates or other nonbarbiturate depressants.

Mechanism of Benzodiazepine Toxicity

Most of the toxic symptoms of overdose by benzodiazepines result from sedative actions on the CNS. At extremely large doses, neuromuscular blockade may occur. Also, following intravenous injection, peripheral vasodilation causes a fall in blood pressure and shock may result.

Within the CNS, the benzodiazepines are selective for polysynaptic pathways. They inhibit presynaptic transmission by stimulating the inhibitory neurotransmitter, GABA. This action is believed to occur because the drugs antagonize a specific protein that normally inhibits the binding of GABA to its receptor site. This effect is also generalized, occurring throughout the CNS. While there is experimental evidence that suggests the benzodiazepines also stimulate or inhibit other brain neurotransmitters, there are more supportive arguments for its effect on GABA.

Respiration is not markedly affected, even with hypnotic doses of most benzodiazepines. Some derivatives may decrease alveolar ventilation (decreased P_{O_2}, increased P_{CO_2}) and thus, induce CO_2 narcosis in persons with preexisting compromised respiratory function (e.g., chronic obstructive pulmonary disease) (24). Benzodiazepines also may potentiate the respiratory depressant effect produced by other sedative drugs taken concomitantly (2,11). Most deaths associated with benzodiazepine overdose following oral ingestion have actually occurred in persons who concurrently ingested ethanol or other CNS-depressant drugs. Intravenous dosing has a greater associated risk of life-threatening hypotension and respiratory depression leading to death (3,7,22).

Characteristics of Benzodiazepine Intoxication

Signs and symptoms of benzodiazepine overdose are presented in Table 4. Effects on motor performance are more prominent than those on cognition. On occasion, severe paranoia, hallucinations, and hypomanic behavior are noted.

Even in large doses, benzodiazepines cause little more than Stage 0 or Stage 1 coma (see Chapter 3, Table 2). The patient can still be aroused. When the victim is not arousable, or cardiovascular and respiratory functions are severely depressed, some other depressant besides a benzodiazepine may also have been ingested (7,20). Serum benzodiazepine levels do not correlate well with toxic signs and symptoms. For diazepam, toxic levels are between 0.5 to 2.0 mg%.

Tolerance to benzodiazepines can occur following chronic ingestion. This may incite cross-tolerance to barbiturates, methaqualone, and ethanol (11). The same may be true for other drugs.

OTHER DEPRESSANTS

Another half-dozen or more CNS-depressant drugs constitute the remainder of the list of

TABLE 4. *Characteristics of benzodiazepine toxicity*

Mild	Moderate	Severe
Ataxia Drowsiness	Responds to verbal stimuli Coma, Stage 0–1	Responds only to deep pain Respiratory depression (rare) Hypotension (rare) Coma, Stage 1–2

those drugs which are still reported to be the occasional cause of toxicity. Toxicity reports involving all but methaqualone have declined in recent years. Methaqualone remains a popular drug of abuse and, consequently, it is a fairly frequent cause of toxicity. However, even it will become less of a problem in future years as it becomes more difficult to obtain on the illicit market.

Chloral Hydrate

Chloral hydrate, as well as chloral betaine and triclofos sodium, are potent CNS sedatives. Chloral hydrate is converted to its active metabolite, trichloroethanol. Chloral betaine and triclofos are converted to chloral hydrate and trichloroethanol, respectively. Chloral hydrate and the metabolites of chloral betaine and triclofos are lipid-soluble and readily enter the CNS. Poisoning resembles barbiturate intoxication. The LD_{50} for chloral hydrate in rats is 200–500 mg/kg. Significant toxicity occurs with doses >2 g, and lethal doses are between 5–10 g.

Chloral hydrate and ethanol in combination are referred to as the infamous "Mickey Finn." Whether the intense CNS depression that results is additive or synergistic to the depressants is not known. It has been suggested that each drug inhibits the metabolism of the other (11). If this is true, the overall effect may be more than additive. The corrosive action of chloral hydrate may cause gastritis, nausea, and vomiting. In addition, it has been shown to be nephrotoxic and hepatotoxic.

Glutethimide, Methyprylon, and Ethchlorvynol

Like other non-barbiturate CNS depressants, glutethimide, methyprylon, and ethchlorvynol produce toxic symptoms similar to barbiturate poisoning. However, these CNS depressants also have characteristic features which are somewhat distinct. For example, they produce significant fluctuations in the depth of coma and the duration of coma is markedly prolonged. Severe hypotension, respiratory depression, bradycardia, hypothermia, and pulmonary edema occur to greater extent than is typically noted with barbiturate poisoning. This probably occurs from a direct action on the vasomotor center. Complications of these actions include hypovolemia secondary to decreased peripheral resistance, and persistant acidosis.

In addition, glutethimide has significant anticholinergic actions resulting in mydriasis, blurred vision, dry mouth, constipation, and hyperthermia (following the initial hypothermia).

The cyclic fluctuation in the depth of coma and wakefulness following overdose with glutethimide may be due to its recycling in the enterohepatic circulation (4), or due to formation and accumulation of an active metabolite, 4-hydroxy-2-ethyl-2-phenyl-glutaramide. This metabolite has a long half-life, and is at least two times more potent than the parent compound (10). Another factor which is unique to glutethimide is that gastric motility may be reduced sufficiently due to its anticholinergic activity, permitting the drug to be metabolized. After a period of time, bowel activity returns and more of the drug is absorbed, and the cycle continues.

Meprobamate

With its introduction into medicine in the 1950s, meprobamate brought with it an alternative means to the barbiturates for reducing anxiety. For nearly two decades, until the advent of the benzodiazepines, meprobamate and its derivatives were the most commonly used nonbarbiturate antianxiety drugs. Meprobamate is not used to the same extent as it was formerly, but it is still a cause of toxicity.

The symptoms of meprobamate overdose are similar to those of barbiturates. Coma has been associated with blood levels between 10.0 to 20.0 mg% for meprobamate. The dosage range for severe toxicity is varied and is probably due to individual differences in the rate of metabolism. Death results from irreversible shock, respiratory depression, and pulmonary edema. Twelve grams was fatal in one instance, whereas other patients have survived doses as high as 40 g (1,13,25).

Victims of meprobamate overdoses have shown apparent recovery from toxic symptoms, only to die later. This may be because meprobamate is only slightly soluble in water and stable at gastric and intestinal pH. Also, the drug will decrease gastrointestinal motility. Thus, there is a great possibility for formation of masses of undissolved tablets (concretions). In some cases, gastrostomy may be necessary to remove these masses (14).

A major difference between meprobamate and barbiturates is that the former has a much wider therapeutic index.

Methaqualone

Methaqualone is a drug of wide abuse. Users of illicit methaqualone report that it increases their interpersonal relations and has aphrodisiac activity.

Its precise mechanism of toxicity is unknown. The depressant action is believed to be similar to that of barbiturates. However, because methaqualone does produce sensual effects that differ from barbiturates, at least part of the activity of these drugs differs. Mild toxic effects include hangover, headache, stupor, restlessness, dry mouth, and blurred vision. With severe overdoses of methaqualone, which are usually consistent with blood levels exceeding 3 mg%, coma is accompanied by pyramidal signs such as hypertomia, hyperreflexia, myoclonus, and convulsions. These effects are usually not observed with other sedative-hypnotic overdoses. Severe hypotension and pulmonary edema are usually absent with methaqualone intoxication, but hemorrhagic tendencies, due to inhibition of platelet aggregation, and peripheral neuropathies are frequently observed.

A distinguishing feature of meprobamate intoxication is the sudden unexpected appearance of hypotension which is due to a direct action of meprobamate on the vasomotor center in the brain. Such hypotension can result in significant decrease in cardiac output, irreversible shock, and cardiac arrhythmias.

Antihistamines

With the introduction in the 1940s of antihistamines into therapy, it was quickly realized that these drugs produced a variety of effects brought about by depression of the CNS. Sedation is the most common side effect in adults (Table 5); and, in massive doses, CNS depression leading to coma may result. However, additional symptoms that resemble anticholinergic actions also may be present. These include: mydriasis, flushing, fever, dry mouth, and blurred vision. Children usually experience central stimulation, with hallucinations, convulsions, and hyperpyrexia, rather than depression.

TREATMENT OF CNS-DEPRESSANT DRUG OVERDOSE

The treatment of CNS-depressant drug overdoses follows the same basic principles, regardless of the drug. Most clinical experience has accumulated with management of barbiturate intoxication. Barbiturate poisoning management is, therefore, the model we will use to help explain the principles of antidoting for all the other CNS depressants discussed in this chapter.

Today, the success rate in saving lives of individuals who ingest a toxic dose of a CNS depressant is such that fewer than 2% succumb. Unfortunately, this has not always been the case.

In the 1930s and 1940s, the primary treatment was directed toward heroic gastric lavage procedures followed by massive treatment with activated charcoal. This practice was replaced in the late 1940s and early 1950s with a protocol that called for administration of large doses of CNS stimulants (analeptics). These drugs in-

TABLE 5. *Characteristics of antihistamine toxicity*

CNS effects		Anticholinergic effects
Children	Adults	
Excitement	Disorientation	Dilated pupils
Tremors	Ataxia	Blurred vision
Hyperactivity	Dizziness	Tachycardia
Hallucinations	Sedation	Warm skin
Hyperreflexia	Coma	Dry mouth
Convulsions		Diminished bowel sounds
		Urinary retention

cluded bemegride (Tegimide®), ethamivan (Emivan®), nikethamide (Coramine®), and caffeine. Morbidity and mortality rates, even with this treatment, ran into the 40 to 50% range. These drugs stimulated respiration sufficiently, but they also increased the brain's demand for oxygen. Added to this was an increased chance for convulsions and cardiac arrhythmias. Today, analeptic drugs are not part of the conventional antidoting protocol.

Vasopressors were formerly given to elevate blood pressure. These agents can significantly reduce the vascular volume if the patient is already hypovolemic and, thus, lessen the victim's chance for survival. They are no longer recommended. Rather, cautious fluid replacement and inotropic agents such as dopamine and dobutamine are preferred.

In the 1960s the "Scandinavian Method" for antidoting barbiturate intoxication was developed because it was recognized that the two most significant pathophysiologic effects of CNS-depressant toxicity were hypoxia and shock. The method (Fig. 1), originating with Scandinavian physicians, stressed support of physio-logical systems, good nursing care, and no analeptic or vasopressor therapy.

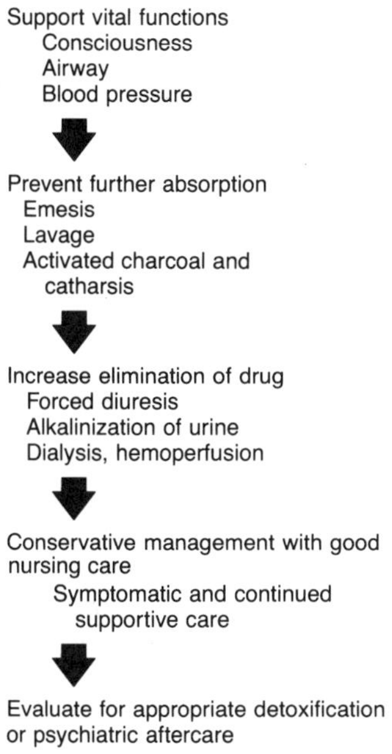

Antidoting Procedure

The highest priority in antidoting any victim of depressant poisoning is to stabilize the respiration and correct anoxia. All other procedures will be of little benefit if the brain suffers damage from insufficient oxygenation.

Oxygen should be given and the patient mechanically ventilated if needed. A cuffed endotracheal tube should be used in Stage 4 coma to decrease the risk of aspiration pneumonia during lavage. To help prevent hypostatic pneumonia, the victim should be frequently turned. Prophylactic antibiotic treatment was at first thought to be beneficial. Now it is considered unnecessary, and can even lead to superinfection. Also, analeptic drugs have no purpose for use in respiratory depression.

Since circulatory collapse is a major threat following ingestion of massive doses of CNS depressants, cardiovascular function must be quickly assessed and deficiencies corrected. The treatment of choice in circulatory shock is volume expansion and dopamine or dobutamine.

Renal failure is responsible for up to one-sixth of all deaths (11). Therefore, kidney function must be constantly monitored. Any signs of uremia may signal that hemoperfusion or hemodialysis is indicated.

Once the supportive measures have been established, blood and urine should be obtained for toxicologic analysis which can aid in the diagnosis and in evaluating the effectiveness of treatment.

Prevent Further Absorption of the Poison

We learned in Chapter 3 that emesis should not be induced in comatose individuals. However, if the victim of a depressant overdose is still alert, responsive, and the gag reflex is present, emesis with syrup of ipecac should be performed. Apomorphine is occasionally recommended based on its shorter time (several minutes at most) for onset of activity. However, because of the additive central depression it

Support vital functions
   Consciousness
   Airway
   Blood pressure

Prevent further absorption
   Emesis
   Lavage
   Activated charcoal and
     catharsis

Increase elimination of drug
   Forced diuresis
   Alkalinization of urine
   Dialysis, hemoperfusion

Conservative management with good nursing care
   Symptomatic and continued
     supportive care

Evaluate for appropriate detoxification or psychiatric aftercare

FIG. 1. Management of acute barbiturate poisoning.

causes, its use is associated with a greater risk for unsuccessful antidoting of the poisoned victim. Apomorphine-induced depression can be successfully terminated with naloxone, if necessary.

In the case of acute CNS depressant intoxication, syrup of ipecac must be given cautiously. Since 30 or more minutes may elapse before emesis occurs, a lethargic patient may become comatose while waiting for emesis to occur. This would increase the chance for aspiration.

In a comatose individual, or if less than 8 hr have elapsed since ingestion, gastric lavage should be considered. Lavage is usually performed with saline solution (castor oil may be used for glutethimide) until a clear return results.

With acute massive ingestion of phenobarbital, meprobamate, and glutethimide, gastric lavage should be repeated several times. If concretions are suspected, endoscopic lavage may be considered. A sample of the gastric aspirate should also be sent to the toxicology laboratory for analysis.

Activated charcoal adsorbs barbiturates as well as all other common CNS-depressant drugs. A slurry can be instilled into the stomach through a nasogastric tube and left there. A saline cathartic may be given to enhance elimination of the remaining drug.

Increase Excretion of Absorbed Drug

Increased excretion of absorbed drug may be accomplished by forced diuresis, dialysis, hemoperfusion, and repeated dosing with activated charcoal.

Forced diuresis, peritoneal dialysis, and hemodialysis are not generally effective in removing sufficient quantities of short-acting or intermediate acting barbiturates and benzodiazepines. Their excretion is enhanced somewhat, but the patient is not significantly benefited. However, forced alkaline diuresis and hemodialysis can effectively remove significant amounts of long-acting barbiturates and some of the non-barbiturate sedative-hypnotics discussed in this chapter (refer to Chapter 3, Tables 7 and 8).

Barbiturates are weak acids, varying from a pKa of 7.2 for phenobarbital, to secobarbital with a pKa value of 8.1. Thus, alkalinization will promote ionization of at least half of the drug in the glomerular filtrate and thus cause it to be excreted more readily. Only the long-acting barbiturates that are eliminated primarily via the renal system will be more significantly eliminated by alkalinization. The short- and intermediate-acting barbiturates rely more on hepatic metabolism for termination of their effects. Phenobarbital excretion is doubled with dialysis, versus a modest 35% increase for short-acting drugs (12).

Addition of 5% albumin or lipid (peanut oil, soybean oil, or cottonseed oil) to the dialysate may help elimination of those drugs that bind to albumin (e.g., short-acting barbiturates, benzodiazepines) or are lipid-soluble (e.g., glutethimide).

Neuvonen and Elonen (19) have shown that multiple doses of activated charcoal starting 10 hr after phenobarbital ingestion in healthy individuals significantly reduce blood levels. Whereas controls had a phenobarbital half-life of 110 hr, activated charcoal reduced this to 20 hr. Phenobarbital is excreted in the enterohepatic circulation (see Chapter 18). It is therefore possible that the charcoal interferes with barbiturate reabsorption. Other workers have also shown similar results with nasogastric administration of activated charcoal (5).

Hemoperfusion, using activated charcoal or a neutral exchange resin (e.g., XAD-2), effectively removes significant amounts of any of the CNS depressants discussed in this chapter. In some cases a greater efficiency may be obtained by using charcoal hemoperfusion over resin hemoperfusion, or vice versa. It must be remembered that these procedures are not without complications and should not be used indiscriminately. It may be beneficial at this time to review the guidelines for use of hemoperfusion as discussed in Chapter 3.

Other Measures

A number of other antidotal measures are also undertaken as needed. For example, if hypothermia is mild (rectal temperature down to 30°C), attention should be directed toward preventing further heat loss. The victim may be wrapped in a blanket and placed in a warm room. If hypothermia is severe (e.g., rectal temperature less than 30°C), the patient is young and otherwise healthy, and the condition is of recent onset, a more aggressive approach to reheating may be indicated, such as placing him in a warm water bath at 40°C.

For older persons, or when hypothermia has persisted over a prolonged period, a slower rewarming of the body is needed. Too rapid heating of the surface temperature may cause cardiac arrhythmias and circulatory failure. For these individuals, warming the inspired air may assist. Wrapping in blankets along with immersing one forearm in water warmed to 43°C has been shown to be effective (17).

An important component of treatment is to assure that victims receive good psychiatric help following their recovery. If the poisoning occurred because of illicit drug use, or was due to intentional overdosing, the situation may be repeated in the future.

SUMMARY

Intoxication with CNS depressants causes a series of predictable effects highlighted by respiratory failure and cardiovascular collapse. Although certain depressant drugs may produce other symptoms of toxicity that are characteristic to those drugs, none take precedence, when treating, over the two mentioned above.

Treatment should be directed toward maintenance of vital functions, prevention of further absorption, and reduction of blood levels of absorbed drug. Good nursing care is an important component of therapy. There are no specific antidotes for CNS depressant drugs.

Case Studies

CASE STUDIES: BARBITURATE OVERDOSE

History: Case 1

A 55-year-old female was found in a deep coma after she had ingested an estimated 30 capsules of a sedative preparation, each containing 100 mg pentobarbital sodium and 260 mg carbromal.

On admission to the hospital, her blood pressure was 80/60 mm Hg, the pulse was 80 beats/min, and respirations were 20/min and shallow. Her pupils were dilated and fixed, no reflexes were present, and she was totally unresponsive to commands or stimuli. She was intubated and kept on a respirator. Large vesicles and bullae containing a clear fluid were present on the dorsal surface of her hands, around both knees, and on her heels.

The initial serum barbiturate blood level was 4.3 mg%. Her condition was deteriorating and respiratory acidosis appeared, so hemodialysis was instituted. After two sessions of 8 to 9 hr each, she awoke on the third hospital day. At this point she was able to breathe without the aid of a respirator. She made an uneventful recovery and was released about 2 weeks after admission.

At the time of this patient's discharge, the skin lesions were healed. The physicians who reported on this case observed that barbiturate was present in these blisters, and implied that the drug had irritated the skin capillaries to cause vesicle formation. However, similar blister formation has also been noted following poisoning with a variety of sedative drugs and chemicals including carbon monoxide. It thus appears that this symptom is nonspecific and should not be used to differentiate one drug from another when attempting to define the nature of the poison. (See ref. 5.)

History: Case 2

A 22-year-old female, who had a history of generalized seizures and schizophrenia, ingested an undetermined quantity of phenobarbital. She had also been taking fluphenazine hydrochloride and benztropine mesylate for her medical conditions. She presented to the emergency room in a comatose state responding only to painful stimuli. Her blood pressure was 110/60 mm Hg, the pulse was 102 beats/min, and the rectal temperature was 37.3°C. Intravenous fluids were instituted. Her respiration was supported artificially.

She was intubated with an endotracheal tube and given gastric lavage. With the nasogastric tube in place, 40 g activated charcoal was administered followed by 20 g sodium sulfate. Activated charcoal (40 g) and magnesium citrate (60 ml) were administered every 4 hr for five additional doses.

Toxicological analysis of the blood for alcohol and other drugs was negative except for phenobarbital.

The initial blood phenobarbital level of 141 μg/ml dropped to 47 μg/ml within 24 hr, during which time her clinical condition rapidly improved. (See ref. 9.)

Discussion

1. A common symptom of severe intoxication with sedative drugs is mydriasis (dilated pupils). This was reported for Patient 1. Why do you think this event occurs? When present, what is the patient's probable prognosis if heroic treatment is not given?

2. The bullous skin lesions present in Patient 1 contained barbiturate. Why should this not surprise you?

3. Patient 2 received an initial dose of sodium sulfate, and magnesium citrate every 4 hr. What was the purpose of these?

CASE STUDY: UNEXPECTED DEATH FROM MEPROBAMATE

History

A 51-year-old female was found unconscious by her husband, after she supposedly ingested 50 400-mg meprobamate tablets. She was a known alcoholic and had previously attempted suicide. Additionally, she was an asthmatic and her medications included prednisone, bronchodilators, and multiple tranquilizers. When she arrived at the hospital, she was unconscious, all reflexes were absent, and she responded only to deep pain. Her blood pressure was 110/60 mm Hg.

Gastric lavage was immediately initiated. Three liters of fluid were necessary before the returned lavage solution failed to show the presence of a white cloudy substance. Gastric lavage was again repeated on two separate occasions, and both resulted in a negligible return of ingested drug.

Further treatment was supportive in nature and 10 hr after she was found unconscious, she was able to speak clearly, her deep-tendon reflexes were normal, and her blood pressure was 140/90 mm Hg.

Toxicological analysis of her blood revealed an initial meprobamate concentration of 14.4 mg%. It was later learned that she had actually ingested 95 400-mg meprobamate tablets, or approximately 38 g of drug.

She continued to show signs of improvement throughout the second hospital day, and at midnight she was resting comfortably. Her blood pressure was 140/80 mm Hg. However, at 1:30 a.m., she was

found unconscious, cyanotic, and with no pulse or respiration. Attempts to revive her were unsuccessful.

Postmortem findings initially provided no evidence or pathological explanation for her death, and why she revealed a moderate degree of pulmonary edema and visceral congestion. Postmortem meprobamate levels included: blood, 18.0 mg%; brain, 14 mg%; kidney, 50 mg%; liver, 30 mg%; and total stomach contents, 25 g. It was then that a large white mass was found in her stomach. (See ref. 14.)

Discussion

1. Why did this patient die? (Hint: What did you learn in Chapter 3 concerning concretion of ingested drugs?)

CASE STUDY: METHYPRYLON INTOXICATION

History

A 57-year-old female was admitted to the hospital after she ingested 22.5 g of methyprylon, 2 to 12 hr previously. She was deeply comatose and not responding to painful stimuli. All reflexes were absent, except for a weak pupillary response to light. Vital signs included: blood pressure, 60/32 mm Hg; pulse rate, 68 beats/min; respirations were slow and shallow.

Treatment was instituted with gastric lavage, during which time the victim's systolic pressure dropped to 30 mm Hg and respirations ceased. She was rapidly intubated, and breathing was maintained with the aid of a respirator. Her blood pressure returned to normal with metaraminol bitartrate (Aramine®).

In order to initiate forced diuresis, hypertonic mannitol and furosemide were given. Intravenous fluids consisting of 5% dextrose and 0.45% saline with potassium chloride were continued.

Four hours after admission, hemodialysis was instituted and within 2 hr following the dialysis procedure, the patient's corneal and deep-tendon reflexes showed signs of responding. Dialysis was continued for another 6.5 hr when a slight muscular twitching movement was noted. She was given phenytoin and diazepam to control these myoclonic movements. The patient also began to breathe and move spontaneously.

The initial methyprylon blood level was 20.9 mg%. Five hours later it was 9.2 mg%, and following dialysis, it was 3.0 mg%. The quantity of drug recovered by gastric lavage was 4.3 g, or about 20% of the ingested dose. It was also estimated that the amount of drug eliminated during the 8.5-hr dialysis period was 3.6 g, which accounted for another 20% of the ingested dose. Approximately 600 mg of drug were excreted in the urine, which accounted for less than 5% of the ingested dose.

By 18 hr after admission, she was fully awake, aware of her environment, and attempting to talk. Over the next few days she remained confused and was treated with meprobamate for suspected withdrawal reactions. The confused state gradually cleared, and she was discharged on the 12th hospital day. (See ref. 15.)

Discussion

1. This patient was recovering from poisoning induced by a CNS sedative, when she was given diazepam, another sedative. Comment on the use of such a therapeutic measure.

CASE STUDIES: MASSIVE DIAZEPAM OVERDOSE

History: Case 1

A 61-year-old female was admitted to the hospital approximately 8 hr following ingestion of 450 to 500 mg diazepam. She was receiving chemotherapy for multiple myeloma, and imipramine for depression, and her drug overdose was an attempt at suicide. On admission, her blood pressure was 110/80 mm Hg, the heart rate was 75 to 80 beats/min, and respirations were 20/min. She was visibly depressed and responsive only to noxious stimuli. Laboratory test results were within the normal limits.

The cause of her intoxication was not initially apparent. Symptoms did not implicate imipramine as the source.

Treatment began with administration of naloxone hydrochloride (Narcan®), 0.4 mg, and 50% dextrose to which she showed no signs of improvement. She was therefore placed under constant monitoring, and further treatment was nonspecific. Fluid administration continued. Other than an isolated incidence of mild hypotension (90/50 mm Hg) which soon resolved, there were no major changes in her clinical state.

She was fully alert and responsive 24 hr after admission and was discharged the following day with no apparent complications. (See ref. 8.)

History: Case 2

A 28-year-old male was brought to the hospital approximately 10 hr after ingesting 2,000 mg diazepam. His vital signs included: blood pressure, 100/60 mm Hg; heart rate, 68 beats/min, and respirations, 16/min. He was responsive to verbal stimuli, and was oriented to time, place, and person.

All laboratory test results were within the normal physiological limits. The initial blood diazepam concentration was approximately 20 μg/ml, which is at least 40 times the minimal effective drug concentration, and this level remained elevated well above the normal therapeutic level for approximately 4 to 5 days.

The patient's initial treatment consisted of intravenously administered 50% dextrose, and naloxone hydrochloride, 0.4 mg, to which his condition did not improve. He was then placed under observation and vital signs were monitored. He was responsive and fully alert within 2 days after ingestion, at which time he was transferred to a psychiatric ward for further evaluation.

Discussion

1. Does it not seem strange that both patients survived these otherwise massive doses of drug? If you disagree, explain why. In neither case did spontaneous emesis occur, nor was it induced. Thus, both victims probably did absorb the entire amount ingested.

2. Why was naloxone used in the initial treatment of both patients? Why was dextrose given?

3. Even though recovery was rapid for Patient 2, diazepam blood levels remained elevated well above the therapeutic range for several days. Why was he fully recovered long before his blood levels were in the therapeutic range (i.e., what factor may account for this discrepancy)?

Review Questions

1. Discuss the meaning of the terms hypnotic and sedative. What can be said about their relative ease at which they may cause a serious toxicity problem?

2. List the important nondrug related factors that must be considered when assessing the probable response that a person will show to an overdose of depressant drug.

3. Which of the following is a true statement?
    A. Most barbiturate poisonings occur by accidental ingestion.
    B. Barbiturates work by blocking GABA release within the brain.
    C. Hypothermia from low-dose barbiturate poisoning occurs by a direct peripheral action on the arterioles.
    D. Barbiturate intoxication occurs when ten or more times the therapeutic dose is ingested.

4. The short-acting barbiturates are said to be more potentially toxic than the long-acting ones. Cite the reasons why this is true.

5. Define the role of GABA in CNS-depressant intoxications. How is GABA classed physiologically and chemically?

6. Hemodialysis would have the greatest effect on reducing blood levels of which of the following?
    A. Secobarbital
    B. Phenobarbital
    C. Pentobarbital
    D. Butabarbital

7. Phenobarbital overdose is best antidoted by forced diuresis that is:
    A. alkaline
    B. acidic

8. Discuss the events that occur to cause the respiration rate to decrease when barbiturates are taken in overdose.

9. Which of the following CNS depressants has the widest therapeutic index?
    A. Methaqualone
    B. Meprobamate
    C. Diazepam
    D. Glutethimide

10. A victim of barbiturate intoxication who is unconscious and not responsive to pain, but has no disturbance in respiration or blood pressure is in which of the following stages?
    A. Coma 1
    B. Coma 2
    C. Coma 3
    D. Coma 4

11. Give a reason why barbiturate-induced skin bullous lesions appear following toxicity. How reliable is their appearance as a diagnostic aid to confirm that poisoning was caused by a barbiturate?

12. Discuss the reliability in using blood levels of barbiturates as a predictor for determining the severity of poisoning.

13. All of the following statements are true about benzodiazepines except:
    A. They are the single most widely used group of CNS sedatives.
    B. Benzodiazepines selectively depress polysynaptic pathways within the CNS.
    C. Effects of benzodiazepine overdose are more prominent on cognition than on motor function.
    D. Cross-tolerance with ethanol and barbiturates may occur.

14. In toxic doses, benzodiazepines depress the respiratory rate to the same extent as equivalent doses of barbiturates.
    A. True
    B. False

15. Cite the reasons expressed in the chapter as to why overdoses of glutethimide induce a cyclic fluctuation in depth of coma.

16. A victim of poisoning with a "Mickey Finn" has ingested a combination of ethanol and:
    A. meprobamate
    B. phenobarbital
    C. chloral hydrate
    D. methaqualone

17. List the various steps that comprise the Scandinavian method for treating CNS-depressant toxicity. What is the purpose of each?

18. Which of the following depressants has significant anticholinergic activity that may require separate antidoting when the drug is taken in toxic overdose?
    A. Meprobamate
    B. Methaqualone
    C. Glutethimide
    D. Pentobarbital

19. All of the following are true statements except:
    A. Prophylactic antibiotic therapy is the treatment for barbiturate poisoning.
    B. Repeated doses of activated charcoal for a day or so after phenobarbital will help lower the blood level of barbiturate.

C. Hypothermia of 30°C may be treated by immersing the patient in water warmed to 40°C.

D. Saline catharsis is beneficial in treating CNS-depressant toxicity.

20. Identify the disadvantages of giving analeptic drugs to CNS-depressant-intoxicated patients.

21. Cite the advantages and disadvantages of using apomorphine to induce emesis following a toxic barbiturate ingestion.

References

1. Allen, M. D., Greenblatt, D. J., and Noel, B. J. (1977): Meprobamate overdosage: A continuing problem. *Clin. Toxicol.*, 11:501–515.

2. Ascione, F. J. (1978): Benzodiazepines with alcohol. *Drug Ther.*, 9:58–71.

3. Baker, A. B. (1969): Induction of anesthesia with diazepam. *Anesthesia*, 24:388–394.

4. Decker, W. J., Thompson, H. L., and Arnesson, L. A. (1970): Glutethimide rebound. *Lancet*, 1:778–779.

5. Goldberg, M. J., and Berlinger, W. G. (1982): Treatment of phenobarbital overdose with activated charcoal. *JAMA*, 247:2400–2401.

6. Goldfrank, L., and Osborn, H. (1982): Barbiturates. In: *Toxicologic Emergencies*, edited by L. S. Goldfrank, pp. 147–152. Appleton-Century-Crofts, New York.

7. Greenblatt, D. J., Allen, M. D., Noel, B. J., and Shader, R. I. (1977): Acute overdosages with benzodiazepine derivatives. *Clin. Pharmacol. Ther.*, 21:497–514.

8. Greenblatt, D. J., Woo, E., Allen, M. D., Orsulak, P. J., and Shader, R. I. (1978): Rapid recovery from massive diazepam overdose. *JAMA*, 240:1872–1874.

9. Groschel, D., Gerstein, A. R., and Rosenbaum, J. M. (1970): Skin lesions as a diagnostic aid in barbiturate poisoning. *N. Engl. J. Med.*, 283:409–410.

10. Hansen, A. R., Kennedy, K. A., Ambre, J. J., and Fischer, L. J. (1975): Glutethimide poisoning: A metabolite contributes to morbidity and mortality. *N. Engl. J. Med.*, 292:250–252.

11. Harvey, S. C. (1980): Hypnotics and sedatives. In: *The Pharmacological Basis of Therapeutics*, 6th ed., edited by A. G. Gilman, L. S. Goodman, and A. Gilman, pp. 339–375. Macmillan, New York.

12. Henderson, L. W., and Merrill, J. P. (1966): Treatment of barbiturate intoxication. *Ann. Intern. Med.*, 64:876–891.

13. Hilstand, E. C. (1956): Overdosage with meprobamate. *Ohio State Med. J.*, 52:1306–1307.

14. Jenis, E. H., Payne, R. J., and Goldbaum, L. R. (1969): Acute meprobamate poisoning: A fatal case following a lucid interval. *JAMA*, 207:361–362.

15. Mandelbaum, J. M., and Simon, N. M. (1971): Severe methyprylon intoxication treated by hemodialysis. *JAMA*, 216:139–140.

16. Matthew, H. (1975): Barbiturates. *Clin. Toxicol.*, 8:495–513.

17. Matthew, H., and Lawson, A. H. (1979): *Treatment of Common Acute Poisonings*, 4th ed. Churchill Livingstone, New York.

18. McCarron, M. M., Schulze, B. W., Walberg, C. B., Thompson, G. A., and Ansari, A. (1982): Short-acting barbiturate overdosage: Correlation of intoxication score with serum barbiturate concentration. *JAMA*, 248:55–61.

19. Neuvonen, P. J., and Elonen, E. (1980): Effect of activated charcoal on absorption and elimination of phenobarbitone, carbamazepine and phenylbutazone in man. *Eur. J. Clin. Pharmacol.*, 17:51–57.

20. Palmer, G. C. (1978): Use, overuse, misuse, and abuse of benzodiazepines. *Ala. J. Med. Sci.*, 15:383–392.

21. Plum, F., and Swanson, A. G. (1957): Barbiturate poisoning treated by physiological methods with observations on effects of betamethylethylglutarimide and electrical stimulation. *JAMA*, 163:827–835.

22. Prensky, A. L., Raff, M. C., Moore, M. J., and Schwab, R. S. (1967): Intravenous diazepam in the treatment of prolonged seizure activity. *N. Engl. J. Med.*, 276:779–784.

23. Price, H. L. (1960): General anesthesia and circulatory homeostasis. *Physiol. Rev.*, 40:189–218.

24. Rao, S., Sherbaniuk, R. W., Prasad, K., Lee, S. J. K., and Sproule, B. J. (1973): Cardiopulmonary effects of diazepam. *Clin. Pharmacol. Ther.*, 14:182–189.

25. Woodward, M. G. (1957): Attempted suicide with meprobamate. *Northwest. Med.*, 56:321–322.

Antipsychotic Agents

17

Several drugs that are widely used to treat the most severe of the psychiatric disorders, the psychoses, are commonly involved in overdosing situations. In addition to their use in mental diseases, they are also used as antiemetics, tranquilizers, and cough suppressants. These drugs (Table 1) are known as antipsychotics, antipsychophrenics, neuroleptics, "major" tranquilizers, psychototropics, and ataractics. We will use the term antipsychotics throughout this chapter.

Poisoning with antipsychotic drugs is commonplace and, in fact, these drugs are included among those that are most generally associated with poisoning. But because of the intense emergency care and heroic antidotal methods most poisoned victims receive, serious morbidity and mortality to overdoses of pure antipsychotic drugs are rare (10). On the other hand, as is the case for intoxication with many other drug classes, a large number of antipsychotic drug poisonings represent mixed poisonings involving a combination of different drugs, rather than a single drug alone. Therefore, great danger still exists.

The reasons for the large number of poisonings are many. To start, antipsychotic drugs are widely prescribed and, indeed, have been largely responsible for emptying the country's mental wards. Since their introduction into clinical medicine in the 1950s, several hundred million patients worldwide have taken them. Today, hundreds of thousands of mental patients that, until a few years ago, would have required institutionalization now receive these drugs as out-

TABLE 1. *Representative antipsychotic drugs*

Antipsychotic drugs	CNS	EPS	ANS
Phenothiazines			
Aliphatic			
Chlorpromazine	+ + + +	+ +	+ + + +
Promazine			
Triflupromazine			
Piperidine	+ +	+	+ + +
Mesoridazine			
Thioridazine			
Piperazine	+	+ + + +	+
Perphenazine			
Fluphenazine			
Prochlorperazine			
Trifluoperazine			
Other			
Haloperidol	+	+ + +	+
Thiothixene	+	+ +	+
Loxapine	+	+ +	+

CNS = central nervous system; EPS = extrapyramidal system; ANS = autonomic nervous system.

Plus system indicates greatest or least activity at a particular site.

patients. The drugs are therefore widely available to a large number of people. Good advice to all persons involved in prescribing or dispensing antipsychotic medication is to permit the patient only enough medication so that if all of it were taken at once, it would be a sublethal dose (14). This might create inconvenience for some, but the potential benefits should prevail.

Whereas the drugs have been nothing short of revolutionary in allowing many of these people to lead fairly normal lives, the average patient is a poor complier when it comes to his medication needs. Many continue to take their drugs faithfully and adhere to their physician's directions. However, too many others, left under minimal supervision, do not. Many patients are also unreliable in what they state to the physician and pharmacist about the dosing of their medication. Psychotic patients are at higher risk than the general population for suicide or self-destruction gestures (5). Furthermore, many of the coated tablet dosage forms resemble candy confections and are attractive to children. Accidental poisoning in young people continues to be a special problem with these types of dosage forms.

The situation is further compounded because, as previously stated, psychotic patients frequently take a large number of a wide variety of medications. The CNS sedative effect produced by antipsychotic agents is at least additive to the sedation caused by other depressant therapy. Their anticholinergic action will likewise be additive to that of the tricyclics. A potentially fatal reaction can therefore occur when these drugs are taken concomitantly. Tricyclic antidepressants are commonly prescribed along with antipsychotic medication. Their potential for toxicity is another special problem that is just as significant as that of the antipsychotics. These drugs will be discussed in detail in Chapter 18.

The drugs listed in Table 1 differ from one another in their milligram potencies. Basically, all have a similar pharmacologic profile and mechanism of action. Likewise, they cause similar toxic reactions that may vary somewhat among the various derivatives. However, there are important differences among the individual members which will be indicated where appropriate. Overdoses of all the antipsychotics are treated by following established principles that are part of essentially the same protocol.

MECHANISM OF ANTIPSYCHOTIC TOXICITY AND CLINICAL MANIFESTATIONS

Overdoses of antipsychotic drugs cause a wide variety of symptoms that involve the central and autonomic nervous systems and the cardiovascular system. To understand how these effects come about and why they develop, and to better understand the principles involved in treating antipsychotic drug intoxication, we will consider the systems individually.

Central Nervous System

All levels of the CNS are affected when the drugs are taken in excess. Of special toxicological interest are the limbic system, hypothalamus, and the basal ganglia.

The *limbic system* is believed to be responsible for controlling a person's behavior and mood. The drugs exert their therapeutic antipsychotic effect by blocking dopaminergic receptors within this system. Those drugs that cause sedation will relax the patient. Those that stimulate or activate will induce an excitatory response.

The amygdala, which is part of the limbic system, may be stimulated by large doses of drug. These lower its seizure threshold so that convulsions occur more readily.

Seizure threshold is lowered by many antipsychotic drugs so that the discharge pattern shown on an EEG resembles that of epilepsy (17). The response is most prominent with the aliphatic phenothiazines (see Table 1) and least prominent with the piperazine phenothiazines and thioxanthenes (i.e., haloperidol, etc.).

The overall activity of the CNS is closely regulated by the *reticular activating system* (RAS). The RAS essentially controls wakefulness. Antipsychotic drugs that are taken in overdosage depress the RAS so that the victim's usual response to toxic doses is sedation, occurring within an hour of ingestion. A wide spectrum of sedative effects is possible ranging from mild lethargy to coma, depending on the characteristics of the particular derivative.

Coma is a common event in acute overdoses of antipsychotic agents with children, but rarely occurs in adults. It resulted in one instance from a 200-mg dose of chlorpromazine that was taken by a 1-year-old child. Another child (a 3-year-old boy) died from ingesting 800 mg chlorpromazine (21). Coma characteristics differ from those caused by barbiturates in that instead of causing a flaccid appearance, the patient frequently displays episodic restlessness, tremors, spasms, and dystonic reactions.

The RAS of the brainstem also helps modulate respiration. Whereas therapeutic doses do not significantly affect the respiration rate, overdoses of antipsychotic agents may cause significant depression. Whyman (21) described an unusual case where a middle-aged female patient, who was being rapidly tranquilized with chlorpromazine, suddenly died from respiratory arrest. There were no other observable signs or symptoms of imminent toxicity that preceded

death. Numerous other cases of respiratory complications, especially in children, have also been reported. For example, Kahn and Blum (15) reported their findings on infants who have died with the sudden infant death syndrome (SIDS). The majority of babies admitted to the hospital with a history of SIDS had taken a phenothiazine-containing syrup prescribed for nasal congestion and/or cough.

The *hypothalamus* moderates a multitude of physiological functions, including control of the vasomotor and temperature regulating systems. Antipsychotic drugs inhibit vasoconstrictor tone, which then induces vasodilation. Hypotension, possibly severe, is the usual outcome. Either hypo- or hyperthermia may result and may be fatal (4,5).

Dopaminergic receptors in the striatum within the *basal ganglia* are blocked with large doses of antipsychotic drugs. This blockade results in the appearance of characteristic effects on the extrapyramidal system (EPS) (Table 2) that are often seen when even therapeutic doses are taken, but which become much more prominent when toxic overdoses are ingested. Ten percent of all antipsychotic drug-intoxicated patients will experience these effects (15). More importantly, their severity cannot be correlated with dosage or the patient's probable extent of poisoning. Some of the EPS effects include involuntary movements such as tremors, tics, athetosis, widespread impairment of voluntary movement, or akinesia, and changes in muscle tone including muscle rigidity and dystonia.

Dystonia (incoordinated spastic movements) is one of the extrapyramidal effects that is often reported to occur with antipsychotic medication, but is readily reversible. However, a limited number of cases in the literature provides strong evidence that it may be persistent in some people (2,9). In both cases, young children with a history of brain disease ingested phenothiazine medications. The dystonic reactions that subsequently developed did not remit over time. One explanation is that individuals with brain damage have a greater predilection to permanent drug-induced neurological damage.

TABLE 2. *Characteristics of phenothiazine toxicity*

Degree of toxicity	CNS	EPS	ANS
Mild	Sedation Ataxia Slurred speech	Minimal	Hypotension Mydriasis Constipation Blurred vision Urinary retention
Moderate	Coma, Stage I, II	Dystonia Akathisia Tardive dyskinesia	Hypotension Mydriasis Constipation Blurred vision Urinary retention
Severe	Coma, Stage II, III	Laryngospasm Hypersalivation Dystonia Stiffness of extremities	Hypotension Shock Arrhythmias Conduction block Renal failure

CNS = central nervous system; EPS = extrapyramidal system; ANS = autonomic nervous system.

Autonomic Nervous System

Antipsychotic drugs induce potent anticholinergic and antiserotonergic actions. These occur in addition to their action on the adrenergic system which may include α-blockade and adrenergic potentiating activities. Anticholinergic potency is variable. Thioridazine has the greatest cholinergic blocking action, chlorpromazine an intermediate action, with the piperazine and haloperidol derivatives having the least. Likewise, a difference can be shown for α-adrenergic blocking effects. We can rank order a few of them as droperidol > triflupromazine > chlorpromazine > thioridazine > fluphenazine > haloperidol > trifluperazine (3). Thus, the overall effect on the autonomic nervous system is complex and frequently unpredictable.

Cardiovascular System

Cardiovascular effects have been reported for almost all the antipsychotic drugs. The responses are both diverse and complex. Not all mechanisms of toxicity are understood, but both peripheral and central sites are involved. A review of 54 deaths due to cardiovascular involvement indicated that two-thirds of them were in men under age 45 (16) (Table 3). These findings suggested that the deaths were drug-related,

TABLE 3. *Deaths due to cardiovascular complications in 5 patients taking phenothiazines[a]*

Age (years)	% Deaths
15–24	5.6
25–34	29.6
35–44	29.5
45–54	24.6
55–64	5.6
> 65	5.6

[a]Total number of patients = 54.
From ref. 16.

rather than from natural effects of aging (i.e., atherosclerotic disease, etc.).

Blood pressure is typically lowered, and occurs with overdoses of practically all antipsychotics (18). Hypotension ensues from central blockade of the vasomotor center, as well as from inhibition of α-adrenergic receptors (3). Recall that epinephrine possesses both α- and β-adrenergic activities. When α-receptors are blocked, as occurs following large doses of antipsychotic drugs, this leaves the β-sites unopposed. The β-agonist component of epinephrine thereby causes a drop in blood pressure. Patients who are clinically hypotensive from antipsychotic overdoses are more prone to develop cardiac arrhythmias.

Antipsychotic drugs produce a local anesthetic effect on the myocardium. This action lengthens the interventricular conduction time, prolongs the refractory period, decreases the sensitivity of the sinoatrial node, and may generate a variety of arrhythmias, and heart block.

The drugs also possess a quinidine-like action which may cause conduction abnormalities. ECG recordings show numerous abnormalities including a prolonged PR and QT interval, a blunted T wave, and a depressed ST-segment. Thioridazine is of particular concern in that it is associated with a greater incidence of T-wave abnormalities. Children are much more susceptible to the cardiotoxic effects of antipsychotic drugs.

Arrhythmias are induced by a host of mechanisms that are not all well understood. Anticholinergic effects or quinidine-like action of phenothiazines and elevated catecholamine levels may be partially responsible for their occurrence.

Antipsychotic drugs also block dopamine receptors at both pre- and postsynaptic sites. α-Adrenergic receptors are blocked only at postsynaptic sites. Leaving the presynaptic α-adrenergic sites unopposed could theoretically induce arrhythmias (7). Other mechanisms may likewise be involved. Those at greatest risk for arrhythmias are persons with hypokalemia and/or preexisting cardiovascular diseases. Most deaths attributed to antipsychotic drug overdoses result from ventricular fibrillation or cardiac arrest (1,8,13). This action may be rapid, with deaths having been reported within 3 to 5 hr of poisoning.

In summary, a typical phenothiazine overdose would result in hypotension, pin-point pupils, coma, hypothermia, respiratory depression, and cardiac arrhythmias.

TREATMENT OF ANTIPSYCHOTIC DRUG TOXICITY

The antipsychotics have a relatively wide therapeutic index which is, at least partially, responsible for their widespread clinical utility. Most can, therefore, be given over a range of doses.

The doses that cause toxic effects are spread over a wide range. A report that reviewed 100 cases of toxicity to chlorpromazine revealed that the average dose for nonsevere intoxication was 1.4 g. The average dose for severe intoxication was 6.2 g. However, survivals of 10 g and even 30 g by adults have been reported (6,11,12).

A patient who has taken a toxic overdose of any antipsychotic drug must be immediately assessed for severity of clinical symptoms, and be constantly monitored for unexpected changes in his condition. Stabilization of the vital signs is the first item of business, and all other procedures take second place. The respiration may require assistance. Basically, management of an antipsychotic drug-intoxicated patient will follow the same basic rules that are also true for the management of most other poisonings. That is, treat the patient's symptoms first.

Phenothiazines are radiopaque. Both whole and partial tablets can be visualized in the gastrointestinal tract. Therefore, this procedure allows for quick determination if it is required to determine whether or not the symptoms are caused by a phenothiazine, or if lavage has accomplished complete removal.

Many patients will be in shock, so elevation of the blood pressure and maintaining a normal blood flow should receive immediate attention. Norepinephrine or dopamine will assist in maintaining an adequate cardiac output. Dopamine is preferred over norepinephrine in that it stimulates β_1-receptors, without causing tachycardia or stimulating β_2-receptors to induce peripheral vasodilation. Thus, an adequate renal perfusion is maintained. The indirect adrenergics (e.g., metaraminol or phenylephrine) are also used. Epinephrine (mixed α- and β-agonist) and isoproterenol (a pure β-agonist) are contraindicated, as both would be expected to lower, rather than raise the blood pressure. Fluids and blood volume expanders should be given.

Phenytoin or lidocaine is appropriate to control phenothiazine-induced arrhythmias because they decrease automaticity and increase conduction velocity. Quinidine or procainamide would be contraindicated. In addition, phenytoin may also help moderate seizure activity. If seizures are not controlled, diazepam should be added. The short-acting barbiturates (e.g., pentobarbital and secobarbital) were, for a long period of time, considered to be a mainstay in controlling convulsant activity. However, their respiratory suppressant action makes them less than ideal. Physostigmine (see Chapter 18) has been used in a limited number of trials to control the anticholinergic effects (20,21). Physostigmine has established itself as a drug of choice for antidoting tricyclic antidepressant toxicity. It is still too early to fully assess its value in antidoting antipsychotic drug intoxication.

Decrease Absorption of the Drug

Once the patient's immediate needs are satisfied, additional measures should be undertaken to reduce further drug absorption. Both emesis and lavage are suitable, preference being dependent on the overall picture of the patient (i.e., whether or not consciousness or seizures are present, etc.). Some references state that emesis is not effective in removing antiemetic agents from the gastrointestinal tract. Recent evidence points to the contrary. Emetics will induce vomiting in a significant number of persons intoxicated with antiemetic medications.

Antipsychotic drugs are not water-soluble and, thus, are not rapidly absorbed from the stomach. Furthermore, their anticholinergic action will delay gastric emptying. Procedures for removing unabsorbed drug from the gastrointestinal tract may, therefore, be effective even if not undertaken for several hours after ingestion (5). A saline cathartic will hasten elimination of the drug from the intestine.

Following emesis or lavage, activated charcoal should be given to adsorb remaining traces of drug. Additionally, these drugs, as is the case with the tricyclic antidepressants, are cycled via the enterohepatic circulation (see Chapter 18). Repeated administration of doses of activated charcoal over the next 24 to 48 hr may be instituted to effectively hasten elimination of the drug from the blood.

Increase Excretion of Absorbed Drug

Forced diuresis has not shown successful results in increasing elimination of antipsychotic

drugs (22). Approximately 70% of a dose is taken up by the liver and, as stated earlier, is excreted via bile.

The dialytic procedures and hemoperfusion have, likewise, failed to show that intoxicated patients are significantly benefited (22). Phenothiazines are highly protein-bound (3).

Treat Other Symptoms

There may be no other serious symptoms that require management. Other times some of the symptoms listed in Table 2 require specific antidoting. For example, the dystonic reactions may be managed with diphenhydramine, or an antiparkinson agent such as benztropine.

SUMMARY

Antipsychotic drug toxicity is commonplace and can be quite severe. Symptoms of overdose are varied and often unpredictable. On the other hand, they can usually be managed if certain principles of therapy are adhered to.

Case Studies

CASE STUDIES: PHENOTHIAZINE TOXICITY

History: Case 1

A 54-year-old female with a 30-year history of manic depressive psychosis was admitted to a psychiatric ward of a hospital. Her vital signs at that time were: temperature, 36.9°C; pulse, 72 beats/min; blood pressure, 136/80 mm Hg; and respirations, 20/min. She was disoriented and talkative. Her physical examination was otherwise unremarkable except for a systolic murmur.

Treatment consisted of thioridazine, 200 mg four times a day; and chlorpromazine, 500 mg at bedtime. Her acute psychosis resolved within 2 weeks. However, during the course of her treatment, she experienced a sudden cardiopulmonary arrest while being attended to in the bathroom. After successful resuscitation, an ECG showed sinus tachycardia, notched broad T waves, and prolongation of the QT interval to 500 msec.

For some unknown reason, she received another 200 mg thioridazine and two more episodes of ventricular arrhythmias developed within 4 hr. Both responded to lidocaine. However, the following day, she experienced five more incidences of ventricular tachycardia, even though she was maintained on a continuous lidocaine drip. In order to convert back to sinus rhythm, it was necessary to give 7 50-mg bolus doses of lidocaine, and 250 mg procainamide every 3 hr. Three direct current cardioconversions were also given.

Lidocaine was discontinued the following day with the QT interval shortening to 380 msec. Procainamide was discontinued 4 days later. Approximately 2 weeks after admission, she was discharged with no apparent cardiac complications. (See ref. 1.)

History: Case 2

A 29-year-old male, with a history of chronic schizophrenia, had been hospitalized periodically for the past 10 years. His medications for the past 5 years included imipramine, 50 mg four times a day; trifluoperazine, 10 mg twice a day; and thioridazine, 200 mg four times a day. About one year prior to his latest hospitalization, he began to experience dyspnea on exertion, orthopnea, and paroxysmal nocturnal dyspnea. He gained 60 pounds.

On admission his blood pressure was 100/78 mm Hg. His pulse was 100 beats/min and regular. A physical examination revealed bilateral basilar rales and mild pitting edema in the lower extremities. A sinus tachycardia of 120/min and nonspecific T-changes were noted on an ECG recording.

Laboratory results included:

P_{CO_2}	= 30 mm Hg
HCO_3^-	= 18 mEq/L
pH	= 7.40
Hb	= 12.7 g
BUN	= 22 mg%
Cholesterol	= 234 mg%
Bromsulphalein	= 19% retention in 45 min
Alkaline phosphatase	= 18.2 U

This patient's treatment consisted of discontinuing the phenothiazines, bed-rest, a salt-restricted diet, and digitalis. He lost 34 pounds within a week.

He was discharged and then reevaluated 15 months later after he had been taking chlorpromazine continuously for 12 months. At this time, signs of congestive heart failure were again present, as were gallop rhythm and cardiomegaly. Recovery this time was less dramatic than previously. (See ref. 19.)

Discussion

1. Patient 1 became intoxicated with antipsychotic medication as an inpatient. Based on the case history, what were the warning signs, if any, that should have contraindicated the use of this medication.

2. Comment on the congestive heart failure in Patient 2. Do you suppose the digitalis he received contributed to his overall condition?

3. Explain why quinidine was not used to treat the ventricular arrhythmias in Case 1.

Review Questions

1. Which of the following chemical classes of phenothiazines is associated with the greatest incidence of extrapyramidal symptoms?
   A. Aliphatic derivatives
   B. Piperazine derivatives
   C. Piperidine derivatives

2. List the major reasons that contribute to the large number of poisonings by antipsychotic medications.

3. The intensity of extrapyramidal symptoms caused by an antipsychotic drug is a good clinical indicator of the extent of poisoning.
   A. True
   B. False

4. Phenothiazines block the dopaminergic receptors in the limbic system.
   A. True
   B. False

5. Discuss a probable mechanism whereby antipsychotic drugs lower the seizure threshold.

6. The inability to regulate the body temperature following phenothiazine overdoses is a result of a toxic action of the drugs on the:
   A. limbic system
   B. reticular activation system
   C. hippocampus
   D. hypothalamus

7. Which of the following is a true statement?
   A. Coma is a common outcome of phenothiazine intoxication in children.
   B. SIDS describes a series of symptoms on the autonomic nervous system that results from overdoses of phenothiazine drugs.

C. Antipsychotic medications stimulate vaso-motor tone.

D. Dystonia is a form of respiratory depression that results from phenothiazine overdoses.

8. Most deaths due to complications on the cardiovascular system by antipsychotic drugs result in men over the age of 65 years.
   A. True
   B. False

9. Phenothiazines cause a variety of effects on the heart that may lead to cardiac arrhythmias. List them and discuss their probable importance to the arrhythmic event.

10. A victim of phenothiazine intoxication presents in shock. Which therapeutic measures should be used, and which should not be used to treat this condition? Discuss your reasoning.

11. Cite how it can be readily determined that an overdose of phenothiazine tablets has been taken, even before symptoms appear.

12. Discuss the rationale for administering each of the following drugs to a victim of phenothiazine intoxication.
    A. Phenytoin
    B. Diazepam
    C. Physostigmine

References

1. Alexander, C. S., and Nino, A. (1969): Cardiovascular complications in young patients taking psychotropic drugs. *Am. Heart J.*, 78:757–769.

2. Angle, C. A., and McIntire, M. S. (1968): Persistent dystonia in a brain-damaged child after ingestion of phenothiazine. *J. Pediatr.*, 73:124–126.

3. Baldessarini, R. J. (1980): Drugs and the treatment of psychiatric disorders. In: *The Pharmacological Basis of Therapeutics*, 6th ed., edited by A. G. Gilman, L. S. Goodman, and A. Gilman, pp. 391–447. Macmillan, New York.

4. Bark, N. M. (1982): Heatstroke in psychiatric patients: Two cases and a review. *J. Clin. Psychiatry*, 43:377–380.

5. Barry, D., Meyskens, F. L., and Becker, C. E. (1973): Phenothiazine poisoning: A review of 48 cases. *Calif. Med.*, 118:1–5.

6. Brophy, J. J. (1967): Suicide attempts with psychotherapeutic drugs. *Arch. Gen. Psychiatry*, 17:652–657.

7. Carlsson, C., Dencker, S. J., Grinby, G., and Haggendal, J. (1966): Noradrenaline in blood-plasma and urine during chlorpromazine treatment. *Lancet*, 1:1208.

8. Crane, G. E. (1970): Cardiac toxicity and psychotropic drugs. *Dis. Nerv. Sys.*, 31:534–539.

9. Dabbous, I. A., and Bergman, A. B. (1966): Neurologic damage associated with phenothiazine. *Am. J. Dis. Child.*, 111:291–292.

10. Dahl, S. G., and Strandjord, R. E. (1977): Pharmacokinetics of chlorpromazine after single and chronic dosage. *Clin. Pharmacol. Ther.*, 21:437–447.

11. Davis, J. M. (1968): Overdosage of psychotropic drugs. *Dis. Nerv. Sys.*, 29:157–164.

12. Douglas, A. D. M., and Bates, T. J. N. (1957): Chlorpromazine as a suicidal agent. *Br. Med. J.*, 1:1514.

13. Greenblatt, D. J., Allen, M. D., Koch-Wesen, J., and Shader, R. I. (1976): Accidental poisoning with psychotropic drugs in children. *Am. J. Dis. Child.*, 130:507–511.

14. Hollister, L. E. (1968): Overdoses of psychotherapeutic drugs. *Clin. Pharmacol. Ther.*, 7:142–144.

15. Kahn, A., and Blum, D. (1979): Possible role of phenothiazines in sudden infant death. *Lancet*, 2:364–365.

16. Leestma, J. E., and Koening, K. L. (1968): Sudden death and phenothiazines. A current controversy. *Arch. Gen. Psychiatry*, 18:137.

17. Logothetis, J. (1967): Spontaneous epileptic seizures and EEG changes in the course of phenothiazine therapy. *Neurology*, 17:869–877.

18. Rivera-Calimlin, L. (1977): Pharmacology and therapeutic application of the phenothiazines. *Ration. Drug Ther.*, 11:1–8.

19. Tri, T. B., and Combs, D. T. (1975): Phenothiazine induced ventricular tachycardia. *West. J. Med.*, 123:412–416.

20. Weisdorf, D., Kramer, J., Goldbarg, A., and Klawans, H. L. (1978): Phenothiazine toxicity. *Clin. Pharmacol. Ther.*, 24:663–667.

21. Whyman, A. (1976): Phenothiazine death: An unusual case report. *J. Nerv. Ment. Dis.*, 163:214–216.

22. Winchester, J. F., Gelfand, M. C., Knepshield, J. H., and Schreiner, G. E. (1977). Dialysis and hemoperfusion of poisons and drugs—Update. *Trans. Am. Soc. Artif. Intern. Organs*, 23:762–842.

Anticholinergic and Tricyclic Drugs

18

Numerous drugs and nondrug substances produce, as their primary toxic symptoms when taken in overdose, an action on the autonomic nervous system. We have already studied plant toxicity (e.g., Jimson weed—anticholinergic effects, and mushrooms—cholinergic or anticholinergic effects); and organophosphate insecticides—cholinergic stimulation. Amphetamine-like drugs that cause stimulation of the adrenergic system are discussed in the following chapter.

Stimulation or blockade of various neuronal pathways within the autonomic nervous system can bring about a wide variety of physiological events. If sufficiently severe, many of these responses can be lethal.

ANTICHOLINERGIC TOXICITY

Numerous drugs have an anticholinergic action and represent a wide variety of pharmacological classes (Table 1). Frequently, the anticholinergic component overshadows other pharmacological actions of the drug when it is taken in toxic amounts.

Anticholinergics competitively inhibit the action of the neurotransmitter, acetylcholine, at central and peripheral receptor sites. Both muscarinic and nicotinic sites are vulnerable, depending on the dose of the compound and whether or not it is a quaternary ammonium analog. For example, quaternary derivatives do not gain access to the CNS to the same extent as nonquaternary derivatives. Consequently, their action

TABLE 1. *Representative substances containing anticholinergic activity*

Antihistamines (H₁ antagonists)
  Brompheniramine
  Chlorpheniramine
  Cyclizine
  Dimenhydrinate
  Diphenhydramine
  Meclizine
  Orphenadrine
  Promethazine
  Tripelennamine
  Pyrilamine

Antiparkinsonian agents
  Benztropine
  Biperiden
  Ethopropazine
  Procyclidine
  Trihexyphenidyl

Antipsychotic agents
  See Chapter 17

Tricyclic antidepressants
  Amitriptyline
  Doxepin
  Imipramine
  Desipramine
  Protriptyline
  Nortriptyline
  Trimipramine

Gastrointestinal anticholinergic and
  antispasmodic agents
  Atropine
  Scopolamine
  Hyoscyamine
  Belladonna (Tr.)
  Methantheline
  Propantheline
  Glycopyrrolate
  Homatropine

Ophthalmic products
  Atropine
  Scopolamine
  Cyclopentolate

Plants
  See Chapter 12

ever (12). These cases usually involve the drug used for nonlegitimate purposes, frequently in association with robbery or sexual assault (4). Whether these reports are generalized, or represent illicit uses confined to isolated geographic areas, remains unknown at this time.

The reason for the decline in toxicity from legitimately used anticholinergics is that these drugs are not employed in therapy now as frequently as in the past. For example, until less than a decade ago, the mainstay treatment for peptic ulcer disease and hyperacidity conditions was large doses of belladonna alkaloids and other atropine-like drugs. These agents have now been largely replaced in therapy with a different class of nontoxic drugs, the histamine-2 blockers (i.e., cimetidine, ranitidine). Atropine, hyoscyamine, and similar alkaloids were also included in numerous proprietary cold and asthma remedies. Their use in medical management of respiratory afflictions has been recently shown to be not only ineffective but also potentially dangerous. Consequently, they are no longer used for these intended purposes. What was once the heyday of anticholinergics in medicine has been modernized with newer forms of therapy.

On the other hand, poisoning from drugs that are not classed pharmacologically as anticholinergics, but which have a potent anticholinergic component, continues to be reported. These drugs include antihistamines, phenothiazines, and the tricyclic antidepressants. Among these classes, the greatest potential for serious poisoning in recent years is from overdoses of the tricyclic antidepressant compounds. Therefore, the remainder of this chapter will discuss the toxic actions associated with tricyclic antidepressants, and their management. Poisoning from other drugs or substances that have anticholinergic action can be expected to exhibit similar symptoms and will be treated in the same manner.

Infants and children are at special risk from anticholinergic drug action (23). Toxicity has been reported following absorption of atropine and similar ophthalmic preparations. Also, doses

is more directed toward peripheral, rather than central, receptor sites. Thus, a wide variety of clinical problems may be manifest.

Today, poisoning by drugs that are classed pharmacologically as anticholinergics (antimuscarinics) is less common than it was in former years. Reports of toxicity to scopolamine, an anticholinergic that has potent CNS sedative activity, is reported to be on the increase, how-of anticholinergic drugs that would be nontoxic to adults may be toxic in children.

Tricyclic Antidepressants

The tricyclic antidepressants have been used in therapy since the late 1950s. Today, they represent the largest group of drugs used for the treatment of depression. They are referred to as tricyclic compounds because of their chemical structures which contain three rings. Recently, a newer compound, maprotiline, was introduced into therapy. Maprotiline is a tetracyclic (four rings) compound that is too new to assess its toxic potential. It possesses the same degree of anticholinergic activity as imipramine, and a greater degree of CNS-sedative activity.

Most reported toxicities occur with amitriptyline (a dibenzocycloheptadiene derivative) or imipramine (a dibenzazepine derivative) (1,5). Toxicities occur as a result of both accidental and suicidal overdosage. Unlike poisoning from antipsychotic drugs (Chapter 17), poisoning by tricyclics is potentially life-threatening. Furthermore, most poisonings involve multiple ingestions with at least one other drug, usually ethanol, diazepam, propoxyphene, or codeine. Thus, there may be additional problems with antidoting in these instances (1,28).

Tricyclic antidepressant drug toxicity has increased to serious proportions in the United States and around the world. It is reported that, in some areas, tricyclics have surpassed CNS depressants as a major cause of poisoning (26). Toxicity problems resulting from these drugs are compounded because of their rapid absorption, tight binding to plasma proteins and tissues, enterohepatic recycling, and low therapeutic index. As with anticholinergics, per se, children are particularly sensitive, with a reported toxic dose of 10 mg/kg, and death resulting from ingestion of 32 mg/kg (29). Large variations in adult toxic doses exist. Death has occurred with 500 mg imipramine while others have survived doses exceeding 1,000 mg (13). It is probably of greater significance to consider the variable physiologic condition of patients as being the most important factor. For example, a patient with preexisting heart disease will probably experience more severe cardiac toxicity than a person with normal cardiovascular function.

Mechanism of Tricyclic Antidepressant Toxicity and Clinical Manifestations

Tricyclics decrease the action of acetylcholine centrally and peripherally and most major symptoms can be explained by this action, but other mechanisms must also be considered. Chorea, for example, is believed to result from an imbalance in acetylcholine and dopamine levels at receptor sites in the basal ganglia (7). Imipramine has a double action—it depresses acetylcholine and enhances dopamine levels. Myoclonus is caused by reduced serotonin uptake with its resultant increase within the synapse. Respiratory dysfunctions and disturbances in body temperature result from a direct action on the respiratory center in the medulla and the thermoregulatory site in the hypothalamus, in addition to the anticholinergic effects such as decreased sweating. Experimental evidence currently suggests a cholinergic component in the reticular activating system as being responsible for maintaining arousal. If this is so, then depression and coma from tricyclic overdosage can be readily explained.

The usual characteristics of tricyclic antidepressant toxicity are summarized in Table 2. Those attributable to the CNS include agitation, delirium, confusion, disorientation, ataxia, visual and auditory hallucinations, loss of short-term memory, seizures, respiratory difficulties, and coma. Their onset may be rapid, occurring within an hour of ingestion (9,16,20). Either hyperthermia or hypothermia may develop. Imipramine more commonly causes hyperthermia, whereas amitriptyline causes hypothermia which is probably due to its CNS-depressant action.

There are quantitative differences among the anticholinergic actions of the various tricyclic antidepressants. Amitriptyline, for example, causes the greatest degree of anticholinergic effects, whereas desipramine has the least amount (3). The peripheral anticholinergic actions listed in Table 2 play a fundamental role in the assessment of a tricyclic antidepressant overdose.

CARDIOVASCULAR EFFECTS

Tricyclic antidepressant agents produce prominent effects on the cardiovascular system, even in therapeutic doses. In toxic doses, the major symptoms of clinical importance are also those on the cardiovascular system. They include tachycardia, arrhythmias, intraventricular conduction disturbances, and hypotension or hypertension. Mechanisms for these cardiac actions are a result of anticholinergic actions on the heart and a quinidine-like myocardial depressant action, as well as inhibition of norepinephrine uptake at adrenergic synapses. The myocardial depressant actions can be visualized on ECG by prolongation of the QT interval and widening of the QRS complex. Blood levels of 100 μg% or greater are associated with significant cardiac effects which are often fatal (2,17).

Tricyclic antidepressants and other anticholinergic agents block the vagus nerve. Recall that vagal stimulation releases acetylcholine which slows the heart rate. Blocking this action leaves the sympathetic action unopposed. Tachyarrhythmias are the usual outcome and, indeed, are the most common cardiovascular complications. Specific ones include atrial tachycardia, fibrillation, and flutter; atrioventricular block; and ventricular tachycardia. Tachycardia may cause numerous effects including decreased cardiac output and hypotension. The quinidine-like actions of tricyclic antidepressants cause a decrease in A-V conduction velocity and establish conditions favorable for re-entry ventricular arrhythmias. Complete heart block may follow massive toxic doses of tricyclic antidepressants.

Additionally, tricyclics prevent neuronal transport and uptake of norepinephrine and/or serotonin into nerve terminals in the sympathetic nervous system (15,31). Uptake of these transmitters is the normal process that terminates their action. Their presence within the synaptic area for a longer period subjects the heart and other systems to increased sympathetic tone.

Arrhythmias may also occur secondarily to an action on the respiratory rate or to metabolic acidosis.

The action on blood pressure is variable. Because tricyclics decrease norepinephrine reuptake into sympathetic neurons, both α- and β-stimulation effects may be present. Initially, α-stimulation causes increased peripheral resistance and β-stimulation increases the heart rate. Both actions contribute to hypertension. However, with time, this excessive norepinephrine is metabolized by catechol-*O*-methyl transferase and monoamine oxidase (within the neuron). The vasopressor and inotropic actions then decrease, leading to hypotension (rather than hypertension). Unless the patient is seen shortly after ingestion, hypotension is the more com-

TABLE 2. *Characteristics of acute tricyclic antidepressant poisoning*

CNS	Cardiovascular	Anticholinergic
Hypothermia	Ventricular rate ≥ 120 beats/min	Mydriasis
Respiratory depression	QRS duration ≥ 100 msec	Blurred vision
Seizures	Arrhythmias	Tachycardia
Abnormal tendon reflexes	Bundle branch block	Vasodilation
Disorientation	Cardiac arrest	Urinary retention
Agitation	Hypotension	Decreased gastrointestinal motility
Myoclonic jerks	Circulatory collapse	Decreased bronchial secretions
Coma		Dry mucous membranes and skin
Pyramidal signs		

mon sequelae. As stated above, tachycardia may also contribute to hypotension. Of special note is that the extent of cardiovascular toxicity cannot be predicted from the severity of the patient's neurologic symptoms (19).

Treatment of Tricyclic Antidepressant Poisoning

Tricyclic antidepressant poisoning is a serious medical emergency, and the poisoned patient must receive immediate treatment if survival is to be assured. Tricyclic poisoning poses a complex medical picture and its treatment is still largely controversial. The most crucial period for cardiac arrhythmias is within the first 12 hr after ingestion (6).

Placement in an intensive care unit is critical. The patient must be constantly monitored for cardiovascular and respiratory functions. Cardiac resuscitation methods must be readily available. Even after the coma phase is terminated and neurological signs appear normal, the chance for delayed life-threatening cardiovascular toxic reactions, often unexpected, still remains (10). Onset of cardiovascular complications has been reported to occur as long as 6 days after ingestion, even after significant clinical improvement (11,25).

Most central and peripheral symptoms of tricyclic poisoning are reversed with physostigmine salicylate (18) (Table 3). This is a reversible acetylcholinesterase inhibitor that binds to acetylcholinesterase and, therefore, produces an action similar to the organophosphate insecticides. The major difference between the two is that physostigmine has a lesser affinity for ace-

tylcholinesterase and thus its action is readily and quickly reversible. It is, therefore, inherently less toxic than the organophosphate insecticides which are generally classed as irreversible.

Physostigmine differs from other drugs such as edrophonium, neostigmine, and pyridostigmine that are also classed as "reversible" acetylcholinesterase inhibitors in that the latter three are quaternary amines. Physostigmine is a tertiary amine. This important chemical difference permits it to cross the blood-brain barrier and thus reach a higher concentration in the CNS. The quaternary derivatives will not reach sufficient levels in the brain to antagonize anticholinergic toxicity that is produced by a central mechanism. The peripheral effects (generally less severe) would be sufficiently antagonized by the quaternaries.

Physostigmine may be given whenever poisoning by any substance that causes anticholinergic effects is suspected. Mild symptoms of peripheral origin generally do not require aggressive therapy. However, those of central origin (e.g., convulsions or coma, severe agitation, hallucinations, or hypertension) must be treated. Also, physostigmine can be used to identify the cause of drug-induced coma, when the cause is unknown (24). For example, a test dose of 2 mg is given by a slow intravenous drip. If no response occurs, a second dose can be administered after about 20 min. If the patient still fails to respond to physostigmine, then poisoning by some means other than by an anticholinergic action should be suspected.

If, however, the patient's response is positive, recovery will normally occur within minutes. Because physostigmine is rapidly metabolized, repeated doses probably will be required at 30- to 90-min intervals given over the next 12 to 24 hr, depending on the dose of poison ingested. Extreme caution must be exercised when physostigmine is used over a period of time since it can produce significant bradycardia and asystole. In addition, it is not uncommon with physostigmine to overshoot the endpoint so that the primary symptoms of toxicity are those of cholinergic stimulation (e.g., salivation, diarrhea, etc.), rather than blockade. For this reason,

TABLE 3. *Treatment of anticholinergic poisoning with physostigmine*

Age group	Test dose	Repeat dose if necessary	Administration[a] (i.v.)
Adult	2.0 mg	1.0–2.0 mg	Over 2–3 min
Child	0.5 mg [b]	0.5 mg	Over 2–3 min

[a]Caution should be exercised with intravenous administration because seizures may occur if administration is too rapid.
[b]Dose every 5 min up to 2.0 mg.

atropine sulfate would be given to "antidote the antidote." It should be stressed that indiscriminant use of physostigmine should be avoided.

Also, relative contraindications to using physostigmine include asthma, cardiovascular disease, gangrene, and mechanical obstruction of the gastrointestinal or urogenital tract (23). Again, atropine will readily reverse its action should complications develop.

When cardiovascular arrhythmias fail to respond adequately to physostigmine, phenytoin or propranolol is indicated. Phenytoin enhances the atrioventricular conduction time, and thus reverses the quinidine-like action (10). Propranolol, a β-adrenergic blocking drug, slows the heart rate by blocking β-stimulant effects on the myocardium, and reduces myocardial susceptibility to generation of action potentials. Some controversy exists over the use of propranolol. Propranolol has increased tricyclic-induced myocardial toxicity in animal studies (21,30). The rationale for use in tricyclic antidepressant poisoning is to reverse the sympathomimetic actions. However, propranolol should be avoided if the patient has asthma, congestive heart failure, or heart block. Other antiarrhythmic drugs (e.g., quinidine and procainamide) should not be given because they may depress cardiac contractility even further.

If hypotension develops, a direct-acting sympathomimetic amine, such as dobutamine or dopamine, should be cautiously used. Indirectly acting pressor amines (e.g., mephentermine, metaraminol) that work by stimulating norepinephrine release are not indicated because their uptake into the adrenergic neurons will be blocked by the presence of the tricyclic.

Potassium chloride and sodium bicarbonate are also routinely used. Sodium bicarbonate is used to increase the blood pH above 7.4. Animal data have shown that the incidence of cardiac arrhythmias increases when the pH is between 7.30 and 7.20 (25,26). Alkalosis, thus, decreases the chance for arrhythmia development (14). Alkalinization also promotes movement of potassium into cardiac muscles (32), so potassium chloride is given. Potassium narrows the width of the QRS complex of the ECG.

Once the patient has been stabilized, emesis or lavage should be undertaken to reduce the possibility of further drug absorption. Emesis is the preferred procedure if ingestion was recent. Lavage is preferred if 1 to 2 hr have elapsed since the poisoning event occurred. After this period, it is doubtful if lavage will be beneficial due to the rapid rate of absorption of tricyclic antidepressants.

Activated charcoal adsorbs tricyclic antidepressants and their metabolites. A portion of tricyclics is secreted directly into the stomach. Continuous aspiration of stomach contents over 24 to 48 hr may remove a significant amount of drug from the body.

Recall, also, that some tricyclics are metabolized to active metabolites. Imipramine is such a drug. One of the means to explain the long pharmacological action of tricyclics is that they are eliminated through the enterohepatic circulation and are then reabsorbed into the blood. This process keeps their blood level elevated and prolongs their effects. Activated charcoal removes from the gastrointestinal tract the active drug before it is absorbed, and metabolites that are cycled through the enterohepatic circulation. For this reason, activated charcoal may be administered in multiple doses over the next 1 to 2 days (22).

A saline cathartic helps facilitate movement through the gastrointestinal tract, and, hence, removal of the drugs from the body. Some thought should be directed to using castor oil rather than a saline cathartic. Castor oil stimulates peristalsis, needed to overcome the ileus caused by tricyclic intoxication. This view is not yet in general acceptance. Assuring that all the drug that is possible has been removed from the gastrointestinal tract is extremely important. Some of the delayed toxicities reported for tricyclics may be due to continued absorption versus an intrinsic "delayed" activity of the drug.

The normal procedures of forced diuresis, hemodialysis, and peritoneal dialysis do not significantly benefit the tricyclic-poisoned patient due to the tight plasma protein binding and limited water solubility (17). Hemoperfusion has been inadequately studied to date, but it does remove tricyclics. In severe intoxication when the prognosis is poor, hemoperfusion may be attempted (17).

Hyperthermia and fever can be treated with ice-water sponging or immersion in cooled water. Phenothiazines should not be used because their own anticholinergic action may potentiate the action of the poison. Seizures are usually adequately controlled with diazepam.

SUMMARY

Poisoning by drugs and plants that cause an anticholinergic response is common. Although the use of drugs that are classed pharmacologically as anticholinergics has declined in recent years, use of other drugs that have this action as a side effect has risen. This certainly holds true for tricyclic antidepressants.

Tricyclic antidepressant medication induces a wide variety of toxic effects that includes cholinergic blockade, as well as other mechanisms. Poisoning is considered to be a medical emergency.

Treatment involves various nonspecific measures, as well as the use of physostigmine, an acetylcholinesterase inhibitor. Physostigmine treatment has been shown to produce a dramatic increase in survival after tricyclic poisoning. However, it is not without toxic actions of its own.

Case Studies

CASE STUDIES: TRICYCLIC ANTIDEPRESSANT OVERDOSE

History: Case 1

A 46-year-old female ingested eight Elavil® (amitriptyline) tablets, 250 mg each, and fifteen Sominex® (scopolamine, methapyrilene, salicylamide) tablets. She was brought to the emergency room in a comatose state, responding only to painful stimuli. She was sweating profusely, was flushed, and her respirations were increased above normal. She displayed occasional myoclonal activity. Her pupils were dilated at 5 mm and were reactive to light.

The patient's vital signs on admission consisted of blood pressure, 140/105 mm Hg; pulse, 100 beats/min; respirations, 20/min; and temperature, 98°F.
Her laboratory results included:

Na^+	= 138 mEq/L
Cl^-	= 104 mEq/L
K^+	= 4.4 mEq/L
HCO_3^-	= 2.6 mEq/L
BUN	= 12 mg%

Arterial blood gasses	
pH	= 7.38
Po_2	= 73 mm Hg
Pco_2	= 58 mm Hg

Treatment consisted of immediate gastric lavage with a 7-L return, oxygen, fluids, and diazepam. She showed occasional PVCs so a lidocaine drip was started. Physostigmine salicylate, 2 mg i.v., was administered about 7 hr after admission.

Almost immediately, the patient awoke and became alert and oriented. In order to maintain her alertness and orientation, additional physostigmine salicylate was required, so doses were administered 4 hr later, and again 3 hr later.

With each dose of physostigmine, she became responsive within seconds. The following day, an additional 2-mg dose of physostigmine was again used, because of the appearance of frequent junctional premature beats. By this time, also, signs of cholinergic stimulation (e.g., nausea, vomiting, diarrhea, and salivation) were apparent. She was discharged 5 days after admission with no apparent residual effects. (See ref. 6.)

History: Case 2

A 32-year-old female was brought to the emergency room 9 hr after ingestion of 1.0 to 1.5 g amitriptyline hydrochloride. On examination, she was stuporous, responding only to deep pain. Her reflexes were normal. Vital signs included blood pressure, 120/80 mm Hg; pulse, 126 beats/min; and respirations 16/min and shallow.

Physical examination revealed a very sick individual who groaned in agony, and thrashed her arms in response to pain. Treatment consisted of 2 mg physostigmine salicylate given intravenously, and within 15 min she had fully awakened. Watery diarrhea occurred, for which she was given 0.4 mg glycopyrrolate. Five hours later her vital signs had stabilized, and she did not require further physostigmine treatments. She still remained sluggish mentally.

Tremors increased over the next few hours and diarrhea and myoclonus persisted, so at 9 hr after admission, another 2-mg dose of physostigmine salicylate was given, along with 2 mg glycopyrrolate. These doses were repeated periodically over the next 8 hr for a total quantity administered of 12 mg physostigmine salicylate, and 1.2 mg glycopyrrolate. Eleven hours after admission, there was a significant decrease in urinary output, so the patient was catheterized.

The following morning, she was alert and tremulous. She was also oriented and responding somewhat better, and no further myoclonus was observed. At this time, physostigmine and glycopyrrolate were discontinued and there were no further problems with urinary retention. She had recovered completely 36 hr after admission.

Toxicological analysis of the patient's blood and urine at the time of admission showed a serum amitriptyline level of less than 0.1 mg%. The urine amitriptyline concentration was 3.8 mg%, with the presence of a metabolite. (See ref. 27.)

History: Case 3

A 38-year-old woman was admitted to the hospital 2 hr after ingesting an estimated 20 to 30 of her mother's 50-mg desipramine tablets. She had also consumed an unknown quantity of alcohol. She was alert, oriented, and able to communicate normally.

On admission her vital signs were: blood pressure, 140/90 mm Hg; pulse rate, 125/min; and respiration, 28/min. Her temperature was not taken. Bowel sounds were present, but hypoactive. No traces of any other drug were found.

The patient received 30 ml syrup of ipecac which resulted in her vomiting fragments of the tablets. Neither activated charcoal nor cathartics were administered.

Over the next 6 hr she remained stabilized. Her blood pressure returned to 120/90 and the ECG was normal. Only tachycardia was evidenced, and this gradually declined. Eight hours postingestion she was fully awake, alert, and able to walk unassisted. Because of this improvement, she was transferred to the psychiatric emergency department for assessment.

Two hours later (10 hr postingestion), her condition was noted to have worsened. Her speech was slurred and she was apparently experiencing auditory hallucinations. She was visibly fearful and agitated. Her respirations became labored, blood pressure was palpable at 60 mm Hg, and her pulse was weak and irregular.

A cardiac tracing showed asystole. Cardiopulmonary resuscitation was initiated but the patient failed to respond. She was pronounced dead 11 hr after drug ingestion. A postmortem blood sample showed a desipramine level of 8.6 μg/ml. Plasma levels of 1.0 μg/ml have been associated with coma, cardiac arrest, and death. (See ref. 8.)

Discussion

1. The onset of cholinergic symptoms in Patient 1 on the second hospital day marked an important event. What was it?

2. Outline the mechanism of activity for physostigmine when used to antidote a tricyclic antidepressant poisoning.

3. In Patient 1, was the cardiovascular response to amitriptyline intoxication expected or unexpected? Outline the mechanism that caused this response.

4. The ingredients in Sominex® tablets surely produced some toxic symptoms of their own. What would you have expected? Did they add to the amitriptyline effects, or partially prevent them from being worse?

5. What actually caused Patient 2 to develop urinary retention? Was this to be expected?

6. Discuss why glycopyrrolate was given to Patient 2. Would atropine sulfate have been better or worse, and why do you think so? (Hint: think in terms of sites of action of these two anticholinergic drugs.)

7. The patient in Case 3 illustrates the fact that death can occur even after symptoms (which were trivial to start) have subsided. What specific measures could have been instituted to reduce the likelihood of this patient dying?

CASE STUDY: ANTICHOLINERGIC POISONING

Case History

A 33-year-old female was brought to the emergency room after being found in her apartment, bound and gagged. On admission she was alert, but could only remember her name. Her vital signs included: blood pressure, 150/100 mm Hg; pulse, 115 beats/min; respirations, 16/min; and rectal temperature, 100°F.

The patient showed no signs of trauma. Her pupils were dilated (8 mm) and were not reactive to light. Heart and lung sounds, and chest X-ray were all normal. An ECG showed a sinus tachycardia at a rate of 120/min, PR interval of 0.18 sec, QRS of 0.08 sec, and a QTc interval of 0.30 sec.

An examination of the abdomen indicated there were no bowel sounds. Furthermore, the abdominal muscles were relaxed and the abdomen was distended. The remainder of the physical examination was unremarkable.

The following laboratory results were obtained:

Na$^+$	= 146 mEq/L
K$^+$	= 4.3 mEq/L
Cl$^-$	= 109 mEq/L
HCO$_3$$^-$	= 22 mEq/L
BUN	= 7 mg%
Glucose	= 94 mg%
Creatinine	= 0.7 mg%

This patient's therapy consisted of oral 50% dextrose in water and 50 g activated charcoal. It was obvious that she had been poisoned, but the identity of the poison could not be determined. She showed no improvement over the next several hours. However, about 12 hr later her mental status began to improve.

It was then revealed that she had been drinking wine from a glass that was very likely contaminated with some anticholinergic substance by a guest, who then robbed her. Toxicological analysis of the patient's blood and urine failed to show the presence of any drug, although a wineglass found in her apartment contained traces of scopolamine.

The source of the scopolamine was never discovered. Scopolamine tablets would have imparted a disagreeable taste to the wine, and would have left a noticeable residue on the side of the glass. Scopolamine powder is not readily available. Eye drops may contain 2.5 mg scopolamine/ml. In a separate toxicity report, a dose of 0.45 mg scopolamine (i.e., 4 drops of a 0.25% scopolamine eye-drop product) caused intense psychosis that persisted for 4 days (2). (See ref. 12.)

Discussion

1. In Chapter 12, a case report of Jimson weed poisoning is reported. With respect to symptoms of toxicity, how did that case compare with this one?

2. This patient apparently ingested a toxic, but sublethal dose of scopolamine. Had she not improved as quickly as she did, what specific antidotal treatment would she have received?

Review Questions

1. Physostigmine is an antidote of choice for treating overdoses of drugs that are:

A. α-Stimulants
B. α-Blockers
C. cholinergic stimulants
D. cholinergic blockers

2. Discuss the dosing schedule for physostigmine when it is used to diagnose the probable cause of a poisoning.

3. If a victim of tricyclic antidepressant drug poisoning goes into shock, how would it be treated? What are the benefits/risks of administering epinephrine?

4. Which of the following is the tricyclic antidepressant that causes the greatest number of poisonings in the United States?
A. Imipramine
B. Amitriptyline
C. Maprotiline

5. Scopolamine causes typical anticholinergic symptoms but, in addition, causes an effect on the CNS that differs from atropine. What is this effect?

6. List all of the major mechanisms by which tricyclic antidepressants cause cardiac complications when they are taken in toxic overdose.

7. All of the following are true statements about tricyclic antidepressant poisoning *except*:
A. myoclonus is caused by reduced uptake with subsequent collection of dopamine in the sympathetic synapses.
B. disturbances in body temperature result in part from a direct action in the thermoregulatory site in the hypothalamus.
C. complete heart block may follow large overdoses.
D. overdoses cause a shortened QT interval.

8. The blood pressure response to a tricyclic overdose is variable over time. Discuss the probable mechanism of this variability.

9. The extent of cardiovascular toxicity from an overdose of tricyclic antidepressants is predictable from the severity of neurologic symptoms.
A. True
B. False

10. Physostigmine is preferred over neostigmine as an antidote for tricyclic poisoning for a very

important reason. What is it? When would neostigmine serve as a suitable antidote in lieu of physostigmine?

11. Theoretically, castor oil should work better as a means to rid the gastrointestinal tract of an overdose of tricyclic antidepressant medicine than a saline cathartic. Explain the reasoning behind this statement.

12. Discuss the rationale for administering each of the following drugs to a victim of a tricyclic antidepressant intoxication.
    A. Sodium bicarbonate
    B. Potassium chloride

References

1. Bailey, D. N., and Shaw, R. F. (1980): Interpretation of blood and tissue concentrations in fatal self-ingested overdose involving amitriptyline: An update (1978–1979). *J. Anal. Toxicol.*, 4:232–236.
2. Biggs, J. T., Spiker, D. G., Petit, J. M., and Ziegler, V. E. (1977): Tricyclic antidepressant overdose. *JAMA*, 238:135–138.
3. Blackwell, B., Stefopoulos, A., and Enders, P. (1978): Anticholinergic activity of two tricyclic antidepressants. *Am. J. Psychiatry*, 135:722–724.
4. Brizer, D. A., and Manning, D. W. (1982): Delirium induced by poisoning with anticholinergic agents. *Am. J. Psychiatry*, 139:1343–1344.
5. Brown, T. C. K., and Leversha, A. (1979): Comparison of the cardiovascular toxicity of three tricyclic antidepressant drugs: Imipramine, amitriptyline, and doxepin. *Clin. Toxicol.*, 14:253–256.
6. Bryan, C. K., Ludy, J. A., Hak, S. H., Roberts, R., and Marshall, W. R. (1976): Overdoses with tricyclic antidepressants. *Drug Intell. Clin. Pharm.*, 10:380–384.
7. Burks, J. S., Walker, J. E., and Rumack, B. H. (1974): Tricyclic antidepressant poisoning: Reversal of coma, choreathetosis, and myoclonus by physostigmine. *JAMA*, 230:1405–1407.
8. Callahan, M. (1982): Admission criteria for tricyclic antidepressant ingestion. *West. J. Med.*, 137:425–429.
9. Crocker, J., and Morton, B. (1969): Tricyclic (antidepressant) drug toxicity. *Clin. Toxicol.*, 2:397.
10. Davies, D. M., and Allaye, R. (1963): Amitriptyline poisoning. *Lancet*, 2:543.
11. Davis, J. M. (1973): Overdose of psychototropic drugs—tricyclic antidepressants. *Psychiatr. Ann.*, 3:6–11.
12. Goldfrank, L., Flomenbaum, N., Lewin, N., Weisman, R., Howland, M. A., and Kaul, B. (1982): Anticholinergic poisoning. *J. Toxicol. Clin. Toxicol.*, 19:17–25.
13. Gosselin, R. E., Hodge, H. H., Smith, R. P., and Gleason, M. N. (1976): *Clinical Toxicology of Commercial Products*. Williams & Wilkins, Baltimore.
14. Jackson, J. E., and Bressler, R. (1982): Prescribing tricyclic antidepressants. Part III: Management of overdose. *Drug Therapy*, 13:175–189.
15. Jefferson, J. W. (1975): A review of the cardiovascular and toxicity of tricyclic antidepressants. *Psychosom. Med.*, 37:160–179.
16. Jick, H., Dinan, B. J., Hunter, J. R., Stergachis, A., Ronning, A., Perera, D. R., Madsen, S., and Nudelman, P. M. (1983): Tricyclic antidepressants and convulsions. *J. Clin. Psychopharmacol.*, 3:182–185.
17. Marshall, J. B., and Forker, A. D. (1982): Cardiovascular effects of tricyclic antidepressant drugs: Therapeutic usage, overdose, and management of complications. *Am. Heart J.*, 103:401–414.
18. Nattel, S., Bayne, L., and Ruedy, J. (1979): Physostigmine in coma due to drug overdosage. *Clin. Pharmacol. Ther.*, 25:96–102.
19. Nicotra, M. B., Rivera, M., Pool, J. L., and Noall, M. W. (1981): Tricyclic antidepressant overdose: Clinical and pharmacological observations. *Clin. Toxicol.*, 18:599–613.
20. Noble, J., and Matthew, H. (1969): Acute poisoning by tricyclic antidepressants: Clinical features and management of 100 patients. *Clin. Toxicol.*, 2:403–421.
21. Nymark, M., and Rasmussen, J. (1966): Effect of certain drugs upon amitriptyline induced electrocardiographic changes. *Acta Pharmacol. Toxicol.*, 24:148–156.
22. Preskorn, S. H., and Irwin, H. A. (1982): Toxicity of tricyclic antidepressants—Kinetics, mechanism, intervention: A review. *J. Clin. Psychiatry*, 43:151–156.
23. Rumack, B. H. (1973): Anticholinergic poisoning: Treatment with physostigmine. *Pediatrics*, 52:449–451.
24. Rumack, B. H. (1976): Physostigmine: Rational use. *J. Am. Coll. Emerg. Phys.*, 5:541–542.
25. Sedal, L., Korman, M. G., Williams, P. O., and Mushin, G. (1972): Overdosage of tricyclic antidepressants. A report of two deaths and a prospective study of 24 patients. *Med. J. Aust.*, 2:74.
26. Skoutakis, V. A. (1982): Tricyclic antidepressants. In: *Clinical Toxicology of Drugs: Principles and Practice*, edited by V. A. Skoutakis, pp. 127–152. Lea & Febiger, Philadelphia.
27. Snyder, B. D., Blonde, L., and McWhirter, W. R. (1974): Reversal of amitriptyline intoxication by physostigmine. *JAMA*, 230:1433–1434.
28. Starkey, I. R., and Lawson, A. A. H. (1980): Poisoning with tricyclics and related antidepressants—A ten-year review. *Quart. J. Med.*, 193:33–49.
29. Steel, C. M. (1967): Clinical effects and treatment of imipramine and amitriptyline poisoning in children. *Br. Med. J.*, 2:663–667.
30. Thorstrand, C., Bergstrom, J., and Castenfors, J. (1976): Cardiac effects of amitriptyline in rats. *Scand. J. Lab. Invest.*, 36:7–15.
31. Vohra, J. K. (1975): Cardiovascular abnormalities following tricyclic antidepressant drug overdosage. *Drugs*, 7:323–325.
32. Vohra, J., and Burrows, G. D. (1974): Cardiovascular complications of tricyclic antidepressant overdosage. *Drugs*, 8:432–437.

Central Nervous System Stimulants: Convulsants

19

A large number of drugs (Table 1) cause intense stimulation of the CNS when they are ingested in toxic amounts. While we traditionally consider items such as amphetamine and strychnine to exert strong convulsant activity, our ability to identify many other drugs as CNS stimulants is perhaps less secure. Stimulants represent a diverse group of substances that are chemically and pharmacologically dissimilar, and when they are ingested in sufficient dosage they cause a wide variety of effects related to central stimulation. They are also antidoted in much the same manner, with a few exceptions, as is noted later in this chapter.

The specific stimulants considered in this chapter include amphetamine and its derivatives, strychnine, camphor, and cocaine. They are representative of all other stimulants. Some of the hallucinogenic stimulants [e.g., lysergic acid diethylamide (LSD), 3,4-methylenedioxyamphetamine (MDA), 2,5-dimethoxy-4-methylamphetamine (DOM)] will be covered in Chapter 20. The principles of toxicity and antidotal therapy that are outlined in this chapter form the basis for antidoting almost all other

TABLE 1. *Drug compounds with CNS-stimulant activity*

Amphetamine
  See Table 2

Anorexiants
  See Table 2

Analeptics
  Doxapram
  Methylphenidate
  Nikethamide
  Pentylenetetrazol
  Picrotoxin
  Strychnine

Xanthines
  Caffeine
  Theobromine

Local anesthetics
  Camphor
  Cocaine

Nonprescription diet aids
  Phenylpropanolamine

Psychotomimetics
  See Chapter 20

chemicals that cause CNS stimulation as their major toxic effect.

We should also be reminded that our discussion of stimulant toxicity in this chapter is limited to acute convulsive effects and their medical management. Another area of study, the psychology of abuse of amphetamine and cocaine, and the physiological effects of chronic use, is left for textbooks of pharmacology and psychology.

AMPHETAMINE

Numerous derivatives of amphetamine have been used over the years to modify a wide variety of medical conditions, legitimate or otherwise. Today, however, their official use is restricted to management of narcolepsy, hyperkinesis (hyperactivity) in children, and to the short-term treatment of obesity. Many states have officially banned their medical use within these states in weight-control programs, so legal amphetamine sales have declined significantly. Amphetamine use by the intravenous route (illicit use) has also been reported to have decreased in the United States compared to a decade ago (17). However, in all states, even with tightened control and decreased intravenous use, amphetamine abuse, and therefore toxicity, is still ranked overall as a very significant medical problem.

We will still consider all of the drugs that have amphetamine-like activity together, and refer to the group simply as amphetamine. Some of the more common drugs are listed in Table 2. The drugs mentioned in this table are not all important causes of intoxication, but they are

TABLE 2. *Drugs with amphetamine-like activity*

Amphetamine
Benzphetamine
Chlorphentermine
Dextroamphetamine
Diethylpropion
Methamphetamine
Phendimetrazine tartrate
Phenmetrazine
Phentermine

included here to keep the discussion complete. Also, it is speculated that as amphetamine and methamphetamine (Table 3) become even more difficult to obtain, these drugs, and even other derivatives, may emerge as important causes of toxic reactions. We have already seen this happen with several of them. The toxic actions seen on overdose are, for the most part, qualitatively similar to each other. Their actions do differ quantitatively from those of the other congeners, however.

Mechanism of Amphetamine Toxicity

Amphetamine induces intense stimulation of the CNS, mainly by causing release of catecholamines (epinephrine, norepinephrine, dopamine) into central synaptic spaces and inhibiting their reuptake into nerve endings (32). In this manner, the endogenous neurotransmitters remain present within the synapses in higher concentration and for a longer than normal period of time. All neurons that normally respond to their stimulation are, therefore, positively affected.

One of the problems frequently encountered by amphetamine users is that tolerance develops to some of the central effects (e.g., the anorectic and euphoric actions) (17). Therefore, users may increase the dose to several hundred milligrams daily. Tolerance does not occur to all of the central actions, however. A toxic psychosis may appear after months of continued use. In these individuals, if amphetamine use is continued, the convulsive threshold may actually be lowered, so that lethal toxicity becomes a real problem (17).

Characteristics of Amphetamine Poisoning

Amphetamine causes a variety of signs and symptoms depending on the dose ingested. Most toxic effects are actually extensions of its pharmacologic actions. Table 4 lists some of the more prominent features seen and ranks them according to their severity. Symptoms noted as $1+$ and $2+$ may be experienced even with therapeutic doses and are generally not causes of great concern. The conditions listed as $3+$ and $4+$ reflect severe CNS stimulation and require immediate attention.

Amphetamine-induced psychosis with euphoria and hallucinations is common. Euphoria may account for the widespread abuse potential of amphetamine. Hallucinations, when they occur, however, are generally perceived as unpleasant. These may be auditory in nature (mostly in patients using amphetamines chronically), or visual (more common following a single large dose) (22). Tactile hallucinations are also occasionally experienced. Psychosis generally disappears within a week after onset, with hallucinations clearing first.

Respiratory and cardiovascular functions are both stimulated with tachypnea, tachycardia, and hypertension resulting. Flushing and diaphoresis (sweating) appear. This stimulation can eventually lead to depression of both systems, if toxicity is sufficiently severe to cause convulsions (explained later).

Hyperpyrexia may be significantly severe, with temperatures above 109°F having been reported. Temperatures this high are obviously incompatible with life and are a contributing cause of death. No doubt, hyperpyrexia is one of the causes of death following intense exercise

TABLE 3. *Chemical formulae for amphetamine and methamphetamine*

Chemical name	Substitutions				R_1—⟨benzene⟩—CH-CH-NH with R_2 R_3 R_4
	R_1	R_2	R_3	R_4	
Amphetamine	H	H	CH_3	H	
Methamphetamine	H	H	CH_3	CH_3	

TABLE 4. *Characteristics of amphetamine toxicity grouped by severity*

Signs and symptoms	Severity[a]
Restlessness, irritability, insomnia, tremor, hyperreflexia, sweating, mydriasis	1+
Hyperactivity, confusion, hypertension, tachypnea, tachycardia, mild fever, hyperpyrexia	2+
Delirium, mania, self-injury, intense hypertension, tachycardia, arrhythmias and hyperpyrexia	3+
All of the above, plus convulsions, coma, circulatory collapse, and death	4+

[a]For explanation, see text.
From ref. 9.

in a person who previously consumed amphetamine. In one example, a bicyclist ingested 105 mg amphetamine prior to a race. He eventually collapsed from heat exhaustion, and despite heroic measures to resuscitate him, he died of cardiovascular collapse (6). Hyperpyrexia is believed to be caused peripherally by drug-induced vasoconstriction, but whether lethal hyperpyrexia is produced centrally or peripherally is not known at this time.

The dose of amphetamine needed to produce acute lethal toxicity varies widely. For example, severe toxic reactions have occurred with doses of 30 mg, whereas a female using amphetamine, in whom tolerance had not yet developed, survived a 200-mg dose (15). The acute lethal dose in adults has been reported as 20 to 25 mg/kg, and in children as 5 mg/kg (2,37). Death from as little as 1.5 mg/kg of amphetamine in an adult has also been noted (37). Therapeutic, toxic, and lethal blood levels of amphetamine are listed in Table 3 in the Appendix.

STRYCHNINE

Strychnine, in doses of 0.5 to 1.0 mg, was formerly used in a variety of medications intended for internal stimulant use. While it is no longer employed in medicine to the same extent as previously, some of these older remedies may still remain in home medicine cabinets and pharmacy back-room shelves. Today, its legitimate use is mainly confined to a variety of products which are intended to control destructive rodents. Strychnine, therefore, is still an important substance involved in accidental poisoning in children, and intentional (suicidal) poisoning in adults.

Mechanism of Strychnine Toxicity

Strychnine causes a generalized stimulation of all portions of the CNS, both in the spinal column and brain. It brings about this activity, not through direct activation of stimulatory neurons, but by depressing the inhibitory pathways (11). This effect is only seen at postsynaptic sites. Therefore, excitatory neuronal activity is no longer checked by inhibitory forces, and it proceeds unrestrained. In essence, strychnine converts normal reflex neural activity into explosive convulsive force. The slightest sensory stimuli (e.g., tactile, auditory, visual) may induce convulsions after strychnine.

Glycine is a postsynaptic inhibitory transmitter in the brain and spinal cord. Strychnine acts as a competitive inhibitor of the glycine receptor (18). This probably explains how the stimulant poison can exert its convulsant activity. In fact, a rare disorder called nonketotic hyperglycemia is modestly treated with strychnine (7,35). In this disorder, glycine is not metabolized and accumulates in the brain, resulting in severe neurologic deficiency. Because strychnine competes with glycine at the receptor site, glycine's activity is decreased.

Characteristics of Strychnine Toxicity

The major effects of strychnine intoxication result from generalized stimulation of the CNS (Table 5). The victim of strychnine-induced convulsions assumes a characteristic pattern during seizure, with the exact nature defined by whichever of the body's muscles are the strongest. In other words, the stronger muscle of a set of extensor/flexor muscles will be maximally stimulated in tonic fashion. This usually involves massive extension. (Interestingly, the sloth's flexor muscles are the stronger, so, as

TABLE 5. *Characteristics of strychnine toxicity*

Stiffness of facial and neck muscles
Hyperreactive reflexes
Lactic acidosis
Opisthotonos
Tetanic convulsions
Respiratory paralysis
Asphyxia
Death

expected, strychnine causes the animal to curl up!)

The back will be arched in hyperextension, a position termed opisthotonos (Fig. 1). In this position, only the crown of the head and the feet touch the ground.

Following the tonic phase of seizure, a period of symmetrical extensor bursts occurs. This is followed by a period of postictal depression in which the victim may sleep. This depends on the number of convulsive episodes, their strength, and the dose of convulsant ingested. However, bursts of sensory stimulation may initiate outbursts of repeated symmetrical thrashing.

The muscles of the face and neck are the first to become stimulated and contract. They stiffen and the person's face assumes a characteristic grimace. The victim soon becomes generally hyperactive. A slight sensory stimulus may initiate symmetrical extensions, or, in more advanced stages of poisoning, a full-blown convulsion. All voluntary muscles, including the diaphragm, abdominal and thoracic muscles, will be fully contracted. Consequently, respiration which is increased initially due to the central stimulant effect, ceases during the convulsive episode. Convulsive periods may recur, with each episode inciting increased depression following its termination. These contractions require a great expenditure of energy. Also, since respiration ceases during episodes, the cause of central hypoxia becomes obvious. Between episodes, the victim's muscles are extremely painful and consciousness is not lost.

A single large dose of strychnine may be sufficient to cause death from a massive convulsive episode. Most victims, however, will sustain two to five convulsive episodes before death occurs.

Blood lactate levels may increase to cause metabolic acidosis. Lactic acid is a by-product of muscular activity, and during periods of strenuous contraction, lactic acid production is enhanced.

The heart rate and blood pressure are raised slightly during a convulsive episode. This is due partly to a massive sympathetic discharge, but also to the extensive skeletal muscular contractions. These effects are variable, however, and may or may not be manifest in any particular victim of strychnine poisoning.

Small quantities of strychnine impart an extremely bitter taste to the mouth and cause reflex gastric secretion. This was the basis for its inclusion in many of the old remedies used to stimulate the appetite. Strychnine has no activity on the intestine in nonconvulsive doses, so its inclusion in old-time preparations (i.e., aloin, strychnine, and belladonna tablets) was without therapeutic merit.

Death is caused by medullary paralysis. It is due to asphyxia which is related to the periods of intense muscle contraction which interferes with respiration. In fact, if a victim of strychnine is given a skeletal muscle relaxant to prevent the tonic seizures, and is artificially ventilated, asphyxiation does not occur (30). The lethal dose of strychnine is reported to be approximately 15 mg for children and 30 to 100 mg for adults (11).

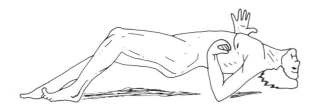

FIG. 1. Opisthotonos from a toxic overdose of strychnine. The body's weight is supported entirely by the head and feet.

COCAINE

Cocaine is not generally thought of as being included among the central stimulant poisons. However, central stimulation is one of its major pharmacological, as well as toxicological, effects. The euphoria, which is caused by stimulation of the cerebral cortex, is the reason why cocaine abuse is so widespread. Even though cocaine has been used (abused) for hundreds of years, the use of cocaine has recently increased in the United States. Twenty-five metric tons of illicit cocaine were reportedly brought into the United States in 1978, with a street value exceeding $16 billion. At least 6,500,000 Americans used cocaine during that year (5). So, there is no doubt that toxicity from overdoses will continue to be a major problem for many years into the future.

Mechanisms of Cocaine Toxicity

Cocaine interferes with the reuptake process that returns norepinephrine into the adrenergic nerve endings and, thereby, terminates its action. Consequently, norepinephrine accumulates within the synaptic spaces and causes stimulation of systems innervated by adrenergic neurons. Cocaine is the only local anesthetic known to produce such an action. Cocaine has also been shown to block reuptake of dopamine and interfere with serotonin activity.

Characteristics of Cocaine Toxicity

The variety of signs and symptoms of toxicity that can be traced to cocaine overdose are listed in Table 6 according to the specific organ system affected.

As previously stated, cocaine causes generalized CNS stimulation. The individual normally feels euphoric, although dysphoria may occur on occasion. Restlessness, excitement, and garrulousness can accompany euphoria. Motor coordination is not usually hampered when smaller doses are taken. With large doses, however, the lower motor centers and cord reflexes are stimulated. Muscular twitching is first noted and clonic-tonic convulsions result later. Convulsions resulting from an acute oral toxic dose generally appear within 30 to 60 min after ingestion. Because the vomiting center may also be stimulated, emesis is common.

As with other central stimulants that cause massive convulsive episodes and, consequently, suppression of respiration, cocaine-induced contractions are followed by central depression. Death from massive doses is usually a result of respiratory failure.

The sympathetic nervous system is stimulated, both centrally and peripherally. This action accounts for many of the CNS and cardiovascular effects, as well as the other manifestations of cocaine intoxication that are listed in Table 6.

The most prominent cardiovascular feature of toxic doses of cocaine is tachycardia which, depending on the overall cardiovascular health of the victim, may lead to arrhythmias. Sinus tachycardia is most commonly reported, along with ventricular dysrhythmias. The toxic actions on the heart are related to the stimulant action on the sympathetic nervous system. A direct toxic action on the myocardium has occasionally been shown following massive intravenous doses of cocaine (4,28).

Since the sympathetic nervous system innervates the vasculature, vasoconstriction occurs. This effect, along with an increased heart rate, causes the blood pressure to increase. Following an initial period of hypertension, though, the blood pressure falls and cardiac depression ensues.

Hyperpyrexia may occur, and as stated earlier, this action may be responsible for death. It probably results from an interaction of at least three forces. Because stimulation causes increased muscular activity, body heat production is increased. Additionally, vasoconstriction restricts heat loss. Finally, cocaine is believed to cause direct stimulation of the heat-regulation center.

The effect of cocaine on the respiratory system follows the same progression; there is an initial stimulation resulting in tachypnea followed by dyspnea and, eventually, respiratory failure.

TABLE 6. *Characteristics of cocaine intoxication ("Caine reaction")*

Phases	CNS	Circulatory system	Respiratory system
Early stimulative	Excitement Apprehension Headache Nausea, vomiting Twitching of small facial muscles, fingers	Pulse variations; usually will slow Blood pressure: elevation, decrease Skin pallor	Increased respiratory rate and depth
Advanced stimulative	Seizures; tonic, clonic Hyperkinesis	Increased pulse Increased blood pressure	Cyanosis Dyspnea Rapid or irregular respirations
Depressive	Muscle paralysis Loss of reflexes Unconsciousness Loss of vital functions Death	Circulatory failure Death	Respiratory failure Cyanosis Death

From ref. 27.

CAMPHOR

Camphor-containing products are also not generally thought of by nonmedical persons as being toxic. Indeed, camphor has long been employed for external application as a rubefacient, mild analgesic, antipruritic, and counter-irritant. Its medical uses were described by Marco Polo in the 13th Century. As recently as the early 20th Century, it was still listed in the American and European literature as a cardiovascular stimulant (16). Even in the 1940s its oral and subcutaneous use was promoted to treat cardiac or respiratory collapse and fainting.

Internal and parenteral preparations of camphor are no longer available. However, the wide variety of proprietary products that do contain this drug (Table 7) attest to the substance's current popularity.

Over the years numerous cases of toxicity to camphor have been reported, but not until recently has the serious potential for camphor poisoning been realized. No doubt, the overall incidence will decrease in the next few years, since the Food and Drug Administration banned camphorated oil (180 mg camphor/ml) from sale in the United States (10). Camphorated oil has been the largest single cause of camphor-related poisonings. Most poisonings have occurred because the victims mistook camphorated oil for castor oil, or other remedies that

TABLE 7. *Representative proprietary products that contain camphor*

Acne products
  Komed
  Microsyn

Analgesic (external) products
  Analbalm
  Banalg
  Dencorub
  Emul-O-Balm
  Heet
  Mentholatum
  Panalgesic
  Sloan's Liniment

Antitussive; congestion products
  Vicks VapoRub
  Vicks Vapo Steam
  Va-Tro-Nol Nose Drops

Diaper rash and prickly heat products
  Mexsana Medicated Powder

Hemorrhoidal products
  Pazo
  Tanicaine Ointment

Insect sting and bite products
  Campho-Phenique
  Chiggerex
  Obtundia products

either sound or look like camphorated oil, and ingested an unsuspected toxic dose (34).

One teaspoonful of camphorated oil may result in serious toxicity in adults, although recovery has occurred following ingestion of 1.5 ounces

(12). Recall that the average volume of a swallow is 5 ml for a child, and 14 to 21 ml for an adult (19). A fatal dose, especially in a child, could easily be ingested with a single swallow.

Mechanism of Camphor Toxicity

Camphor is absorbed from all sites, but the precise mechanism for inducing toxic symptoms is elusive. It stimulates the brain at all levels. Necropsy of a 19-month-old child who died from 1 g camphor revealed profuse dermal, bowel, stomach, and kidney hemorrhaging, and extensive degenerative changes in central neurons, especially in Sommer's section of the hippocampus (31). Similar pathology has also been noted in other reports. This neuronal damage could explain the symptoms of severe CNS stimulation. The liver and kidneys may show fatty degeneration if death is delayed.

Characteristics of Camphor Poisoning

Signs and symptoms of poisoning may appear within 5 to 15 min following ingestion, or be delayed for several hours if food is present in the stomach. Because it is highly lipid-soluble, camphor quickly enters into the CNS. The clinical manifestations associated with camphor intoxication appear in the order shown in Table 8, although vomiting may follow the other symptoms. Any odor of camphor on the breath or in the urine should be considered positive for camphor poisoning. Death is from status epilepticus or postictal respiratory failure. If the

TABLE 8. *Characteristics for camphor ingestion*

Nausea, vomiting
Burning in mouth, throat, and stomach
Dizziness
Delirium, hallucinations
Dyspnea
Cold, clammy skin
Face alternately pale and flushed
Pulse rapid and weak
Irritation, excitement, convulsions
Depression following CNS stimulation
Muscle tremors and rigidity
Urinary retention, anuria
Transient hepatic damage

---

victim survives, there are usually no residual problems extending beyond the initial encounter.

TREATMENT OF TOXICITY

Treatment of toxicity from CNS stimulants is directed primarily toward management of hyperthermia, convulsive episodes (and, hence, preservation of respiration), normalization of the blood pressure, and protection of the heart against arrhythmia. Additionally, individual measures are taken to minimize further absorption of the drug from the gastrointestinal tract, enhance its excretion, and to treat other symptoms when necessary (refer to Chapter 3 for specific details). For most central stimulants, antidoting is nonspecific and directed toward controlling symptoms. However, certain specific procedures are also undertaken for individual compounds. Table 9 summarizes many of the clinical manifestations associated with CNS stimulants, and Fig. 2 outlines the procedures generally used in the treatment of stimulant poisonings.

Amphetamines

Because of the wide range in potentially toxic doses, toxic amphetamine ingestion must be treated without hesitation. The problem is further compounded by the fact that a toxic ingestion frequently involves one of the delayed-action dosage forms such as timed-release tablets or capsules. Whereas symptoms of toxicity would normally be expected to occur within a few hours of ingestion, their onset could be delayed for many more hours following ingestion of a timed-release product. This lack of appearance of symptoms within the expected time might be falsely interpreted as a belief that the victim is in a less critical state.

This same "disadvantage," on the other hand, may also prove to be beneficial. Emergency personnel have a better chance to remove unabsorbed drug from the gastrointestinal tract before it causes further toxic problems.

Phenothiazines are usually recommended for treatment of amphetamine-induced psychosis which is due to an excess of dopamine. Chlor-

TABLE 9. *Summary of the clinical manifestations of CNS-stimulant toxicity*

Degree of toxicity	CVS	CNS	Other
Mild	Tachycardia Palpitations Hypertension	Increased activity Insomnia Anxiety Blank stare Hyperthermia Hyperreflexia Mydriasis Blurred vision Psychotic state	Goose bumps Choreoathetoid movements Rapid shallow respirations Urinary retention Delayed gastric emptying time

Moderate	Pallor
	Anginal pain
		Delirium
		Confusion
		Psychotic state
		Pupils—dilated,
		   sluggish
		   reaction to
		   light
		Nystagmus
		Tremors
			Diaphoresis

Severe	Hypertensive
	  crisis
	Ventricular
	  fibrillation
	Circulatory
	  collapse
	Death
		Convulsions
		Pupils—dilated,
		   nonreactive to
		   light
		Hyperthermia
		  (> 109°F)
		Coma
		Death
			Aspiration of vomitus
			Asphyxia
			Respiratory failure
			Death

promazine also has been shown to reverse hyperthermia, convulsions, and hypertension associated with amphetamine toxicity without causing depression. The dose is repeated every 30 min as needed. Haloperidol has also been advocated, since it is thought that it produces less respiratory depression and a reduced chance for sustained hypotension and reflex tachycardia (13). Both of these drugs are direct antagonists to amphetamine. Barbiturates antagonize amphetamine, but only when given in anesthetic doses.

Recalling from Chapter 17 that one of the potentially toxic effects of chlorpromazine and haloperidol is to lower the convulsive seizure threshold, administration of these drugs to a victim of massive amphetamine toxicity could prove detrimental. Therefore, diazepam may be the preferred antidote to control extremely excited states. But to counter this suggestion is the fact that, as stated above, chlorpromazine and haloperidol are direct antagonists of am-

phetamine. Therefore, these agents exert significant antidotal action on amphetamine toxic effects such as hyperthermia.

Convulsions are usually associated with increased body temperature. Therefore, this condition must be vigorously treated. The patient may be placed in a cool room and kept as quiet as possible, and a hypothermic blanket used. Depending on the case, salicylates may be administered concurrently with phenothiazines to aid in temperature reduction.

Reduction of Absorption and Forced Excretion

Once the victim is stabilized, an attempt should be made, if possible, to remove any remaining drug from the gastrointestinal tract. Recall that one of the general contraindications to use of emetics (and lavage) is poisoning by a convulsant. For amphetamine, the situation may be potentially worsened if a phenothiazine that has antiemetic activity has been given. On the other

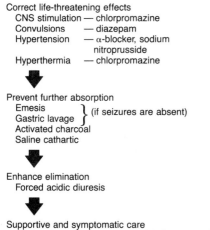

Correct life-threatening effects
    CNS stimulation — chlorpromazine
    Convulsions   — diazepam
    Hypertension   — α-blocker, sodium
                          nitroprusside
    Hyperthermia   — chlorpromazine

Prevent further absorption
    Emesis   } (if seizures are absent)
    Gastric lavage }
    Activated charcoal
    Saline cathartic

Enhance elimination
    Forced acidic diuresis

Supportive and symptomatic care
    Cool, quiet environment— to minimize external stimuli
    Monitor electrolytes
    Monitor vital functions
    Obtain psychiatric consult

FIG. 2. Management of acute CNS stimulant poisoning.

hand, most medical experts agree that emesis can still be induced, even in the presence of a phenothiazine.

A rule of thumb is that if ingestion of amphetamine occurred within 4 hr, emesis may be initiated. Syrup of ipecac is indicated, as long as the patient is alert. If the victim is comatose, gastric lavage should be undertaken. After 4 hr, activated charcoal is preferred over emesis.

Renal clearance of amphetamine is enhanced by forced diuresis with furosemide or mannitol, and acidification of the urine with ammonium chloride. In a study to demonstrate the effect of urine pH on amphetamine excretion, a urinary pH of 5.0 produced a 55% excretion of a dose of *d*-amphetamine within 16 hr, compared with a 3% excretion at a pH of 8.0 (3). In other words, the plasma half-life of amphetamine can be decreased to 7–8 hr with acidification. Ascorbic acid is occasionally used to acidify the urine, but its use produces inconsistent effects and should not be relied on for this purpose.

When the patient fails to respond to these measures, dialysis may be performed. Both hemodialysis and peritoneal dialysis will remove amphetamine from the blood.

Additional Measures

General measures of supportive care must also be applied. The victim should be placed in a quiet environment, away from sensory stimulation, as this may precipitate further convulsions. He should be protected from self-inflicted harm by providing padded bed rails and using physical restraints if necessary.

Strychnine

Strychnine poisoning is managed in similar fashion to other acute stimulant poisonings. All efforts at antidoting strychnine must be directed toward prevention of convulsions. If the victim of strychnine poisoning is attended to at once, the prognosis for complete, uneventful recovery is good (Table 10). The alkaloid is rapidly excreted through the kidney with 70% excretion being reported within 6 hr (33). In fact, a patient could theoretically take approximately two lethal doses over a 24-hr period without experiencing cumulative effects (11). Therefore, if the patient can be successfully managed for the first few hours, survival is likely.

Diazepam is far ahead in therapeutic appeal of other sedative drugs that have been used in the past to antidote strychnine. It provides superior control of massive tonic convulsions without potentiating postictal depression. On occasion, a patient will experience severely depressed respiration with diazepam, but this is rare (20). Thus, the patient must be constantly monitored, even after diazepam has been given. The benzodiazepines are known to increase the

TABLE 10. *Laboratory values of a victim of strychnine poisoning*[a]

	Admission to ER	Hours after arrival		
		0.5	1	3
Sodium (mmol/l)	148	139	139	142
Potassium (mm/l)	3.5	4.2	3.5	4.1
Chloride (mmol/l)	103	102	103	109
Bicarbonate (mmol/l)	9	4	18	24
Anion gap (mmol/l)	36	33	20	9
pH	—	7.02	7.33	7.41

[a]Modified from ref. 21.

affinity of γ-aminobutyric acid (GABA) receptors in the CNS. GABA is an inhibitory neurotransmitter, and thus synaptic inhibitory transmission is enhanced.

Keeping the victim quiet and away from all forms of sensory stimulation is an extremely important part of treatment of strychnine and other convulsants. The slightest stimulation can evoke a full-blown convulsive reaction with opisthotonos.

Reduction of Absorption and Forced Excretion

Strychnine is rapidly absorbed from the gastrointestinal tract. Seizure activity may be seen within several minutes and tonic convulsions within 15 to 30 min. Therefore, measures toward removing the alkaloid from the gastrointestinal tract must be initiated shortly after ingestion. Prior to convulsant activity, emetics or lavage may be used. Potassium permanganate is an oxidizing agent and reacts with strychnine (and many other organic substances) to destroy them. Activated charcoal also adsorbs strychnine. Forced diuresis or dialysis measures are probably of minimal value since strychnine is normally so rapidly cleared from the blood.

Cocaine

Therapeutic measures for antidoting cocaine toxicity involve many of the same procedures as described for amphetamine. The patient's condition must be quickly assessed and emergency measures undertaken to stabilize the vital signs.

Diazepam is currently considered to be the drug of first choice to control cocaine-induced seizures. When seizure control is inadequate, phenobarbital may be substituted.

Cardiovascular effects must be aggressively treated. Propranolol, a β-adrenergic blocking agent, will normally reverse and control both hypertension and tachycardia (25–27). Intravenous doses, up to a total of 8 mg, will restore the blood pressure and heart rate to normal within several minutes.

If the victim is in the depression stage of poisoning (hypotension), attention must be immediately directed toward raising the blood pressure. Intravenous fluids and vasopressors such as dopamine are indicated at this point.

Hyperthermia must also be controlled. Procedures discussed for amphetamine will be undertaken for victims of cocaine poisoning.

Cocaine-induced psychosis with hallucinations, paranoia, and hyperexcitability requires treatment. Neuroleptic agents have been used with success. More recently, lithium has been used (29).

Reduction of Absorption and Forced Excretion

As for amphetamine ingestion, if less than 4 hr have elapsed since ingestion, emesis or lavage may be undertaken. After this period, or if the victim displays signs of convulsive episodes, activated charcoal should be used in place of evacuation procedures.

It is important to determine the route by which the cocaine was used. Most cocaine use occurs by the intravenous or nasal routes, rather than by oral ingestion. Therefore, procedures designed to remove cocaine from the gastrointestinal tract, if none is present, may only subject the patient to unnecessary trauma.

Although some studies imply that forced diuresis with acidification of the urine enhances cocaine excretion, neither procedure is universally accepted. Dialysis and hemoperfusion are also ineffective for enhancing excretion.

Camphor

Camphor must be removed from the stomach as quickly as possible. Immediate emesis or gastric lavage is indicated (before convulsions and generalized stimulation occur). Activated charcoal should follow this removal, by lavaging and withdrawing it until the odor of camphor is no longer detected in the return. Or, an appropriate quantity of charcoal can be instilled into the stomach and left there.

Barbiturates have long been used to control convulsions, but diazepam is generally preferred because it produces less respiratory depression. Hemodialysis with oil will hasten removal of camphor from the blood. Succinyl-choline may be used to help control muscular rigidity and spasm. As for any other CNS stim-ulant, the patient must be kept quiet and at minimum sensory input. No oily cathartic or alcohol should be given as these will promote absorption of camphor into the blood.

SUMMARY

A large variety of drugs can cause intense stimulation of the CNS leading to convulsions. Many of these drugs are well known as con-vulsants. Others, however, are not generally recognized by the public as stimulants; their toxic potential is therefore greater.

Antidotal procedures for treatment of con-vulsive states are mostly nonspecific, directed toward controlling symptoms. Review these once again, following the steps outlined in Fig. 2.

Case Studies

CASE STUDIES: CAMPHOR INTOXICATION

History: Cases 1,2

Male and female twins, aged 39 months, were found by their mother at 1:45 a.m., 15 min after the family had returned home from an evening of visiting friends. The boy was on the floor convulsing, the girl was holding an empty bottle that had contained camphorated oil. Both children smelled of camphor, so they were rushed to the hospital.

Upon admission, both children were lavaged and given intravenous diazepam and phenobarbital to control convulsions. The boy spontaneously vomited, revealing a quantity of undigested food. He was again lavaged and the returning solution revealed a strong odor of camphor. Shortly thereafter, he experienced respiratory arrest, but his breathing was supported artificially. Over the next 24 hr, he experienced three additional seizures.

The sister was convulsing by the time she arrived at the hospital. She also spontaneously vomited un-digested food. Lavage revealed a thick, yellow, oily

material that smelled of camphor. She later experi-enced another convulsion, and following a 24-hr pe-riod of intense neuromuscular irritability, resumed normal activity.

Both children were discharged after 4 days of intensive care. The quantity of poison ingested by either child was not determined. (See ref. 1.)

History: Case 3

A 3-year-old girl suffering from generalized sei-zures was brought to the emergency room. Two hours before, she had projectile vomiting and complained of intense gastric discomfort. Upon admission, se-cobarbital was given intramuscularly, and within 30 min the seizures were controlled.

The victim's vital signs included: respiration, 28/min; pulse, 126 beats/min; temperature, 36.4°C; blood pressure, 120/90 mm Hg. The only other immediate finding was a distinct odor of camphor on her breath.

The mother revealed that she had been applying Vicks VapoRub® (4.81% camphor) intranasally, twice a day for 5 months, because of the child's persistent rhinorrhea. Two hours before the convulsion, the child was found with an open jar of the product. An estimated tablespoonful (0.7 g camphor) was miss-ing. Previously, the child enjoyed the taste, often sucking on the cotton-tipped applicator used to apply it.

All laboratory tests for pathology were negative. Serum concentration of camphor was determined to be 1.95 mg/100 ml. The child was discharged 24 hr after admission. A follow-up examination with an EEG 15 days later was normal. (See ref. 24.)

Discussion

1. Comment on the fact that Patients 1 and 2 had food in their stomachs. Did this most likely increase or decrease absorption of the poison, and on what information do you base your answer?

2. What was stated about Patient 3 that leads you to suspect she also had food in her stomach at the time of poisoning?

3. Assuming that these three patients had not re-sponded positively to the treatment they received, what would have been the next step?

CASE STUDIES: COCAINE INTOXICATION

History: Case 1

This case involved a 38-year-old male who had a history of light cigarette smoking (40 packs per year).

He did not suffer from diabetes mellitus, hypertension, or hyperlipidemia, and had never experienced a myocardial infarction. There also was no family history of any of these conditions. On a routine medical examination, he was found to be slightly overweight. He had a pulse rate of 68 beats/min and his blood pressure was 120/80 mm Hg. The physical condition of this patient was otherwise normal, as well as were all laboratory test results, chest X-rays, and ECG recording.

Approximately one year later, he was admitted to a hospital complaining of dizziness and a feeling of "heaviness" in his left arm. On examination, a subendocardial anterolateral myocardial infarction was discovered. Isoenzyme studies revealed an increased serum creatinine phosphokinase (CPK) level of 310 IU/L (normal: 2–83) with elevated MB bands.

He recovered from this infarction and was eventually able to walk 3 miles a day without difficulty. He remained symptom-free until approximately 3 years later.

At that time he experienced pain in his chest and left neck area, dyspnea, diaphoresis, and felt anxious and nervous after snorting (inhaling) approximately 500 mg cocaine. His blood pressure was 152/98 mm Hg, and his pulse rate was 88 beats/min. His ECG failed to reveal any abnormalities, and the chest pain was relieved with nitroglycerin. His diagnosis was angina, and he was sent home.

He abstained from cocaine use for about 6 months, but after again snorting cocaine he experienced substernal chest pressure radiating to the left arm, as well as dyspnea and sweating.

On admission to the emergency room, his blood pressure was 130/90 mm Hg, pulse rate was 96 beats/min, and an S_1 gallop rhythm was noted. The ECG showed an elevated S-T segment and a flattened T wave. Pain was alleviated with nitrates and morphine sulfate. An inferolateral subendocardial myocardial infarction was noted on ECG examination.

The patient stopped using cocaine after that incident and has remained symptom-free. He has also returned to work full-time without apparent sequelae. (See ref. 8.)

History: Case 2

A 25-year-old male had been admitted to a hospital for psychiatric care on two previous occasions as a result of drug abuse problems. He was admitted again, this time in a psychotic state due to the use of large quantities of cocaine.

The patient believed he had special powers which could solve the current world problems, and he felt he was in constant communication with government agencies, including the FBI and CIA. He also claimed he was writing a book about his experiences which would be the salvation to mankind. Overall, he was grandiose, paranoid, and hyperactive.

Treatment consisted of neuroleptic agents, but when side-effects developed, he refused further medication. Lithium therapy was therefore initiated, and when serum levels reached 0.7 mEq/L, his psychotic behavior subsided. He then started to attend group psychotherapy and was soon released from the hospital. He became productive in society without recurrence of his former psychotic episode. (See ref. 29.)

History: Case 3

A 26-year-old male boarded an airplane in Colombia, which was destined for the United States. About 45 min after takeoff, he began to experience nausea. Oxygen was administered by flight attendants. However, 75 min later he experienced a generalized seizure and died.

On autopsy, 27 rubber condoms measuring approximately 2 cm in diameter were found in his stomach. Each contained approximately 5 g of a white powder, consisting of 35% cocaine. The bags were tied closed with string. One of these bags had ruptured.

Gross examination of the patient's tissues revealed pulmonary congestion and edema, hepatic congestion, and gastric hyperemia. (See ref. 36.)

Discussion

1. Explain the probable origin of the heart irregularities displayed by the patient in Case 1.

2. Do the symptoms experienced by Patient 2 sound like they were caused by cocaine? Characterize cocaine symptoms.

3. Discuss how cocaine caused Patient 3 to convulse.

CASE STUDIES: AMPHETAMINE TOXICITY

History: Case 1

A 16-year-old female was taken to the emergency room, an hour after confessing to her mother that she had ingested a "large handful" of what was supposedly mescaline tablets. Instead, she actually consumed amphetamine (total dose unknown). Gastric lavage was immediately performed and the victim was admitted. Shortly thereafter, however, she became agitated, experienced auditory hallucinations and insomnia which persisted for 2 days. She was discharged on the third day after showing constant improvement.

Two days later, she began experiencing auditory hallucinations again, this time with delusions. Also, she showed signs of stereotypic behavior by playing with the control dials on a television for two consecutive hours. She claimed to be conversing with deceased relatives, to have been appointed by God as a church elder, and that Satan had fathered her 16-month-old child.

She was readmitted to the hospital where she was treated with haloperidol, hydroxyzine, flurazepam, propoxyphene, and chlorpromazine at bedtime. Approximately 8 to 10 days later, she was no longer experiencing psychotic symptoms and was discharged on the 14th hospital day. (See ref. 23.)

History: Case 2

A 21-year-old male was brought to the emergency room following ingestion of an estimated 2.2 g amphetamine sulfate that he took in a suicide gesture.

On examination 1 hr after ingestion, he was fully oriented and agitated. He quickly became hyperkinetic and incoherent.

Physical findings included a pulse of 168 beats/min, blood pressure 160/80 mm Hg, rectal temperature of 108.4°F, and respirations were rapid and shallow at 48/min. His skin was blanched and slightly moist. Pupils were dilated to about 6 mm, and reacted minimally to light. The conjunctivae were edematous and became injected during the first hour. It was not possible to move his head in any direction, but all extremities were easily moved and reflexes were normally reactive.

Laboratory report revealed the following:

Hematocrit	= 50%
WBC	= 16,700/mm^3
Na$^+$	= 151 mEq/L
K$^+$	= 5.8 mEq/L
Cl$^-$	= 108 mEq/L
Glucose	= 95 mg%

His treatment consisted of vigorous gastric lavage, followed by chlorpromazine and pentobarbital. Following chlorpromazine, he became hypotensive (60 mm Hg systolic) but resumed an adequate blood

pressure when fluids were given. His temperature decreased to 101.6°F following immersion in an ice bath and massage. By 12 hr after admission, his temperature had returned to normal.

Twelve hours after admission, petechiae were noted over his lower extremities. His hematocrit fell twenty points over the next 5 days. He also developed acute renal failure. The patient responded slowly to all treatment, but eventually improved. He was discharged on the 37th hospital day. (See ref. 14.)

Discussion

1. When Patient 1 was first brought into the hospital, the cause of intoxication was unknown. What studies could have been done, or symptoms looked for to designate amphetamine as the probable cause of poisoning?

2. Comment on the hallucinations that Patient 1 experienced. Were they expected?

3. What are some of the reasons why Patient 2 did not succumb to the dose of amphetamine he allegedly ingested.

4. What events led into Patient 2's reduction in hematocrit? To what does the hematocrit refer?

CASE STUDY: STRYCHNINE POISONING

Case History

The patient was a 34-year-old female who had a medical history of personality disorders and attempted suicides. She was brought to the hospital approximately 30 min after ingesting a rodenticide product containing approximately 340 mg strychnine sulfate.

Upon admission the patient was alert, and displayed continuous spontaneous muscular twitches. While she was being examined, she experienced a generalized tonic seizure with opisthotonos positioning. All the while she remained fully aware of her surroundings and was frightened. She maintained full voluntary respiration and showed no signs of cyanosis.

Treatment. The victim's seizures were controlled with intravenous diazepam and succinylcholine. Thiopental sodium was administered to induce generalized anesthesia.

A nasogastric tube was then positioned and gastric lavage with saline performed. A slurry of activated charcoal and potassium permanganate (1:5000) was then instilled through the tube.

Laboratory values are presented in Table 10. Treatment with diazepam was continued. Phenytoin, sodium bicarbonate, and potassium chloride were added to her drug regimen. Diuresis was forced with saline.

The patient awoke in a quiet, darkened room. She continued to display spastic contractions of the muscles of her limbs, back, and neck for the next several hours. However, 6 hr after admission, she had fully recovered and no further spastic activity was noted. (See ref. 21.)

Discussion

1. Was the quantity of strychnine ingested a lethal dose?

2. Cite the reason why this patient was acidotic, and had an anion gap value of 33. Would a similar condition exist for other patients poisoned with (a) strychnine, and (b) other convulsants?

3. Comment on why this patient was placed in a quiet, darkened recovery room.

4. It appears that the victim was not lavaged until after she was under generalized anesthesia. Why did the treating physicians wait so long?

5. Within 6 hr after admission the patient had recovered. Did you expect her symptoms to persist longer? If they had, would dialysis procedures have been beneficial?

Review Questions

1. The occurrence of toxic reactions to the drugs listed in Table 2 (except for amphetamines, per se) is expected to increase in the future. Discuss why this statement is made.

2. A toxic dose of amphetamine would be expected to produce which of the following symptoms of poisoning: tachypnea (I), hypertension (II), or tachycardia (III)?
   A. II only
   B. III only
   C. I and II only
   D. II and III only
   E. I, II, and III

3. Toxic doses of amphetamine may cause hallucinations in certain individuals. Describe these reactions and relate their occurrence to the victim's dosing history.

4. Tolerance occurs to the CNS actions of amphetamine drugs, when the drugs are taken over a period of time.
   A. True
   B. False

5. Cite the pharmacological basis for strychnine-induced CNS stimulation. How does this differ from the mechanism of action of amphetamine?

6. Diazepam is the drug of first choice for controlling convulsive episodes caused by strychnine. Cite the reasons why it is preferred.

7. All of the following are true statements *except:*
   A. Cocaine causes direct stimulation of the heat-regulation center.
   B. Death from camphor poisoning is caused by hemorrhage into the gastrointestinal tract.
   C. Opisthotonos is a characteristic symptom of strychnine poisoning.
   D. Amphetamine excretion is enhanced by forced diuresis and urine acidification.

8. Victims of strychnine poisoning must be closely monitored for several days because of a chance for recurrence of convulsions due to the drug's long half-life.
   A. True
   B. False

9. Which of the following convulsants is a cause of euphoria, along with its other manifestations of CNS stimulation: strychnine (I), camphor (II), or cocaine (III)?
   A. II only
   B. III only
   C. I and II only
   D. II and III only
   E. I, II, and III

10. What is postictal depression? What causes it, and what is its toxic significance?

11. Explain the genesis of strychnine-induced hypertension and tachycardia.

12. Toxic symptoms on the cardiovascular system caused by cocaine are bi-phasic. Discuss the usual patterns and tell how these come about.

13. Discuss the medical significance of amphetamine-induced hyperpyrexia.

14. Explain what is meant by the following state-

ment: "Strychnine causes a characteristic convulsive pattern, but it may differ in various people."

15. Which of the following is a true statement?
    A. The largest single cause of camphor poisoning has been camphorated oil.
    B. Motor coordination is adversely affected at minimal doses of cocaine which cause euphoria.
    C. Strychnine action on the CNS is restricted to the motor cortex.
    D. The acute lethal adult dose for amphetamine is 5 mg/kg.

16. Chlorpromazine and haloperidol are commonly used to calm a victim of amphetamine toxicity. These drugs may have a major disadvantage, however. Discuss the problem and cite an alternative drug that can be used.

17. In Chapter 3 we learned that emesis was contraindicated in poisonings where convulsants were involved. However, in this chapter we are now told that emesis may be undertaken. Discuss the issue and cite any restrictions to this general statement.

18. A 1982 regulatory action by the Food and Drug Administration was directed at curtailing camphor-related poisonings. What was this action?

References

1. Aronow, R., and Spigiel, R. W. (1976): Implications of camphor poisoning. *Drug Intell. Clin. Pharm.*, 10:631–634.
2. Baldessarini, R. J. (1972): Pharmacology of the amphetamines. *Pediatrics*, 49:694–701.
3. Beckett, A. H., Rowland, M., and Tutner, P. (1965): Influence of urinary pH on excretion of amphetamine. *Lancet*, 1:303.
4. Benchimol, A., Bartall, H., and Desser, K. B. (1978): Accelerated ventricular rhythm and cocaine abuse. *Ann. Intern. Med.*, 88:519–520.
5. Bensinger, P. B. (1979): Statement before the Permanent Subcommittee on Investigation. *U.S. Senate*, December 7, 1979.
6. Bernheim, J., and Cox, J. N. (1960): Amphetamine overdosage in an athlete. *Br. Med. J.*, 2:590 (abstract).
7. Bruner, D. A., Page, T., Grego, C., Sweetman, L., Kulovich, S., and Nyhan, W. L. (1981): Progressive neurodegenerative disorder in a patient with nonketotic hyperglycinemia. *J. Pediatr.*, 98:272–275.

8. Coleman, D., Ross, T. F., and Naughton, J. L. (1982): Myocardial ischemia and infarction related to recreational cocaine use. *West. J. Med.*, 136:444–446.
9. Espelin, D. E., and Done, A. K. (1968): Amphetamine poisoning. *N. Engl. J. Med.*, 278:1361–1365.
10. Federal Register (1982): *Federal Register*, September 21, Vol. 47, p. 41716.
11. Franz, D. N. (1980): Central nervous system stimulants. In: *The Pharmacological Basis of Therapeutics*, 6th ed., edited by A. G. Gilman, L. S. Goodman, and A. Gilman, pp. 585–607. Macmillan, New York.
12. Gaft, H. H. (1925): Camphor liniment poisoning. *JAMA*, 84:1571.
13. Gary, N. E. (1978): Methamphetamine intoxication: A speedy new treatment. *Am. J. Med.*, 64:537–540.
14. Ginsberg, M. D., Hertzman, M., and Schmidt-Nowara, W. W. (1970): Amphetamine intoxication with coagulopathy, hyperthermia, and reversible renal failure. *Ann. Int. Med.*, 73:81–85.
15. Greenwood, R., and Peachey, R. S. (1957): Acute amphetamine poisoning, an account of 3 cases. *Br. Med. J.*, 1:742–744.
16. Heard, J. D., and Brooks, R. C. (1913): Clinical and experimental investigation of the therapeutic value of camphor. *Am. J. Med. Sci.*, 145:238–253.
17. Jaffe, J. H. (1980): Drug addiction and drug abuse. In: *The Pharmacological Basis of Therapeutics*, 6th ed., edited by A. G. Gilman, L. S. Goodman, and A. Gilman, pp. 535–584. Macmillan, New York.
18. Johnston, G. A. R. (1978): Neuropharmacology of amino acid inhibitory transmitters. *Ann. Rev. Pharmacol. Toxicol.*, 18:269–289.
19. Jones, D. V., and Work, C. E. (1961): Volume of a swallow. *Am. J. Med. Child.*, 102:427.
20. Jordan, C., Lehane, J. R., and Jones, J. G. (1980): Respiratory depression following diazepam: reversal with high-dose naloxone. *Anesthesiology*, 53:293–298.
21. Lambert, J. R., Byrick, R. J., and Hammeke, M. D. (1981): Management of acute strychnine poisoning. *CMA Journal*, 124:1268–1270.
22. Oderta, G. M., and Klein-Schwartz, W. (1982): Central nervous system stimulants. In: *Clinical Toxicology of Drugs: Principles and Practice*, edited by V. A. Skoutakis, pp. 183–199. Lea & Febiger, Philadelphia.
23. Perry, P. J., and Tuhl, R. P. (1977): Amphetamine psychosis. *Am. J. Hosp. Pharm.*, 34:883–885.
24. Phelan, W. J. (1976): Camphor poisoning: Over-the-counter dangers. *Pediatrics*, 57:428–431.
25. Rappolt, R. T., Gay, G. R., and Inaba, D. S. (1976): Propranolol in the treatment of cardiopressor effects of cocaine. *N. Engl. J. Med.*, 295:448.
26. Rappolt, R. T., Gay, G. R., Inaba, D. S., and Rappolt, N. R. (1976): Propranolol in cocaine toxicity. *Lancet*, 2:640–641.
27. Rappolt, R. T., Gay, G. R., Inaba, D. S., and Rappolt, N. R. (1978): Use of Inderol (propranolol—Ayerst) in a I-a (early stimulative) and I-b (advanced stimulative) classification of cocaine and other sympathomimetic reactions. *Clin. Toxicol.*, 13:325–332.
28. Ritchie, J. M., and Greene, N. M. (1980): Local anesthetics. In: *The Pharmacological Basis of Therapeutics*, 6th ed., edited by A. G. Gilman, L. S. Goodman, and A. Gilman, pp. 300–320. Macmillan, New York.

29. Scott, M. E., and Mullaly, R. W. (1981): Lithium therapy for cocaine-induced psychosis: A clinical perspective. *South. Med. J.,* 74:1475–1477.

30. Slater, I. H. (1971): Strychnine, pictotoxin, pentylenetetrazol, and miscellaneous drugs. In: *Pharmacology in Medicine,* 4th ed., edited by J. R. DiPalma, pp. 517–532. McGraw-Hill, New York.

31. Smith, A., and Margolis, G. (1954): Camphor poisoning. *Am. J. Pathol.,* 30:857.

32. Snyder, S. H. (1972): Catecholamines in the brain as mediators of amphetamine psychosis. *Arch. Gen. Psychiatry,* 27:169–179.

33. Teitelbaum, D. T., and Ott, J. E. (1970): Acute strychnine intoxication. *Clin. Toxicol.,* 3:267–273.

34. Trestrail, J. H., and Spartz, M. E. (1977): Camphorated and castor oil confusion and its toxic results. *Clin. Toxicol.,* 11:151–158.

35. von Wendt, L., Simila, S., Saukkonen, A. L., Koivisto, M., and Kouvalainen, K. (1981): Prenatal brain damage in nonketotic hyperglycinemia. *Am. J. Dis. Child.,* 135:1072.

36. Wetli, C. V., and Mittleman, R. E. (1980): The "body packer syndrome"—Toxicity following ingestion of illicit drugs packaged for transportation. *J. Forensic Sci.,* 26:492–500.

37. Zalis, E. G., and Parmley, L. F. (1963): Fatal amphetamine poisoning. *Arch. Intern. Med.,* 112:822–826.

Hallucinogens: Psychotomimetics

20

Hallucinogens are chemicals which, when taken in toxic doses, produce changes in perception, thought, and mood. The drugs and chemicals discussed in this chapter are also referred to as psychotomimetic agents, psychedelics ("mind-magnifying"), psycholytics ("mind-releasing"), or psychotogens.

Bear in mind that there is a fine line of distinction in this definition. Several classes of legitimate drugs (e.g., the anticholinergics, opioids, corticosteroids, etc.) can also cause euphoria and distort the vision when taken in sufficient dosage.

Hallucinogens can be derived from natural products, or produced synthetically. The classification we will follow is based on their chemical structure. Table 1 outlines the major chemical categories and lists representative examples of each.

TABLE 1. *Psychotomimetic agents: classification*

Ergot alkaloids
Lysergic acid diethylamide (LSD-25)
Tryptamine derivatives
DMT, *N,N*-dimethyltryptamine
DET, diethyltryptamine
Bufotenine, 5-hydroxy-*N,N*-dimethyltryptamine
Psilocybin and psilocin
Phenethylamine derivatives
Mescaline
DOM, STP, 2,5-dimethoxy-4-methylamphetamine
MDA, 3,4-methylenedioxyamphetamine
Miscellaneous
Phencyclidine, PCP

ERGOT ALKALOIDS

Lysergic Acid Diethylamide

In 1938, lysergic acid diethylamide (LSD-25) (Fig. 1) was inadvertently synthesized in a Swiss laboratory (14). Nearly a decade later, the first report of its effects in humans was released. As little as 25 to 50 ng (10^{-9} g) given orally produced marked behavioral effects. When LSD first came to light, it appeared that it might be useful in elucidating an etiology for schizophrenia (10), but after several years of intensive study and LSD misuse, the conclusion was reached that there is no legitimate medical use for this substance.

LSD is an extremely potent, odorless, colorless, and tasteless compound. It appears on the street in many dosage forms. For example, the liquid form is sometimes placed on sugar cubes or pieces of blotter paper. Solid dosage forms consist of extremely small, colorful "micro-dot" tablets. The average dose of LSD is 100 µg, but doses as high as 1,500 µg have been reported to cause no toxicity, and there have been reports of chronic users ingesting doses as high as 10,000 µg without suffering serious complications. The reason for an abuser of LSD to use such a high dose may be because tachyphylaxis, or rapid production of tolerance, occurs with repeated daily doses. A significant increase in dose may be necessary in 3 to 4 days after continued use, but physical dependence does not occur. An interesting element in LSD abuse is that recovery from the tolerance is just as rapid. Therefore, using a constant dose of LSD is possible, if only used on weekends or recreationally. Cross-tolerance with both mescaline and psilocybin has been shown to occur.

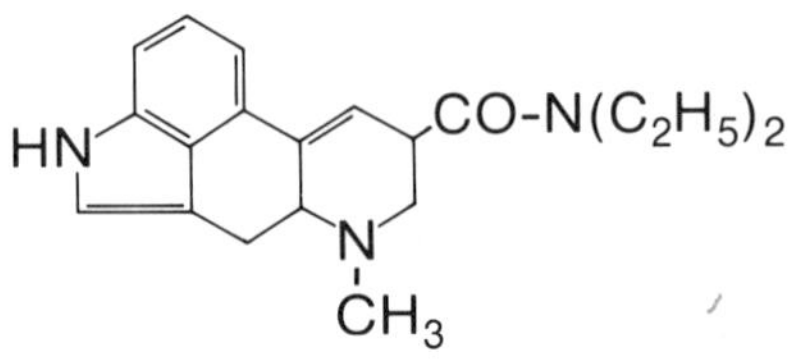

FIG. 1. Chemical structure of LSD (lysergic acid diethylamide).

The primary actions of LSD are on the CNS, with changes in mood and behavior being commonplace. The psychological effects can last 6 to 12 hr following an average dose. It affects both the pyramidal and extrapyramidal systems.

Mood changes range from euphoria to dysphoria. For example, the LSD user may feel euphoric, displaying hilarious laughter at some times, and then the mood swiftly changing to sadness with crying episodes. These mood swings tend to be influenced by small changes in the environment.

LSD acutely affects sensory perception. Although LSD acts on the auditory, tactile, olfactory, and gustatory senses, the most marked effects are on visual perception. Colors of objects become more intense. Flat surfaces assume a depth. Fixed objects begin to undulate and flow. Since there is an alteration of time perception, these visual changes seem to continue forever. LSD also causes disruption of ego function and the fear of self-destruction. Body parts may feel unnatural or foreign.

In addition to its effects on the CNS, LSD affects both the sympathetic nervous system and the parasympathetic nervous system, but sympathetic activities predominate. Therefore, as a sympathomimetic agent, some of the characteristics of LSD would include marked mydriasis, hyperthermia, piloerection, hyperglycemia, tachycardia, and hypertension.

Acute Lysergic Acid Diethylamide Toxicity

The toxicity of LSD has been studied in animals, and varies from species to species. Mice can tolerate the highest doses, and rabbits are the most sensitive. By extrapolation of animal data, the LD_{50} value of LSD for humans is estimated to be 0.2 mg/kg. Therefore, an average adult weighing 150 pounds would require a single oral dose of about 14 mg to achieve the LD_{50}. Thus, it could be stated that LSD has a high therapeutic index. Also, because large dose variations can be tolerated without significant physiologic consequences, variations in dose of street preparations of LSD do not seem as critical on a potential toxicity basis when compared to other street drugs such as phencyclidine (PCP). The major concern regarding street forms of LSD, as well as any other preparation manufactured in someone's basement, is the possibility of contaminants or impurities being present and, in some cases, the adulterant being used to dilute the drug. These problems are discussed later in the treatment of hallucinogenic substances.

When hallucinogens such as LSD are taken in a so-called "therapeutic" dose, a temporary psychotic state or "trip" results. Usually, an experienced user is knowledgable about adjusting the amount of drug needed to obtain this desired experience. On occasion, hallucinogens produce "bad trips" or adverse reactions. This has been attributed to the first-time user's lack of experience in relating the effects observed as being pleasurable. Other times, adverse reactions occur from contaminants or impurities because the drug may have been synthesized in a clandestine laboratory which lacks quality control assurance measures. Also, the mental state of the user has a definite influence on the incidence of adverse effects. These effects tend to fall into three categories: acute panic reactions, flashbacks, and prolonged psychoses.

Panic reactions are often seen at some stage of LSD usage, but rarely result in any major complications. This reaction is often described as a feeling of losing control. The person is no longer thinking rationally and feels he will not be able to come to grips with himself. It is important during these episodes that the person be reminded that what he is experiencing is drug-induced, and the "bad trip" will not last forever. For the panicked hallucinogen user, he may feel that his body and the chair he is sitting on are one and the same, and continued reassurance that he is a real person is helpful. Repeating the person's name and the present location and surroundings may help alleviate some of the anxiety associated with these panic reactions.

One of the more widely publicized chronic reactions to LSD use is the *flashback*. It is impossible to predict who will experience flashbacks, but the incidence is usually stated as one of every twenty users. They appear to occur more frequently in those users who have previously experienced "bad trips" and consistently abuse this drug, but flashbacks have also been reported to occur following a single LSD exposure. There are no set patterns of frequency or intensity, and flashbacks can be brief or last for several hours. One study has shown that flashbacks occur more frequently just before going to sleep and while under severe stress (17).

Three categories of flashbacks have been described: *perceptual*—seeing vivid colors, hearing sounds from previous trips; *somatic*—paresthesias, tachycardia; *emotional*—feelings of loneliness, panic, and depression. The most serious form is the emotional type, because the persistent feelings of fear, loneliness, and other emotions can lead to suicide.

Treatment of flashbacks is basically the same as for the acute panic reactions. The surroundings should be quiet. The person should be reassured that the condition is temporary and will not lead to permanent brain damage. If sedation is necessary, diazepam is recommended. A lighted room at bedtime may decrease the incidence of the flashback in some individuals.

Another danger that has plagued the hallucinogen abuser is the occurrence of prolonged psychosis or neurosis. States of paranoia and schizophrenia have been reported to occur, even after the general state of intoxication had subsided (8).

TRYPTAMINE DERIVATIVES

Hallucinogenic effects are also produced by a variety of tryptamine derivatives. Their names, chemical structures, and sources are listed in Table 2. These compounds do not differ greatly, chemically speaking, from one another. Likewise, their pharmacologic and toxicologic profiles are similar. The major difference is in their potency. Psilocybin will be used as a prototype for this group because it is the most commonly encountered hallucinogen in this category.

TABLE 2. *Chemical formulae for various derivatives of tryptamine*

Chemical name	Substitutions	R_1	R_2	R_3	R_4
DMT (*N,N*-dimethyltryptamine)		CH_3	CH_3	—	—
DET (diethyltryptamine)		CH_2-CH_3	CH_2-CH_3	—	—
Bufotenin (5-hydroxy-DMT)		CH_3	CH_3	—	OH
Psilocybin (O-phosphoryl-4-hydroxy-DMT)		CH_3	CH_3	OPO_3H	—
Psilocin (4-hydroxy-DMT)		CH_3	CH_3	OH	—
Serotonin (5-hydroxytryptamine)		H	H	—	OH

Psilocybin and Psilocin

Psilocybin occurs naturally in several species of mushrooms (Fig. 2), notably *Psilocybe mexicana*. Teonanacatl ("food of the Gods") has been used by the Indians of Mexico and Central America for centuries (9). The custom of incorporating the sacred mushroom into a semireligious ceremony dates back to 1500 B.C. In 1958, Hoffman, the discoverer of LSD, successfully isolated two alkaloids from *Psilocybe mexicana*: psilocybin, identified as the major constituent, and psilocin, which was shown to be equally as active but present in small quantities. These alkaloids are also present in numerous other varieties of mushrooms belonging to the genus *Psilocybe*, as well as in other mushroom species. Psilocybin is an unstable compound and is converted to psilocin in the body.

Pharmacological Effects of Psilocybin

As a hallucinogen, psilocybin exhibits a range of effects similar to LSD and mescaline. However, the potency of LSD is considerably greater than psilocybin, which, in turn, is more potent than mescaline. Twenty milligrams of psilocybin is equivalent to the usual dose (100 μg) for an LSD "trip." Therefore, LSD appears to be approximately 150 to 200 times more potent than psilocybin which is 1 to 5 times weaker than psilocin.

Oral doses of 60 to 200 μg/kg produce symptoms including weakness, nausea, anxiety, dreamy states, dizziness, blurred vision, dilated pupils, and increased deep tendon reflexes. The visual effects consist of brighter colors, longer afterimages, sharp definition of objects, and colored patterns and shapes that are generally pleasing, but sometimes frightening. The duration of action is usually about 3 hr.

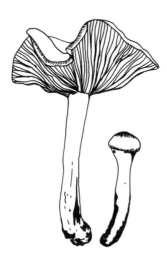

FIG. 2. Drawing of the psilocybe mushroom—source of psilocybin and psilocin.

Psilocybin Toxicity

Toxicological studies with psilocybin are limited. The LD_{50} in mice is 280 mg/kg. There have been no reports of toxic effects produced by psilocybin in humans when used under controlled experiments. The Indians' use of the drug in its natural form provides little information as to its cumulative toxicity since the mushrooms are not ingested chronically. However, there have been a few case reports of *Psilocybe* poisonings.

PHENETHYLAMINE DERIVATIVES

The phenethylamine group of hallucinogenic compounds (Table 3) represents a larger portion of those hallucinogens found in street use. Except for mescaline, the other members are synthetic analogs of amphetamine. The pharmacological actions of these drugs are similar to those of epinephrine and norepinephrine. This group of hallucinogens does not contain the indole nucleus; therefore, they are structurally dissimilar to the ergot alkaloids (LSD) and tryptamine derivatives (e.g., psilocybin).

Mescaline

One of the best documented hallucinogenic plants is the Peyote cactus, *Lophophora wil-liamsii*, which contains mescaline as its primary active ingredient. This plant has been used by Indians in northern Mexico as an adjunct to religious ceremonies since earliest recorded history (4). Individuals have also used the mescaline-containing buttons to relieve fatigue and hunger, and for treatment and prevention of various diseases. The peyote cult was largely confined to Mexico until the 19th Century when a number of tribes and tribal segments migrated north across the Rio Grande into the United States, and promoted the use of the plant.

Interest in peyote for nonreligious purposes began around 1890. A tincture was prepared to be used in the treatment of angina pectoris and pneumothorax, and as a depressant, respiratory stimulant, and cardiac tonic. The *National Standard Dispensatory* of 1905 devoted an entire page to peyote and its tinctures.

Pharmacological Actions of Mescaline

Mescaline is a phenethylamine derivative which belongs to the structural class of tetrahydroisoquinoline alkaloids and differs structurally from LSD, psilocybin, and other hallucinogenic drugs. Mescaline is a close chemical relative to epinephrine and norepinephrine.

When taken orally, at 5 mg/kg, mescaline produces unusual psychic effects and sensory

TABLE 3. *Chemical formulae for various phenylethylamine derivatives*

R_3, R_2, R_4, R_5 substituted benzene ring with -CH_2-CH(R_1)-NH_2 side chain

β-phenethylamine

Chemical name	R_1	R_2	R_3	R_4	R_5
Mescaline (3,4,5-trimethoxyphenethylamine)	H	H	OCH_3	OCH_3	OCH_3
Amphetamine	CH_3	H	H	H	H
DOM, STP (2,5-dimethoxy-4-methyl amphetamine)	CH_3	OCH_3	H	CH_3	OCH_3
MDA, XTC (3,4-methylenedioxyamphetamine)	CH_3	H	CH_2 (O—O)		H

alterations similar to those caused by small doses of LSD or psilocybin. The dose required for mescaline is about 4,000 to 5,000 times higher than that of LSD. The pupil size increases, pulse rate is also increased, and blood pressure is elevated. Deep tendon reflex thresholds are decreased by mescaline. Hallucinations are usually visual, consisting of bright, colored lights, geometric designs, animals, and sometimes people.

Mescaline is readily absorbed from the intestinal tract and concentrates in the kidney, liver, and spleen. In man, 60 to 90% of the dose is excreted unchanged; the remainder is eliminated as inactive metabolites. Peak blood levels are achieved about 2 hr after ingestion, with a duration of about 12 hr. The half-life is about 6 hr in man.

Mescaline Toxicity

No known human deaths have yet been reported as a result of taking massive doses of mescaline. Certain drugs, such as insulin, barbiturates, and physostigmine are known to increase the toxicity of mescaline.

2,5-Dimethoxy-4-methylamphetamine

2,5-Dimethoxy-4-methylamphetamine (DOM) is an amphetamine derivative having psychotomimetic effects. It is sometimes referred to as STP which reportedly describes "*serenity, tranquility, and peace.*"

Pharmacological Actions of 2,5-Dimethoxy-4-methylamphetamine

In man, DOM, like other hallucinogens, produces feelings of both euphoria and dysphoria at doses of 5 mg. DOM is 50 to 100 times more active than mescaline, but only one-thirtieth as potent as LSD. After oral administration, initial effects are noted within 90 min with peak effects occurring at about 3 to 4 hr, and hallucinations terminating in 6 to 24 hr. Anxiety is definitely increased at 3 to 6 hr, and obsessive compulsive symptoms are significantly increased after 6 hr.

DOM also causes stimulation of the sympathetic nervous system. This produces increased blood pressure, heart rate, pupillary diameter, and sweating. The CNS effects include nausea, anorexia, increased deep tendon reflexes, an altered EEG, paresthesia, tension, tremors, and fatigue.

2,5-Dimethoxy-4-methylamphetamine Toxicity

The median lethal dose (MLD) of DOM in rats is 60 mg/kg. There have been no deaths yet reported from the direct effects of DOM, but adverse reactions have been reported. These include an "acid trip," and anticholinergic symptoms (e.g., dry mouth, blurred vision, etc.).

3,4-Methylenedioxyamphetamine

3,4-Methylenedioxyamphetamine (MDA, XTC) continues to be a popular illicit drug. Chemically, MDA is related to mescaline and amphetamine. MDA is patented as an anorexiant, but has gained acceptance as a recreational drug due to its perceptual effects. Although the suggested anorectic dose is 8 to 50 mg, the psychotropic dose is closer to 100 mg.

On the street, MDA has been available in liquid form or as a powder which is often incorporated into capsules or tablets. Although MDA is commonly taken orally, it is sometimes inhaled nasally; but rarely injected. Adulterations and varying percentages of purported drugs can often be the source of acute toxicity. As with many drugs obtained illegally, it is never certain that the drug obtained is pure, or if it has been combined with or has been substituted with such items as LSD, amphetamines, atropine, or cocaine.

Pharmacological Actions of 3,4-Methylenedioxyamphetamine

MDA has mild sympathomimetic properties such as mydriasis, and produces stimulatory effects, especially on the respiratory center. MDA produces a sense of physical well-being with heightened tactile sensations. Visual and auditory hallucinations characteristic of an LSD "trip" usually do not occur. MDA is only one-third as potent as amphetamine, and three times as potent as mescaline.

A major distinction between MDA and other psychedelics (e.g., mescaline and LSD) is that MDA causes less distortion of perceptions. Hallucinations seem to manifest themselves when the person is most relaxed. Consequently, the psychic effects of the drug are reported to be more within the control of the user, than they are with the other hallucinogens. MDA produces an "inward, talk experience" in subjects who show interest in interpersonal relationships and an overwhelming desire or need to be with or talk to other people. For this reason it is often referred to as the "Love Drug."

A common undesired effect of MDA is periodic tensing of the muscles in the neck, tightening of the jaw, and grinding of the teeth. Other side effects include erratic behavior, delirium, and temporary amnesia. There have been several deaths related to the use of MDA. The lethal blood levels cited have ranged from 0.4 to 2.6 mg%.

PHENCYCLIDINE

Phencyclidine (PCP, 1-phenylcyclohexyl) piperidine (Fig. 3) was developed in the late 1950s, patented in 1963, and marketed as Sernyl®. Early animal studies showed the drug to have strong analgesic activity and, in 1957, clinical experiments were initiated. Doses of 25 mg/kg given intravenously produced anesthesia sufficient for minor or major surgery. It is chemically related to the dissociative anesthetic ketamine, but is much more toxic. Since in some cases, however, the drug produced postanesthetic confusion and delirium of prolonged duration, clinical investigations were soon dis-

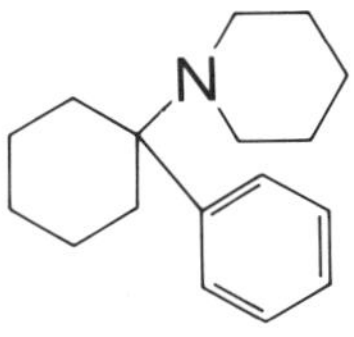

FIG. 3. Chemical structure of phencyclidine (1-phenylcyclohexyl) piperidine.

continued. All legal manufacture of PCP for human use in the United States has ceased.

PCP first began to appear on the streets in the summer of 1967 and was sold on the west coast area as the "*PeaCe Pill*." Many users reported unpleasant experiences, and the drug soon developed a questionable reputation. It disappeared in 1968, only to resurface on the eastern shores as "hog," but there, it also received a bad reputation and soon disappeared. At this time, its popularity has again increased and it is currently one of the most commonly used street drugs (11). It is sold on the street in a variety of different sizes, shapes, and colors of tablets and capsules; and as a white or off-color powder to be sprinkled on pieces of parsley, mint, and marijuana, or other plant material. It appears under a variety of exotic names including Angel Dust, Dust, Crystal, Crystal Joints, CJ, KJ, Peace, and Hog, to name a few.

Pharmacological Actions of Phencyclidine

PCP is taken orally, or used by inhalation, insufflation, and is sometimes injected intravenously. The estimated amount used per episode of smoking is 1.5 to 3.5 mg. The quantity per dose in powders and tablets averages 2 to 6 mg. The onset of subjective effects after smoking is reported to occur within 1 to 5 min and last for 4 to 6 hr. A more rapid onset of 30 sec to 1 min is observed following insufflation of the powder.

Blood levels of PCP as low as 0.10 µg/ml may be associated with behavioral effects leading to injury or death (Table 4). Levels greater than 1.0 µg/ml are associated in most instances with coma, which may result in death due to secondary complications such as seizure and respiratory depression. Doses of PCP resulting in blood concentrations of 2.0 to 2.5 µg/ml and greater are probably uniformly fatal (2).

PCP is an analgesic, with sympathomimetic and CNS stimulant and depressant properties. It has no ganglionic blocking effects, and no anticholinergic or antihistaminic actions.

Neurological signs of PCP at low doses or following chronic administration of less than 10

TABLE 4. *Characteristics of phencyclidine intoxication*

Serum level	Signs and symptoms
20–30 ng/ml	Agitation and irritability, blank stare, catatonia, catalepsy, sweating, flushing, nystagmus, inability to speak, body image changes, disorganized thoughts
30–100 ng/ml	As above; and coma or stupor, vomiting, hypersalivation, repetitive muscular movements, rigidity, shivering, fever, decreased peripheral feelings (pain, touch, etc.), depression, schizophrenia
100 ng/ml	As above, but more intense and prolonged i.e., hypertension, opisthotonos, convulsions, absent peripheral sensations, decreased reflexes, hallucinations, disorientation, loss of memory

From ref. 2.

mg (which gives blood levels up to 100 μg/ml) include: horizontal and vertical nystagmus, variable pupil size with depressed light reflex, and occasional blurred or double vision. Additionally, ataxia, tremors, slurred speech, muscle weakness, drowsiness, and increased respiratory rate and depth are observed (10). Sudden and dramatic mood changes are also seen along with delusion, purposeless talk, disoriented thought process, and sometimes visual hallucinations. As the state of intoxication wears off, the person gradually shifts to a state of mild depression where he is irritable, feels isolated and sometimes paranoid.

The chronic PCP user generally requires 24 to 48 hr to completely return to what he considers normal. Most individuals who have used PCP find the subjective effects difficult to describe, but most agree that the experience is distinctly different from other drug experiences they have encountered. Although many describe the experience as positive, first-time users or those who use PCP unknowingly encounter an unpleasant and often frightening experience.

Psychological dependence and tolerance to the psychic effects of PCP requiring increasing doses to obtain the desired effects are reported by chronic users. Paranoia, auditory hallucinations, violent behavior, severe depression, and anxiety have followed prolonged periods of daily, regular use.

Phencyclidine Toxicity

PCP toxicity is manifested by a stuporous, comatose state in which the patient is responsive only to deep pain. Hypertension and tachycardia are present. Important diagnostic features of PCP intoxication include the presence of vertical and horizontal nystagmus which is associated with hypertension in a comatose individual.

Massive oral overdoses of up to 1 g street-grade PCP have resulted in periods of stupor and coma of several hours to 5 days in duration. Delayed and prolonged respirations and apnea may result. Intoxication is also marked by sustained hypertension and tachycardia, and general motor seizures preceded by muscle tremors and rigidity.

There are numerous reports of PCP-induced psychosis described as an initial violent, aggressive, and/or disorganized behavior with or without paranoia lasting from less than 4 hr to as long as several days. Restless and combative behavior and thought patterns are usually complete in one week, but severe cases may require 12 to 18 months to return to predrug status.

Many deaths associated exclusively with PCP intoxication have been reported in the United States. The manner of death has been accidental, suicidal, and homicidal. In most cases, circumstantial evidence suggested that death was secondary to the behavioral toxicity of PCP (3). In other words, most victims die from trauma, drowning, or similar accidents.

Treatment of Acute Phencyclidine Intoxication

PCP is a common cause of psychotic, drug-related emergency room admissions. The most common diagnostic features for PCP intoxication include horizontal or vertical nystagmus, muscular rigidity and hypertension. The patient may be agitated, psychotic, or comatose, but respirations are not compromised unless PCP was ingested with alcohol, sedatives, or opiates. Since there is no specific antidote for PCP, treatment of acute PCP intoxication is focused on supportive and symptomatic care of the patient. Complete recovery may require several weeks or longer. Also, fluctuations in symptoms are common. A victim may emerge from coma, only to worsen later (6).

There has been some success with placing the agitated, psychotic individual in an attended, quiet, and darkened room, but the "talking down" methods commonly used for LSD and other hallucinogens usually are ineffective.

Diazepam has been successfully used to treat the hyperactivity and agitation of the intoxicated patient. Phenothiazines (e.g., chlorpromazine) and butyrophenones (haloperidol) are not recommended for PCP intoxication because they lower the seizure threshold and may produce severe hypotension.

Unlike the phenethylamine-type of hallucinogens, severe hypertensive crisis is not usually encountered. If present, however, it should be treated with a rapidly-acting vasodilator such as diazoxide or nitroprusside.

Renal damage is sometimes a complication of PCP because of the profound involuntary muscular activity which can lead to diffuse muscle injury and myoglobinuria (5,13). To reduce the possibility of acute renal failure, diuretics such as furosemide have been used. Physical restraint using belts should be used only when necessary to keep muscle injury minimized and, hence, help prevent onset of renal damage (13).

At this point, efforts should be focused on hastening elimination of PCP. It is extremely lipid-soluble, and a weak base with a pKa between 8.6 and 9.4. The drug also undergoes enterohepatic circulation. As a result, when PCP enters the acidic environment of the stomach, it becomes trapped in the ionized form which may be efficiently removed by gastric suction, and adding 30 to 40 g of activated charcoal

every 6 to 8 hr (15). In severe PCP intoxication, acidification of the urine to a pH between 5.0 and 5.5 with ammonium chloride will greatly enhance the elimination of this basic drug. Once urinary pH is approximately 5, furosemide can be given to promote diuresis (1). Decreases in plasma pH have also been shown to aid in removal of PCP from the CNS (10). Because of the small quantities involved, and because the PCP-intoxicated patient often has other drugs in his blood and urine, accurate monitoring of PCP levels is extremely difficult (12,18).

For example, Table 5 illustrates what happens to PCP distribution during plasma and urine acidification. When the urine pH was lowered from 7.5 to 5.0 with ammonium chloride, urinary PCP concentration increased from 43 ng/ml to nearly 4,000 ng/ml. This clearly illustrates that excretion is enhanced. Furthermore, PCP levels in the cerebrospinal fluid were lowered from an initial value of 140 ng/ml to 8 ng/ml.

The treatment of PCP intoxication, as with other hallucinogens, is based on common sense. The principles for antidotal therapy that were established in previous chapters are just as valid for illicit drugs as they are for the licit ones. Common sense should always prevail when an antidoting profile is being established.

TREATMENT OF ADVERSE EFFECTS TO HALLUCINOGENS

The major dilemma encountered in treating psychoactive drug toxicity is being able to get

TABLE 5. *Influence of urine and plasma acidification on phencyclidine distribution*

Body fluid	Before acidification[a]		After acidification	
	pH	PCP (ng/ml)	pH	PCP (ng/ml)
Serum	7.4	66	7.2	50
CSF	—	140	—	8
Urine	7.5	43	5.0	3,997

[a]Acidification performed with ammonium chloride.
From ref. 6.

a rapid, accurate identification of the chemical substance. Substance abuse has taken several forms over the years. The same drug may be found on the street as a fine powder, tablet, or capsule, or it may be disguised in a sugar cube and pieces of blotter paper. In addition, the abuser or experimenter may think he is using a certain drug but, in actuality, the substance may either contain no drug, or an entirely different type of drug. Street drugs have been reported to be "cut" with substances such as mescaline, amphetamine, anticholinergics, and camphor (21). Those compounds that were popular last year may not be this year. The patient's history is often difficult to interpret because of the validity of the circumstances. A scared young teenager is not always ready to tell what he has been enjoying at the concert besides the music. Additionally, he may not even know the identity of his drugs. At one rock concert several years back, 4,000 unidentified doses of illicit drugs were reported to have been taken (20).

Most hallucinogens have a high therapeutic index and, therefore, toxicity due directly to their pharmacologic actions is seldom encountered. It is the psychological manifestations of these compounds that need to be attended to.

In general, the victim who experiences adverse effects to hallucinogens should be placed in a quiet environment to minimize external stimuli which could aggravate their psychotic state. He must not be left unattended, and must be given constant positive assurance.

Other treatment is largely supportive. Increased blood pressure may be a severe problem, especially with the amphetamine-like hallucinogens which have strong sympathomimetic activity. Rapid lowering of blood pressure to normal can be achieved with a vasodilator agent. Convulsions and anxiety are usually managed successfully with diazepam. "Bad trips," panic reactions, and psychotic episodes generally respond well to treatment with chlorpromazine. Following recovery, psychiatric consultation is mandated.

SUMMARY

Hallucinogens are characterized as chemicals which cause intense physiological alterations in very small doses. Poisoning by hallucinogens is a fairly common event. Managing a toxic event following their ingestion is met with numerous obstacles and problems which, at first observation, imply that their antidoting requires a distinct guideline. However, most symptoms can be controlled when basic principles that have been established earlier in this book are implemented.

Case Studies

CASE STUDIES: PHENCYCLIDINE INTOXICATION

History: Case 1

The patient was a 26-year-old female with a history of psychiatric disease. She had no history of abusing either alcohol or other drugs, including PCP.

One evening at a party, she was offered a joint of PCP and smoked approximately one-half of it. Shortly thereafter, she developed paranoia and reported visual and auditory hallucinations.

Two days later she was admitted to a psychiatric hospital for treatment. At this point, both her blood and urine were negative for PCP, but the symptoms persisted.

Her psychosis, which persisted for over 2 weeks, was treated with haloperidol. Eventually she recovered, but she continued to suffer from depression. (See ref. 19.)

History: Case 2

A chronic male abuser of PCP, aged 29 years, was sitting in front of the television, smoking a PCP joint. His wife began nagging him about his habit and his laziness in not having a job. She told him their new baby was sick and she was going to take the child to a doctor. An argument ensued and continued for the next few minutes, at which time the man blacked out.

He awoke to a state of partial consciousness sometime later. He was then observed running naked along the street, covered with blood from self-inflicted wounds. He carried a knife in his hands, yelling, "Hallelujah, I'm Jesus."

Some time later, he entered the house of a strange woman who was pregnant. He killed the woman, her unborn child, and her two-year-old child.

The crazed man was apprehended, and later convicted of murder. He still has no recollection of the event and cannot explain his motives for these actions. (See ref. 19.)

Discussion

1. Outline the series of events these patients might have received to treat PCP intoxication. Shouldn't the patient in Case 1 have been subjected to these procedures?

2. Various experts in treating PCP intoxication agree there is frequently a triggering stimulus for most events that occur as a result of poisoning. What was the event that probably caused the patient in Case 2 to behave as he did?

3. What leads you to suspect that part of the symptoms displayed by Patient 1 were actually due more to her underlying mental illness, rather than to PCP?

CASE STUDIES: LYSERGIC ACID DIETHYLAMIDE INTOXICATION

History: Case 1

A 21-year-old female was admitted to the hospital accompanied by a male friend who was experienced in using LSD. About 30 min after he had convinced her to ingest approximately 200 μg of LSD, she began to experience the effects of the drug and said she felt that the bricks on the wall moved in and out. A panic reaction set in when she was unable to distinguish her body from the chair in which she was sitting, or from her friend's body. Her fears became worsened when she felt she would not be able to get back into herself.

On admission she was hyperexcited and laughed inappropriately. Her talk and reactions to others were disorganized and illogical.

Two days later the panic reaction subsided; however, she was still afraid of the drug and indicated she would never again take it. (See ref. 7.)

History: Case 2

A male in his late twenties was seen at the admitting office in a state of panic. He had at least 15 previous experiences with LSD and other hallucinogens. Most of his prior encounters with LSD were pleasurable except that he had experienced panic reactions twice. During these episodes, he stated that he was losing control and his whole body was disappearing. It had been at least 2 months since he had

taken his last LSD dose, and the problems he experienced now were apparently resulting as a flashback to a prior encounter.

His present experience, on flashback, depicted some of the delusions, perceptual distortions, and feelings of union with things around him which mimicked the kinds of trips he previously encountered. (See ref. 7.)

Discussion

1. Why do flashbacks occur and what provokes them?

2. What is the mode of treatment for a panic reaction as seen in Case 2?

3. Do you suppose the person in Case 1 was sincere in her statement that she would not use LSD again?

CASE STUDY: 3,4-METHYLENEDIOXYAMPHETAMINE MISUSE

Case History

A 24-year-old male arrived at a party around 7:30 p.m. He ingested one Quaalude® tablet containing 300 mg methaqualone. Approximately 15 min later he ingested 500 mg of a white powder which was believed to contain a mixture of LSD, morphine, and amphetamine. The powder was wrapped in a tissue and formed into a ball which he swallowed. At 11:00 p.m. he ingested an additional 700 mg of the powder.

Within an hour he complained of being extremely "high" and needed to calm down. While resting, he was sweating profusely and speaking irrationally.

For the next hour or so, he was totally incoherent and was thrashing violently. His hands were continually moving as if he were trying to pick up things. Finally, the victim's eyes rolled back and he swallowed his tongue.

He was immediately attended to by guests at the party. They pulled his tongue back and initiated mouth-to-mouth resuscitation, and he seemed to improve. He then became very calm and slept, but at 2:30 a.m. he was found completely unresponsive and was rushed to the hospital. On admission, his pupils were dilated and fixed, and the ECG showed no signs of cardiac activity. He was pronounced dead at 4:00 a.m.

Autopsy findings were unremarkable except for visceral coagulation and signs of anoxia. Toxicity findings confirmed ingestion of methaqualone by the presence of its metabolite in the urine, but failed to demonstrate the presence of amphetamine or morphine. However, thin-layer chromatographic analysis of the urine did reveal an unusual amine compound identified, by using more specific analytical instruments, as 3,4-methylenedioxyamphetamine (MDA). (See ref. 16.)

Discussion

1. Explain the patient's "thrashing" about. How did MDA cause this?

2. Following an episode of apparent hyperexcitability, the victim became sedated and slept. What is the most likely explanation for this?

3. Comment on the probable cause of death.

Review Questions

1. Discuss the toxic meaning of the terms, psychedelics, psycholytics, psychotomimetics, and psychotogens.

2. Defend or rebuke the statement: "Used properly, LSD has a legitimate place in medicine." Cite the reasons you chose your point of view.

3. List each of the following in decreasing order of toxicity: LSD, PCP, mescaline, psilocybin, psilocin, and DOM.

4. Explain the physiological origin of LSD-induced tachycardia and hypertension. How do these come about?

5. Describe the pharmacological/toxicological effects an individual using psilocybin would experience.

6. A victim of DOM toxicity should receive treatment directed toward:
   A. Increasing the blood pressure
   B. Decreasing the blood pressure

7. A patient experiencing a toxic reaction to PCP should expect symptoms referrable to which of the following pharmacological actions: ganglionic blocking effect (I), sympathomimetic action (II), or anticholinergic action (III).
   A. II only
   B. III only
   C. I and II only

D. II and III only
E. I, II, and III

8. Tolerance to LSD develops rapidly; recovery from this tolerance occurs slowly.
   A. True
   B. False

9. Flashbacks are an important toxicologic consequence of LSD therapy and the victim experiencing them must be carefully managed. Discuss the forms these flashbacks may take, and their danger to the victim.

10. The phenethylamine derivatives mimic effects of some naturally occurring endogenous neurotransmitters. What are these neurotransmitters, and, overall, what are the symptoms of poisoning these drugs cause?

11. Describe the presenting symptoms that would most likely be noted in a victim of STP poisoning.

12. List the major reasons why it is often difficult to effectively antidote a person who presents at the emergency room with symptoms of toxicity from an unknown psychotomimetic agent.

13. Describe the treatment protocol and objectives for PCP intoxication. Why are phenothiazines and butyrophenones not recommended as antidotes?

14. Most hallucinogens have a low therapeutic index.
    A. True
    B. False

References

1. Aronow, R., and Done, A. K. (1978): Phencyclidine overdose: An emerging concept in management. *J. Am. Coll. Emerg. Physicians*, 7:56–59.
2. Aronow, R., Miceli, J. N., and Done, A. K. (1980): A therapeutic approach to the acutely overdosed PCP patient. *J. Psychedelic Drugs*, 12:259–267.
3. Beeson, H. A. (1982): Intracranial hemorrhage associated with phencyclidine abuse. *JAMA*, 248:585–586.
4. Bergman, R. L. (1971): Navajo peyote use: Its apparent safety. *Am. J. Psychiatry*, 128:51–60.
5. Cogen, F. C., Regg, G., and Simmons, J. L. (1978): Phencyclidine-associated acute rhabdomyolysis. *Ann. Int. Med.*, 88:210–212.
6. Done, A. K., Aronow, R., and Miceli, J. N. (1980): Pharmacokinetic bases for the diagnosis and treatment

of acute PCP intoxication. *J. Psychedelic Drugs*, 12:253–258.

7. Frosch, W. A., Robbins, E. S., and Stern, M. (1965): Untoward reactions to lysergic acid diethylamide (LSD) resulting in hospitalization. *N. Engl. J. Med.*, 273:1235–1239.

8. Hatrick, J. A., and Dewhurst, K. (1970): Delayed psychosis due to LSD. *Lancet*, 2:742–744.

9. Hofmann, A. (1961): Chemical, pharmacological and medical aspects of psychotomimetics. *J. Exp. Med. Sci.*, 5:40.

10. Jaffee, J. H. (1980): Drug addiction and drug use. In: *The Pharmacological Basis of Therapeutics*, 6th ed., edited by A. G. Gilman, L. S. Goodman, and A. Gilman, pp. 535–584. Macmillan, New York.

11. Karp, H. N., Kaufman, N. D., and Anand, S. K. (1980): Phencyclidine poisoning in young children. *J. Pediatr.*, 97:1006–1009.

12. Khajawall, A. M., and Simpson, G. M. (1982–83): Peculiarities of phencyclidine urinary excretion and monitoring. *J. Toxicol.: Clin. Toxicol.*, 19:835–842.

13. Lahmeyer, H. W., and Stock, P. G. (1983): Phency-clidine intoxication, physical restraint, and acute renal failure: Case report. *J. Clin. Psychiatry*, 44:184–185.

14. Mace, S. (1979): LSD. *Clin. Toxicol.*, 15:219–224.

15. Picchioni, A. I., and Conroe, P. F. (1979): Activated charcoal—a phencyclidine antidote, or hog in dogs. *N. Engl. J. Med.*, 300:202.

16. Poklis, A., Mackell, M. A., and Drake, W. K. (1979): Fatal intoxication from 3,4-methylenedioxyamphetamine. *J. Forensic Sci.*, 24:70–75.

17. Shick, J. F. E., and Smith, D. E. (1970): Analysis of the LSD flashback. *J. Psychedelic Drugs*, 3:13–19.

18. Simpson, G. M., Khajawall, A. M., Alatorre, E., and Staples, F. R. (1982–83): Urinary phencyclidine excretion in chronic abusers. *J. Toxicol.: Clin. Toxicol.*, 19:1051–1059.

19. Smith, D. E., and Wesson, D. R. (1980): PCP abuse: Diagnostic and psychopharmacological treatment approaches. *J. Psychedelic Drugs*, 12:293–299.

20. Taylor, R. L., Maurer, J. I., and Tinklenberg, J. R. (1970): Management of "bad trips" in an evolving drug scene. *JAMA*, 213:422–425.

21. Unwin, J. R. (1968): Illicit drug use among Canadian youth. *Can. Med. Assoc. J.*, 98:449–454.

Vitamins

21

Accidental poisoning by vitamin products currently ranks as a major cause of poisoning in children under the age of five. Similar toxic reactions also occur in adults, and reports of such poisonings have increased since the advent of the megadose concept. Luckily, few deaths are reported since symptoms of severe poisoning appear quickly and sufficient time is usually available to seek antidotal assistance.

The consumption of vitamins (and minerals) has increased in the United States over the past several years due to our heightened interest in good health and nutrition, exercise, and preventive medicine. It is also a time of interest in fad diets, and a generalized belief that vitamins will prevent many of the major diseases from occurring. While this trend has contributed to the decrease seen in vitamin deficiency diseases, this same expanded consumption has also increased the unnecessary potential toxicity to these substances and, indeed, most reported cases result from accidental, rather than intentional administration (4,156 of 4,580 cases reported for 1978) (18). They can also be purchased without a prescription in nonpharmacy outlets in dosage strengths that often require a prescription when purchased from pharmacy outlets. Because of their intense advertising promotions in consumer-oriented publications and direct mail announcements, excessive self-dosing is not uncommon and now is expected to increase to even greater heights. A long battle to gain control of vitamin regulation for American consumers appears to finally have ended in 1981, when the Food and Drug Administration put this issue to rest (8). With governmental pressure off vitamin product manufacturers and promoters, at least for the present, advertising campaigns and, ultimately, increased use, rational and irrational, is expected. Additionally, many health professionals lack sound scientific knowledge and good judgment regarding the absolute benefits of vitamins and their potential for toxicity and may fail to adequately advise their patients about these issues.

Only rarely is an acute vitamin toxicity reaction reported. Most cases involve chronic utilization of vitamins over months to years. Generally, symptoms appear slowly over a period of time so that early recognition usually occurs allowing the victim to seek medical help before the event causes serious, irreversible damage. In some instances, there is no doubt that many of the reported cases of toxicity to "vitamins" are actually due to iron contained in the product, or even to some other mineral.

MEGADOSING

A vitamin megadose is defined as a dose that is ten or more times the recommended daily allowance (RDA) (9). This differs from most "therapeutic formulae" which include vitamins at 2 to 5 times the RDA. Most people who advocate the use of megadoses report that they personally feel better when these large doses are consumed. They strongly argue that if a little is good, more is better. Rarely do they take megadoses of any vitamin because of a true diagnosed vitamin deficiency state. Vitamin overdosing (megadosing) can produce toxic reactions and may produce confusing symptoms which lead to expensive and inappropriate laboratory tests, and to severely toxic reactions.

Toxic manifestations of vitamin overingestion are more commonly seen with the fat-soluble vitamins A and D. Fat-soluble vitamin K has been less frequently reported to induce toxicities, probably because it is not available for self-administration without a prescription. Vitamin E is practically nontoxic, at least according to current knowledge. For the most part, the water-soluble B complex and vitamin C are eliminated in the urine when taken in overdose. While they do produce some minor reactions and may be the cause of a drug interaction or modification of a laboratory value, these generally cannot be considered to be life-threatening. An exception is vitamin C which induces serious renal toxicity in a small number of susceptible individuals. Because of the *potential* seriousness of vitamins A, D, and C in overdoses, their toxicity is discussed in more detail than the other vitamins.

Vitamin A

Vitamin A toxicity was first reported by Arctic explorers in 1857 when they consumed large quantities of polar bear liver. Numerous accounts of toxicity have since continued to appear in the literature (6). Whereas modern, sophisticated techniques and instrumentation continue to provide a wealth of detailed knowledge on the overall problem, there is little factual information concerning the exact pathogenesis of vitamin A-induced toxicity.

Vitamin A poisoning is usually due to over-ambitious prophylactic vitamin therapy from extended self-medication. Hypervitaminosis A has also resulted from overingestion of animal liver by hunters. It has resulted from food faddism, and, unfortunately, from solicitous parents who have inadvertently given overdoses to children. Hypervitaminosis A has also occurred in patients receiving large doses to treat certain skin diseases, such as ichthyosis, acne, and Darier's disease (a genetically-transmitted disease in which the skin becomes extremely crusty).

Chronic renal disease may also result in a state of relative hypervitaminosis A. This is compounded in patients on hemodialysis because of the failure of this procedure to remove vitamin A from the blood. The practice of prescribing vitamins for patients undergoing hemodialysis is common, but it is suggested that these patients avoid supplementing their diets with products containing vitamin A (25).

Mechanisms of Vitamin A Toxicity

The mechanism of vitamin A toxicity to the CNS is unclear. A *"retinol-binding" protein* in the CNS is involved in transport of the vitamin across lipid membranes. Clinical toxicity resulting in hypervitaminosis A occurs when this protein becomes saturated with the vitamin. Cellular membranes are thus exposed to unbound vitamin which then causes degradation of the membrane structure (27). This same mechanism may be responsible for the increased cerebral spinal fluid pressure that is characteristic of vitamin A toxicity (5).

The exact pathogenesis of vitamin A-induced liver damage is, likewise, not clear. Strong evidence suggests that excessive hepatic levels lead to fibrosis, sclerosis of the central hepatic veins,

and destruction of sinusoidal spaces with subsequent portal hypertension and ascites (2,16).

Vitamin A significantly elevates serum parathyroid hormone levels in otherwise healthy men, at doses as low as 25,000 units. Toxic symptoms resulting from hypercalcemia, bony changes, and premature epiphyseal closure are felt to be due to this action (3).

Symptoms of Vitamin A Toxicity

Vitamin A-induced symptoms of toxicity are summarized in Table 1. While these outcomes at first appear to be widely diverse, they are readily categorized into several subheadings. A patient intoxicated with vitamin A may not show

TABLE 1. *Signs and symptoms of vitamin A intoxication*

Gastrointestinal
  Nausea/vomiting, anorexia, gingivitis, mouth fissures, abdominal cramping

Central nervous system
  Headache, irritability and restlessness, fatigue, nystagmus, increased intracranial pressure, hydrocephalus, neurological symptoms and psychiatric disturbances, paresthesias (arms and legs), vision changes, dizziness, sluggishness, bulging fontanels

Skin
  Dry, pruritic skin; rash; desquamation; alopecia

Muscle and joints
  Myalgia; muscle fasciculations; tender, deep and hard swellings on extremities and occipital area of head; joint and muscle pain

Bone
  Hyperostoses

Other
  Hepatosplenomegaly, lymph node enlargement, hepatic fibrosis, bleeding, chronic fever, hypercalcemia, sensitivity reactions, cirrhosis, rodent teratology

all of these symptoms, and since many of them are nonspecific, early suspicion and diagnosis of toxicity may be missed.

Another problem is that detection of vitamin A toxicity is occasionally missed because many of the symptoms of poisoning are similar to those of the underlying condition for which the vitamin was taken.

Most toxicity reports indicate that daily doses of vitamin A in the range of 300,000 to 600,000 units (given over a period from a few months to several years) are required to produce symptoms. However, lesser doses are occasionally reported to be toxic. Daily doses averaging 40,000 units or more in adults (given over several months to a few years) have caused toxicity symptoms (1). Ingestion of as little as 25,000 to 50,000 units of retinol daily for 30 days has induced signs of increased intracranial pressure in infants (15).

Treatment of Vitamin A Intoxication

Treatment of vitamin A intoxication includes immediate discontinuation of the substance. Most signs and symptoms will disappear within a week or two. Hyperostoses may remain evident for several months after clinical recovery. However, if symptoms are ignored and the vitamin is not withdrawn, irreversible hepatic damage, including cirrhosis, may result.

Vitamin E is occasionally reported to protect against hypervitaminosis A. While some papers state that vitamin E offers a degree of protection against toxicity, others show that vitamin E may actually enhance tissue uptake of vitamin A. If significant, this latter effect could answer why previous reports state that vitamin E lowers vitamin A blood levels.

Vitamin D

Vitamin D is the most toxic of all vitamins. A large number of cases of toxicity has been reported in people using vitamin D to treat arthritis, muscle cramps, cold hands and feet, and a variety of other real or imagined disorders. Additionally, the vitamin is occasionally used in excess to treat various nutritional disorders in persons of all ages. Because excessive and repeated doses are frequently taken, reports of toxicity to this vitamin have increased in recent years (6).

Vitamin D misuse in Britain and the European continent, with intakes averaging 300,000 to 400,000 units daily, is believed to have been responsible for the idiopathic hypercalcemia of infancy that was frequently reported during and immediately following World War II. At that time, ambitious supplementation of food with vitamins reached a peak and was often far in excess of what was needed. The disorder was clinically characterized by hypercalcemia and skeletal abnormalities, as well as premature hardening of the arteries, irreversible mental retardation, and early death, usually before puberty. The disease became rare after the dietary intake of vitamin D was reduced to less than 1,500 units daily (19).

Mechanisms of Vitamin D Toxicity

All of the clinically significant problems inherent in vitamin D toxicity are caused by its effect to elevate plasma calcium levels. The vitamin, per se, does not elevate calcium. Rather, this is dependent on conversion of vitamin D through a succession of steps, to 1,25-dihydroxycholecalciferol as shown in Fig. 1. Once formed, 1,25-dihydroxycholecalciferol exerts

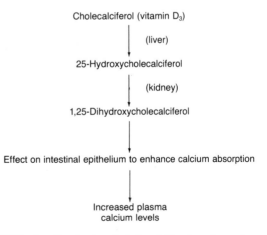

FIG. 1. Synthesis of cholecalciferol to its active form, 1,25-dihydroxycholecalciferol.

effects at several sites, including the intestinal epithelium, to promote calcium absorption. Vitamin D toxicity would be expected to be more severe in an individual whose thyroid has been removed, since the counter-hormone, calcitonin, is synthesized within the parafollicular cells of this gland. Calcitonin normally exerts a negative effect on plasma calcium levels. In its deficient state, however, the control for calcium is reduced, and plasma levels rise unchecked.

Symptoms of Vitamin D Toxicity

Symptoms of vitamin D toxicity are largely referable to hypercalcemia and are listed in Table 2. Deaths occurring after acute toxic doses are usually attributed to this finding. Toxic effects from chronic use are due to deposition of calcium in the body's soft tissues, especially in the kidneys and heart. Aortic valvular stenosis (narrowing) and nephrocalcinosis with calcification of other soft tissues are characteristic findings. Renal function may be severely and irreversibly impaired and normal cardiac rhythm may become abnormal following prolonged deposition of calcium salts within the myofibrils of the heart. X-ray examination of patients poisoned with vitamin D shows metastatic calcification and generalized osteoporosis of bone. A single episode of moderately severe hypercalcemia may arrest the growth of children

TABLE 2. *Signs and symptoms of vitamin D intoxication*

Hypercalcemia (weakness, fatigue, lassitude, headache, nausea/vomiting, diarrhea)
Impaired renal function (polyuria, polydipsia, nocturia, decreased urinary concentrating ability, proteinuria)
Deposition of calcium salts in soft tissues (nephrolithiasis and nephrocalcinosis)
Hypertension
Decreased plasma cholesterol
Osteoporosis, skeletal abnormalities
Supravalvular aortic stenosis
Premature hardening of the arteries
Irreversible mental retardation
Anorexia
Hypotonia
Constipation
Arrested growth

---

completely for 6 months or more and physicians often report that this deficit in height may never be fully corrected (21).

A large single dose of vitamin D_3 or D_4 generally does not cause toxicity. Vitamin D intoxication can occur after chronic oral ingestion of large doses of vitamin D_2 or D_3 (usually in excess of 50,000–100,000 units daily) taken for several months (11). These excessive quantities are stored in body fat later to be released slowly into the blood.

A study compared vitamin D consumption in patients who suffered from angina pectoris, previous myocardial infarction, or degenerative joint disease (14). It specifically correlated men with different dietary intakes of vitamin D over many years to their incidence of myocardial infarction. The result suggested that high doses of vitamin D (dietary consumption of 12,000 units or more per day) might be a precipitating cause of myocardial infarction. The data were only inferential and no objective evidence was presented to prove this theory. Daily doses of vitamin D ranging from 700 to 2,500 units in adults are associated with increased plasma cholesterol levels, but the significance of this finding is unknown.

Treatment of Vitamin D Toxicity

Hypervitaminosis D treatment consists of immediately discontinuing the vitamin, reducing calcium intake, administering glucocorticoids, and assuring a generous fluid intake.

If hypercalcemia occurs, it may persist for weeks to months after termination of ingestion. However, cessation of the vitamin and lowering of oral calcium intake normally leads to rapid disappearance of symptoms. When they persist, a glucocorticoid such as prednisone (20–40 mg or more orally per day) can be given to reduce intestinal absorption, control hypercalcemia, and prevent irreversible renal damage and ectopic calcification. In this manner, a dramatic lowering of calcium to normal levels may be accomplished within days.

Vitamin K

No fad uses for vitamin K have developed since it is not a component of over the counter remedies. Thus, there are few cases of toxicity reported in the literature.

Symptoms and Mechanism of Vitamin K Toxicity

The major toxicity is associated with water-soluble synthetic analogs such as menadione. These derivatives are oxidants and may cause erythrocytic membranes to rupture with resultant cell hemolysis, jaundice, and kernicterus. This occurs more prevalently in persons with glucose-6-phosphate dehydrogenase deficiency and at doses exceeding 10 mg (29). Vitamin K_1 (phytonadione) generally does not lead to hyperbilirubinemia and for this reason is the preferred form.

Vitamin E

At present, vitamin E is believed to be nontoxic. Research is under way to determine its toxic potential. Reported undesirable side effects of megadoses of vitamin E include headaches, nausea, fatigue, dizziness, blurred vision (perhaps related to the fact that large doses may antagonize the action of vitamin A), inflammation of the mouth, chafing of the lips, gastrointestinal disturbances, muscle weakness, low blood sugar, increased bleeding tendencies, degenerative changes, and emotional disorders (12). Also reported are disturbances in growth, thyroid function, mitochondrial respiration rate and bone calcification, and a decreased hematocrit. In a limited study of 28 adults who took up to 800 units daily for a period of 3 years, no serious toxicity was demonstrated (7).

In man and in experimental animals, it is believed that vitamin E may interfere with vitamin K metabolism resulting in a prolonged prothrombin time. Excessive vitamin E intake in experimental animals decreases the rate of wound healing and in man results in gastrointestinal symptoms and creatinuria.

Vitamin C

Serious toxicity to vitamin C administration is uncommon. However, numerous untoward effects may occur when it is taken in overdose, or by persons susceptible to the vitamin. Vitamin C toxicity is not a cause of death. Major symptoms of toxicity are summarized in Table 3.

Several controversial points should be examined. It is often reported that large doses of vitamin C destroy substantial amounts of vitamin B_{12}, and, therefore, retard the latter's absorption to reduce its level in the blood. However, megadoses of vitamin C would be required over a period of several years before this destruction of vitamin B_{12} would be significant to produce symptoms of megaloblastic anemia (5,10).

Other reports state that vitamin C will acidify the urine. While this is not an absolute toxicity, per se, these reports must be considered because of the implication that concurrently administered drugs may be made more or less active. Current consensus is that doses up to 6 g/day (and in some studies, up to 12 g/day), will not significantly alter urine pH (17). This opinion is contrary to earlier reports indicating that doses of 1 g or more per day will acidify the urine.

Large doses of the vitamin taken during pregnancy may cause scurvy in some newborns. The effect is reported to occur in some women who have ingested as little as 400 mg ascorbic acid daily throughout pregnancy. One suggestion is that the vitamin enhances development of fetal liver microsomal enzymes which cause scurvy because of enhanced destruction of the vitamin after birth (15). Another theory states that the fetal body recognizes the danger of increased vitamin C levels and increases its own metabolic

TABLE 3. *Side effects of vitamin C administration*

Interference with urine and stool testing
  Negate occult blood tests
  Cause false-negative reaction with glucose
    oxidase tests
Decrease absorption of vitamin B_{12}
Rebound scurvy following prolonged administration
  of megadoses
Increased urinary oxalate, cysteine and uric acid
Acidification of urine
Diarrhea; occasional nausea

rate to destroy the excess substance. Following birth, this increased destruction of the vitamin continues so that symptoms of scurvy are seen shortly after delivery. A similar, but less dangerous, rebound scurvy is occasionally reported in adults who suddenly withdraw from large doses. For these reasons, it is considered wise to taper megadoses of vitamin C by about 10 to 20% daily, rather than to abruptly discontinue them (9).

Kidney Stone Formation

Ascorbic acid increases renal excretion of oxalate, uric acid, and calcium. These then may increase the potential for stone formation in the kidney and bladder. This potential seems to be governed by genetic factors and only occurs in a small segment of the population. When it does occur, however, susceptible individuals may experience the problem with ascorbic acid doses of 1 g or more daily. The toxicologic problems with oxalate on the kidney were discussed in Chapter 4.

Vitamin B₁

Numerous toxicities were reported in the 1940s and 1950s to parenterally administered vitamin B_1 (thiamine). These ranged from nervousness, convulsions, weakness, trembling, headache, and neuromuscular paralysis, to cardiovascular disorders including rapid pulse, anaphylactic shock, peripheral vasodilation, arrhythmia, and edema. Sensitivity reactions to injectable doses of 100 times the RDA were reported. However, with the subsequent decline in use of thiamine in its parenteral form, there have been fewer toxicities reported and it is no longer considered to possess a major toxicological threat.

Niacin

In single doses of 50 mg niacin (nicotinic acid), intense flushing and pruritus have been reported. When the practice of giving niacin, ranging upwards to 30 g or more a day was advocated, more serious toxicity became increasingly common. These effects included intense flushing and unbearable pruritus, skin rash, heartburn, nausea and vomiting, diarrhea, ulcer activation, abnormal liver function, hypotension, tachycardia, fainting, hyperglycemia, hyperbilirubinemia and jaundice, dermatoses, hyperuricemia, elevated serum enzymes, and hyperkeratosis of the skin. A greater incidence of atrial fibrillation and other cardiac arrhythmias is seen in persons taking niacin (4).

The most common serious toxicities reported for niacin include abnormal liver function and jaundice. The body uses niacin for NAD and NADH formation which then serve as coenzymes for various dehydrogenase enzymes in oxidation-reduction reactions. Many of these enzymes are found in the liver and modulation of their activity with megadoses of niacin may explain the abnormal hepatic functions.

Vitamin B₆

Vitamin B_6 (pyridoxine)-induced reactions are rare. Convulsive disorders have occurred due both to vitamin excess, as well as to a deficiency state (24). Oral doses of up to 1 g daily have not shown adverse reactions, although doses of 200 mg daily followed by abrupt withdrawal have caused symptoms of dependency.

Vitamin B₁₂

Vitamin B_{12} (cyanocobalamin) is associated on rare occasions with allergic reactions to the injectable products. Symptoms of edema of the face, urticaria, shivering, bronchospasm, rash, dyspnea, aphonia, and, on occasion, anaphylaxis have appeared, but only after years of continuous vitamin administration.

Consideration has been given to preservatives and other substances contained in the preparations as being the cause of these symptoms. However, patients have continued to experience such reactions when purified cyanocobalamin was injected, or when another commercial brand was substituted.

Folic Acid

Folic acid is relatively nontoxic with oral doses as high as 15 mg daily showing no substantial reports of adverse effects. A few sensitivity reactions have been recorded. Long-term folic acid therapy may increase seizure frequency in some epileptics and may precipitate vitamin B_{12} deficiency neuropathy in some cases of megaloblastic anemias (22). It is also suspected of inducing mild psychological disorders in normal subjects. While not a direct toxicity, folic acid can mask symptoms of pernicious anemia. In doses exceeding 0.4 to 1 mg/day, the hematological warning signs of pernicious anemia are masked by folic acid, but the life-threatening neurological toxicities continue undetected until it may be too late to adequately treat the condition.

TREATMENT OF VITAMIN TOXICITIES AND ADVERSE EFFECTS

In the majority of cases, vitamin-induced toxicities and adverse effects are best managed by discontinuing the vitamin and treating the specific symptoms, if needed. With the exception of vitamin D-induced hypercalcemia, rarely are other measures necessary.

SUMMARY

Vitamin-induced toxicity often manifests only after prolonged vitamin A or vitamin ingestion. Vitamin C taken in megadoses may also inflict toxic problems, again, usually after chronic therapy. We should remember that any given product containing multiple vitamins may also contain iron and, as we learned in Chapter 10, iron can be extremely toxic in overdose. Thus, care must always be taken when drawing a conclusion on a "vitamin product" ingestion, to assure that iron is not a constituent.

Case Studies

CASE STUDY: GLUCOCORTICOID MODIFICATION OF VITAMIN D INTOXICATION

History

We are presented with a 49-year-old female who had undergone a subtotal thyroidectomy 16 years

earlier. She received thyroid replacement therapy and was directed to consume a high calcium diet.

Six years after her thyroid operation, dihydrotachysterol was added. Two years later, vitamin D was substituted for dihydrotachysterol, and she was given calcium supplements to go along with her high calcium diet. At no time thus far was her serum calcium level above 9.7 mg% (normal, 8.5–10.5 mg%).

Two years later, the patient passed a kidney stone, and calcium supplementation was stopped. Vitamin D (100,000 units/day) was continued.

After another 2 years, the serum calcium level measured 14.2 mg%. The patient reported weight loss and anorexia, intense itching, back pain, and bone pain. Vitamin supplementation was discontinued, but the serum calcium level remained elevated. Three years prior to this present interview, two renal stones were discovered by intravenous pyelography.

The patient was put on prednisone therapy, 10 mg every 6 hr, and dietary calcium intake was limited. Serum calcium levels decreased from 12.2 mg% to 9.1 mg%. Fecal calcium excretion was only minimally affected. (See ref. 28.)

Discussion

1. The patient had a subtotal thyroidectomy years before. However, she was receiving thyroid hormone treatment. Was removal of her thyroid gland, therefore, of probable significance or insignificance? Explain why you arrived at your answer.

2. The fact that serum calcium levels decreased while fecal calcium excretion remained unchanged with prednisone therapy suggests a possible site of glucocorticoid activity. What is it?

3. What was the cause of back pain and bone pain?

CASE STUDY: MEGAVITAMIN DOSE

History

A 4-year-old boy was brought to the hospital by his grandmother, the owner of a health food store. She was concerned about his persistent fever and irritability which had continued over the past 4 months, but recently became more severe.

The boy had been previously examined on two different occasions for hyperkinetic activity. One physician recommended megavitamin therapy, but his grandmother denied giving her grandson any vitamins.

Physical examination revealed a febrile (39.5°C) and very irritable child. His lips were irritated, and fissures were present at the corners of his mouth. He had a slight murmur, and his liver was palpable 3 cm below the right costal margin. Neurological examination was normal, but he refused to walk stating it pained him to do so.

Laboratory results were unremarkable, except for an SGOT level of 93 units/ml (normal, 15–35 units/ml) and LDH of 1,100 units/ml (normal, 200–600 units/ml). Computerized tomography of the brain showed mild enlargement of the lateral ventricles; the echocardiogram was normal. Laboratory results also showed a vitamin A level of 1,430 mg%.

His grandmother continued to deny that she gave him vitamins, although it was later found that his nursery school teacher observed him ingesting vitamin tablets throughout the day during nursery school.

His hospital stay lasted 4 weeks, during which time no more vitamins were given, and his vitamin A level decreased to 320 mg% in 1 week. Liver function tests remained abnormal and a liver biopsy revealed mild fatty infiltration. The child was released to the care of foster parents. (See ref. 26.)

Discussion

1. Two primary sites of vitamin A intoxication were evident in this young patient. What were they? Was this what you anticipated?

2. The child's symptoms were those of vitamin A overdose. Assuming he took a "multiple vitamin" preparation, why did symptoms of poisoning from the other vitamins not show up?

3. Fever is not usually mentioned in most vitamin A intoxication reports. What could have caused this child's fever?

CASE STUDY: VITAMINS A AND D INTOXICATION

History

A male farmer, aged 62 years, ingested 8 ml of a veterinary preparation containing vitamins A and D (500,000 units/ml vitamin A, and 50,000 units/ml vitamin D). The contents of the vial was intended for parenteral use at a dose of 1 ml/600 pounds. He reported no immediate ill effects, but developed a severe headache, became nauseous, and vomited over the next several hours.

During the night he continued to suffer from a severe generalized headache, as well as blurred vision

and scotomas (areas of absent vision within the usual visual area). When the headaches became increasingly severe, he went to the hospital.

On admission, his physical examination was generally unremarkable. Laboratory results consisted of: Hct 37%, WBC 4,500/cu mm, and serum Ca^{2+} 9.0 mg% (normal, 8.5–10.5 mg%). His electrolytes, glucose, and creatinine concentrations were all normal.

During his 5-day hospital stay, he continued to experience photophobia, scotomas, nausea, and headaches. These symptoms subsided on the fourth hospital day, but at that time, exfoliation of the skin on the face and hands occurred. Also during his hospital stay, vitamin A levels (normal, 15–60 µg%) were determined, and are listed below:

Day	Levels (µg%)
1	340
3	126
4	101
5	106

Liver function tests were within normal limits, but thyroid function studies underwent some complex changes during his hospital stay. The patient had an uneventful recovery over several months. (See ref. 13.)

Discussion

1. Does the patient in this case study manifest the typical signs and symptoms of vitamin A toxicity?

2. What is the major mode of toxicity for vitamin D? Was vitamin D toxicity clinically significant in this patient?

CASE STUDY: VITAMIN D-INDUCED BLADDER STONE

History

A 2-year-old female had been given an excessive intake of calcium and vitamin D since the age of 9 months because she refused to eat the quantity of meat her mother felt was necessary for normal body growth. She was therefore given large quantities of cheese and a minimum of 36 oz of vitamin D-fortified milk each day, as well as daily vitamin supplements. It was estimated that her daily intake for calcium was 2 g and 400 to 600 units of vitamin D.

She was hospitalized for treatment of a urinary tract infection, when an abdominal X-ray revealed calcification in the bladder. Urinalysis for electrolytes and other excreted compounds was normal except for excessive excretion of the amino acids cystine, lysine, and ornithine. The calculus, composed of calcium and cystine was surgically removed and the child had an uneventful recovery. (See ref. 20.)

Discussion

1. This patient experienced a classical vitamin D intoxication that was caused by well-meaning parents. What particular food substance do you suppose actually contributed most to this reaction?

CASE STUDY: VITAMIN C INGESTION AND RENAL STONES

History

A 21-year-old male had a calcium oxalate kidney stone removed after it was discovered by a urologist. The man had complained of flank pain. Physical examination was unremarkable and his family history did not show previous renal disease.

Laboratory results showed that the serum and 24-hr urine levels of calcium, phosphorus, and uric acid were normal, but urine oxalate level was 126 mg/24 hr (normal, less than 40 mg/24 hr).

When it was revealed that he had been taking 1 g vitamin C each day for many months to prevent colds, he was advised to discontinue the vitamin. He did so, and his urinary oxalate level decreased to 56 mg/24 hr 18 days later. (See ref. 23.)

Discussion

1. Outline the mechanism of formation of a calcium oxalate renal stone. How could vitamin C cause its appearance?

2. What advice should a patient who is contemplating taking large doses of vitamin C be given?

Review Questions

1. All of the following are true statements about vitamin A intoxication *except*:
   A. Its occurrence is usually due to overambitious prophylactic use.
   B. Chronic renal disease is more likely to result in its occurrence than when kidney function is normal.
   C. Hepatic damage occurs from destruction of sinusoidal spaces.

D. Brain damage occurs when the vitamin binds to the "retinol-binding" protein.

2. Most "therapeutic formulae" of vitamin product mixtures contain these substances at 10 times their RDA.
   A. True
   B. False

3. Vitamin K shares an important feature with vitamins A and D (i.e., all are fat-soluble). Still, vitamin K toxicity is only rarely seen. Why?

4. Daily consumption of vitamin D ranging from 700 to 2,500 units is associated with:
   A. increased plasma cholesterol levels.
   B. decreased plasma cholesterol levels.

5. State the reasons why vitamin D intoxication could logically be expected to be more severe in a person with a previous complete thyroidectomy.

6. Cite the pros and cons in giving vitamin E to antidote a person experiencing symptoms of hypervitaminosis A.

7. Which of the following would be contraindicated in a patient who ingested an acute vitamin D overdose?
   A. Forced fluids
   B. Calcium lactate
   C. Ascorbic acid
   D. Prednisone

8. All of the following are symptoms of vitamin A intoxication *except*:
   A. myalgia
   B. headache
   C. muscle pain
   D. weight gain

9. Vitamin D, per se, is not toxic but, rather, is converted to an active substance. What is it?

10. Give a plausible explanation why a neonate, whose mother took large doses of vitamin C during pregnancy, may develop scurvy following birth.

11. A symptom of vitamin A intoxication is *hyperostosis*. What is this, and why do you think it occurs?

12. All clinically significant symptoms of acute vi-

tamin D intoxication can be traced to elevated blood levels of what specific mineral?

13. Which of the following results from ingestion of vitamin A in doses as low as 25,000 units?
    A. Increased serum parathyroid hormone
    B. Decreased serum parathyroid hormone

14. Following ingestion of a toxic dose of many poisons, the event may be missed, or the presenting symptoms misdiagnosed. This also may occur with vitamin A. Why does it occur with the vitamin?

15. Ascorbic acid increases renal excretion of which of the following: oxalate (I), uric acid (II), or calcium (III)?
    A. II only
    B. III only
    C. I and II only
    D. II and III only
    E. I, II, and III

References

1. Avery, G. S., Heel, R. C., and Speight, T. M. (1980): Guide to adverse drug reactions. In: *Drug Treatment: Principles and Practice of Clinical Pharmacology and Therapeutics*, 2nd ed., edited by G. S. Avery, pp. 1225–1251. Publishing Sciences Group, Littleton.
2. Babb, R. R., and Kieraldo, J. H. (1978): Cirrhosis due to hypervitaminosis A. *West. J. Med.*, 128:244–246.
3. Chertow, B. S., Williams, G. A., and Kiani, R. (1974): The interactions between vitamin A, vinblastine, and cytochalasin B in parathyroid hormone secretion. *Pro. Soc. Exp. Biol. Med.*, 147:16–27.
4. Coronary Drug Project Research Group (1975): Clofibrate and niacin in coronary heart disease. *JAMA*, 231:360–381.
5. DiPalma, J. (1978): Vitamin toxicity. *Am. Fam. Physician*, 10:106.
6. DiPalma, J. R., and Ritchie, D. M. (1977): Vitamin toxicity. *Ann. Rev. Pharmacol. Toxicol.*, 17:133–148.
7. Farrell, P. M., and Bieri, J. G. (1975): Megavitamin E supplementation in man. *Am. J. Clin. Nutr.*, 28:1381–1386.
8. FDA Consumer, (1981): 15:2.
9. Herbert, V. D. (1979): Megavitamin therapy. *NY J. Med.*, February, p. 278.
10. Herbert, V. D., and Jacob, E. (1974): Destruction of vitamin B_{12} by ascorbic acid. *JAMA*, 230:241–242.
11. Holick, M. F., and Potts, J. T. (1980): Vitamin D. In: *Principles of Internal Medicine*, edited by K. J. Isselbacher, R. D. Adams, E. Brawnwald, R. G. Petersdorf, and J. D. Wilson, pp. 1843–1849. McGraw-Hill, New York.
12. Kligman, A. M. (1982): Vitamin E toxicity. *Arch. Dermatol.*, 118:280.
13. LaMantia, R. S., and Andrews, C. E. (1981): Acute vitamin A intoxication. *South. Med. J.*, 74:1012–1014.
14. Linden, V. (1974): Vitamin D and myocardial infarction. *Br. Med. J.*, 3:647–649.
15. Mandel, H. G., and Cohn, V. H. (1980): Fat-soluble vitamins. In: *The Pharmacological Basis of Therapeutics*, 6th ed., edited by A. G. Gilman, L. S. Goodman, and A. Gilman, pp. 1583–1601. Macmillan, New York.
16. Muenter, M. D., Perry, H. O., and Ludwig, J. (1971): Chronic hypervitaminosis A intoxication in adults. *Am. J. Med.*, 50:129–136.
17. Nahata, M. C., Shimp, L., Lampman, T., and McLeod, D. C. (1977): Effect of ascorbic acid on urine pH in man. *Am. J. Hosp. Pharm.*, 34:1234.
18. National Clearinghouse for Poison Control Centers Bulletin, (1980): *US Dept. Health Services, Rockville*, 24:3.
19. National Research Council, Food and Nutrition Board, (1975): Hazards of overuse of vitamin D. *Am. J. Clin. Nutr.*, 28:512–513.
20. O'Regan, S., Robitaille, P., Mongeau, J. C., and Homsy, Y. (1980): Cystine calcium bladder calculus in a 2-year-old child. *J. Urology*, 123:770.
21. Parfitt, A. M. (1972): Hypophosphatemic vitamin D refractory rickets and osteomalacia. *Orthop. Clin. North Am.*, 3:653–680.
22. Reynolds, E. H. (1973): Anticonvulsants, folic acid, and epilepsy. *Lancet*, 1:1376–1378.
23. Roth, D. A., and Breitenfield, R. V. (1977): Vitamin C and oxalate stones. *JAMA*, 237:768.
24. Schaumburg, H., Kaplan, J., Windebank, A., Vick, N., Rasmus, S., Pleasure, D., and Brown, M. J. (1983): Sensory neuropathy from pyridoxine abuse. *N. Engl. J. Med.*, 309:445–448.
25. Schmunes, E. (1979): Hypervitaminosis A in a patient with alopecia receiving renal dialysis. *Arch. Dermatol.*, 115:882–883.
26. Shaywitz, B. A., Siegel, N. J., and Pearson, H. A. (1977): Megavitamins for minimal brain dysfunction. *JAMA*, 238:1749–1750.
27. Smith, F. R., and Goodman, D. S. (1976): Vitamin A transport in human vitamin A toxicity. *N. Engl. J. Med.*, 294:805–808.
28. Streck, W. F., Waterhouse, C., and Haddad, J. C. (1979): Glucocorticoid effects in vitamin D intoxication. *Arch. Intern. Med.*, 139:974–977.
29. Zinkham, W. H., and Childs, B. (1957): Effect of vitamin K and naphthalene metabolites on glutathione metabolism of erythrocytes from normal newborns and patients with naphthalene hemolytic anemia. *Am. J. Dis. Child.*, 94:420–423.

Appendix

TABLE 1. Vital signs

TABLE 2. Normal clinical laboratory values: blood

TABLE 3. Therapeutic, toxic, and lethal blood levels

References

The data listed in the following tables are *not* absolute values. Many of the figures are dependent on intralaboratory variations and the sensitivity of analytical methods used in their determination. The values are to be used only for reference when comparing data presented in the text or the case studies that follow the chapters.

TABLE 1. *Vital signs*

Respiration	
Adult	12–18/min
Child	20–50/min
Pulse	
Adult	60–90 beats/min
Child	80–160 beats/min
Blood pressure	
Adult	
Systolic	100–140 mm Hg
Diastolic	60–90 mm Hg
Child	
Systolic	80 (+ 2 × age in years)
Diastolic	2/3 of systolic
Temperature	98.6°F (96.8–99.3°F)
	37°C (36–37.4°C)

TABLE 2. *Normal clinical laboratory values: blood*

Test	Normal value
δ-Aminolevulinic acid	0.01–0.03 mg%
Base, total	145–160 mEq/L
Bicarbonate	24–28 mEq/L (24–28 mM/L)
Bilirubin, serum	
Total	0.1–1.2 mg%
Direct	0.1–0.3 mg%
Indirect	0.1–1.0 mg%
Blood gases	
pH	7.35–7.45 (arterial)
	7.36–7.41 (venous)
P_{CO_2}	35–45 mm Hg (arterial)
P_{O_2}	95–100 mm Hg (arterial)
BUN—see Urea nitrogen	
Calcium	
Serum	8.5–10.5 mg%
Total	4.2–5.2 mEq/L
Carbon dioxide, serum	
Content	24–29 mEq/L (24–29 mM/L)
Combining power	24–30 mEq/L (24–30 mM/L)
Tension, P_{CO_2}	35–45 mm Hg
Chloride	95–106 mEq/L (95–106 mM/L)
Creatinine	0.8–1.2 mg%
Glucose (fasting)	65–110 mg%
Hemoglobin—whole blood	
Female	12.0–16.0 gm%
Male	13.5–18.0 gm%
Iron	
Total	50–175 μg% (9–31.3 μM/L)
Binding capacity	250–450 μg%
Percent saturation	20–55%
Lactate dehydrogenase (LDH)	110–250 IU/ml
Osmolality, serum	275–295 mOsm/kg water
Oxygen	
Capacity	16–24 vol% (varies with Hb)
Content	15–23 vol% (arterial)
Saturation	94–100% of capacity
Tension, P_{O_2}	95–100 mm Hg (arterial)
P_{CO_2}	35–45 mm Hg (arterial)
pH	7.35–7.45 (arterial)
Phosphatase, alkaline	5–13 units% (King-Armstrong)
Potassium	3.5–5.0 mEq/L
Sodium	136–145 mEq/L
Transaminases	
SGOT (aspartate aminotransferase)	8–40 units/ml
SGPT (alanine aminotransferase)	1–36 units/ml
Urea nitrogen (BUN)	8–25 mg% (2.9–8.9 mM/L)
Vitamin A	15–60 μg%
Vitamin B_{12}	200–1,025 pg/ml
Vitamin D	
25-hydroxycholecalciferol	10–80 ng/ml
1,25-dihydroxycholecalciferol	21–45 pg/ml

TABLE 3. *Therapeutic, toxic, and lethal blood levels*

Substance	Therapeutic or normal	Toxic	Lethal
Alcohols			
Ethanol	—	100 mg% (legal intoxication)	>350 mg%
Ethylene glycol	—	150 mg%	200–400 mg%
Isopranol	—	340 mg%	—
Methanol	—	20–80 mg%	>80 mg%
Antidepressants			
Amitriptyline	5–20 μg%	>50 μg%	1–2 mg%
Desipramine	15–30 μg%	>50 μg%	1–2 mg%
Doxepin	10–25 μg%	50–200 μg%	1–2 mg%
Imipramine	15–25 μg%	50–150 μg%	>200 μg%
CNS depressants			
Barbiturates			
Short-acting	0.01–0.1 mg%	0.7–1.0 mg%	>1.0 mg%
Intermediate-acting	0.1–0.5 mg%	1.0–3.0 mg%	>3.0 mg%
Long-acting	1.5–5.0 mg%	4.0–6.0 mg%	8–15 mg%
Benzodiazepines	0.01–0.3 mg%	0.5–2.0 mg%	—
Chloral hydrate	0.2–1.0 mg%	10 mg%	25 mg%
Ethchlorvynol	0.05–0.5 mg%	2–10 mg%	15 mg%
Glutethimide	0.02–0.08 mg%	1–8 mg%	3–10 mg%
Meprobamate	0.8–2.4 mg%	6–10 mg%	14–35 mg%
Methaqualone	0.3–0.6 mg%	1–3 mg%	>3.0 mg%
Methyprylon	0.5–1.5 mg%	3–6 mg%	10 mg%
CNS stimulants			
Amphetamine	2–3 μg%	50 μg%	200 μg%
Caffeine	0.5–1.0 mg%	—	>10 mg%
Cocaine	5–15 μg%	90 μg%	0.1–2.0 mg%
Diethylproprion	0.7–20 μg%	—	—
Methamphetamine	20–60 μg%	60–500 μg%	1–4 mg%
Methylphenidate	1–6 μg%	80 μg%	230 μg%
Strychnine	—	0.2 mg%	0.9–1.2 mg%
Metals			
Arsenic	0.0–2.0 μg%	100 μg%	1.5 mg%
Cadmium	0.01–0.02 μg%	5 μg%	—
Copper	100–150 μg%	540 μg%	—
Iron	65–175 μg%	500–600 μg%	2–5 mg%
Lead	0–30 μg%	130 μg%	>200 μg%
Mercury	0–8 μg%	100 μg%	> 600 μg%
Narcotics			
Codeine	1–12 μg%	20–50 μg%	>60 μg%
Diphenoxylate	1 μg%	—	—
Hydromorphone	0.1–3 μg%	10–200 μg%	> 300 μg%
Meperidine	30–100 μg%	500 μg%	1–3 mg%
Methadone	30–110 μg%	200 μg%	> 400 μg%
Morphine	1–7 μg%	10–100 μg%	> 400 μg%
Oxycodone	1–10 μg%	20–500 μg%	—
Pentazocine	10–60 μg%	200–500 μg%	1–2 mg%
Propoxyphene	5–20 μg%	30–60 μg%	80–200 μg%

TABLE 3. *(continued)*

Substance	Therapeutic or normal	Toxic	Lethal
Nonnarcotic analgesics			
Acetaminophen	0.5–2.0 mg%	12–30 mg%	150 mg%
Acetylsalicylic acid	2–10 mg%	15–30 mg%	>55 mg%
Ibuprofen	50–420 μg%	—	—
Phenothiazines			
Chlorpromazine	50 μg%	100–200 μg%	0.3–1.2 mg%
Haloperidol	0.05–0.9 μg%	100–400 μg%	—
Perphenazine	0.5 μg%	100 μg%	—
Promazine	—	100 μg%	—
Prochlorperazine	—	100 μg%	—
Thioridazine	100–150 μg%	1.0 mg%	2–8 mg%
Thiothixene	1.0 μg%	—	—
Trifluoperazine	80 μg%	120–300 μg%	0.3–0.8 mg%
Psychotomimetics			
LSD	—	0.1–0.4 μg%	—
MDA	—	—	0.4–1.0 mg%
Phencyclidine	—	0.7–24 μg%	100–500 μg%

References

Baselt, R. C., and Cravey, R. H. (1977): A compendium of therapeutic and toxic concentrations of toxicologically significant drugs in human biofluids. *J. Anal. Tox.*, 1:81–103.

McBay, A. T. (1973): Toxicological findings in fatal poisonings. *Clin. Chem.*, 19:361–365.

Henry, J. B. (editor) (1981): *Clinical Diagnosis and Management by Laboratory Methods*, 16th ed. Saunders, Philadelphia.

Scully, R. E. (1978): Normal reference laboratory values: Case records of the Massachusetts General Hospital. *N. Engl. J. Med.*, 298:34.

Winek, C. L. (1976): Tabulations of therapeutic, toxic, and lethal concentrations of drugs and chemicals in blood. *Clin. Chem.*, 22:832–836.

Subject Index

fatigue, 160
hyperkeratosis in, 160
irritability in, 160
Mee's lines in, 160
neuropathy in, 160
pancytopenia in, 161
weakness in, 160
weight loss in, 160
diarrhea in, 34
mechanism of, 158–159
salivation in, 34
treatment, dimercaprol, 156, 161
uses, 158
Arsenical, pentavalent, 21
Arsine gas, 158
Arylamino compounds, 79
Arylnitro compounds, 79
Asphalt, 106,107
Aspirin; *see also* Salicylates
dialyzability, 48
toxicity, 6
for zinc toxicity, 178
Asthma, 137
Ataxia
in toxicity, 34
acetone, 195
alcohol, 34
antihistamine, 266
barbiturate, 34
benzodiazepine, 264
bromide, 34
ethanol, 64
ethylene glycol, 69
hallucinogens, 34
heavy metal, 34
hydrocarbon, 108
organophosphate, 131
phenothiazine, 277
phenytoin, 34
solvents, 34
Atropa belladonna, 211
Atropine
as an antidote, 50
cardiotoxicity, 34
combined with pralidoxime, 133
diphenoxylate combined with, 248
toxicity
mydriasis in, 34
xerostomia in, 34
for toxicity
adrenergic blocking agents, 225
nicotine, 138
organophosphate, 133
Attapulgite, 40
Automatism, 261

Baby product cosmetics, 7
Back pain
in methanol toxicity, 66
BAL, *see* Dimercaprol
Ballpoint pen ink, 7
Barbital, 48,263

Barbiturate(s)
acetylcholine interaction with, 261
γ-aminobutyric acid release and, 261
classification of, 261,263
elimination kinetics, 262
mescaline toxicity and, 314
norepinephrine interaction with, 261
propoxyphene toxicity and, 250
suicide poisonings and, 261
toxicity
ataxia in, 34
bullous lesions in, 262
coma in, 34,263
convulsions in, 34
drowsiness in, 34,263
ethanol and, 262
fasciculation in, 34
hypothermia in, 261
long- vs short-acting, 262
mechanism, 261–262
mydriasis in, 34
nystagmus in, 34
respiratory failure in, 261
shock, 262
stupor, 263
treatment of, Scandinavian method, 267
for toxicity
camphor, 302
Bath oil, 7
Bathtub floating toys, 7
Battery (dry cell), 7
Battery acid, 115
Beer
absorption of, 61
tyramine in, 23
Beeswax, 7
Bentonite, 140
Benzene, 21
Benzodiazepines, 259,263–264
γ-aminobutyric acid and, 264
concomitant use with other drugs, 264
therapeutic index, 264
tolerance, 264
toxicity
ataxia in, 264
coma in, 264
drowsiness in, 264
hallucination in, 264
mechanism of, 264
Benzphetamine, 293
Beryllium, 156
Bipyridyl compounds, 139–141
Bladder perforation, 47
Bleach, 7,191–192
acidic agents and, 192
alkalosis and, 192
ingestion of, 191–192
perborates in, 192
peroxides in, 192
toxicity, treatment, 192

Bleeding, intraperitoneal, 47
Blindness
in methanol toxicity, 67
Blood
toxicological analysis in poison, 33,49–50
Blood brain barrier
permeability to
ethanol, 61
mercury compounds, 172
Blood coagulation, 141,142
Blood dyscrasia
in toxicity
arsenic, 160
ipecac, 38
Body conditioners, 7
Body fluids
toxicological analysis in, 31
Boric acid
adsorption by activated charcoal, 41
dialyzability, 48
infant death from, 196
as an insecticide, 196
nephrotoxicity, 196
toxicity
convulsions in, 196
cyanosis in, 196
diarrhea in, 196
emesis, 34
hyperpyrexia in, 196
hypotension in, 196
jaundice in, 196
lethargy in, 196
skin rash in, 196
tremor in, 196
weakness in, 196
Botulinus toxin
lethal dose, 5
toxicity
hallucinations in, 34
paralysis in, 34
Bougienage
for corrosive ingestion, 123
Bradycardia
in toxicity, 34
ipecac, 38
narcotic, 251
nicotine, 138
organophosphate, 131,132
Breath odor
in toxicity
ammonia, 34
arsenic, 34
chloral hydrate, 34
cyanide, 34
ethyl alcohol, 34
ethyl chlorvinyl, 34
gasoline, 34
isopropranol, 34
kerosene, 34
methyl salicylate, 34
nail polish remover, 34
organophosphate, 34